NEUROANATOMY

4TH EDITION

BOARD
REVIEW
SERIES

NEUROANATOMY

4TH EDITION

James D. Fix, Ph.D.
Professor Emeritus of Anatomy
Marshall University School of Medicine
Huntington, West Virginia

Questions Contributor:
Deon M. Harvey, Ph.D.

Wolters Kluwer | Lippincott Williams & Wilkins
Health
Philadelphia · Baltimore · New York · London
Buenos Aires · Hong Kong · Sydney · Tokyo

Acquisitions Editor: Crystal Taylor
Managing Editor: Kelly Horvath
Marketing Manager: Emilie J. Moyer
Production Editor: Beth Martz
Design Coordinator: Holly Reid McLaughlin
Compositor: Aptara

351 West Camden Street
Baltimore, Maryland 21201-2436 USA

530 Walnut Street
Philadelphia, Pennsylvania 19106 USA

Printed in India

Library of Congress Cataloging-in-Publication Data
Fix, James D.
 Neuroanatomy / James D. Fix.—4th ed.
   p. ; cm. — (Board review series)
 Includes bibliographical references and index.
 ISBN 0-7817-7245-1
   1. Neuroanatomy—Examinations, questions, etc. I. Title. II. Series.
   [DNLM: 1. Neuroanatomy—Examination Questions. WL 18.2 F566n 2002]
   QM451 .F59 2002
   611'.8'076—dc21

                                                                        2001037710

We'd like to hear from you! If you have comments or suggestions regarding this Lippincott Williams & Wilkins title, please contact us at the appropriate customer service number listed below, or send correspondence to **book_comments@lww.com.** If possible, please remember to include your mailing address, phone number, and a reference to the book title and author in your message. To purchase additional copies of this book call our customer service department at **(800) 638-3030** or fax orders to **(301) 824-7390.** International customers should call **(301) 714-2324.**

1 2 3 4 5 6 7 8 9 10

To Ilse, for her constant support and understanding.

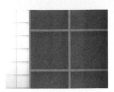

Preface

BRS Neuroanatomy, fourth edition, is a concise review of human neuroanatomy intended primarily for medical and dental students preparing for the United States Medical Licensing Examination (USMLE) Step 1 and other examinations. It presents the essentials of human neuroanatomy in a concise, tightly outlined, well-illustrated format. There are over 600 board-type questions with complete answers and explanations, some included at the end of each chapter and some in a comprehensive examination at the end of the book.

New to This Edition
- Magnetic resonance angiograms
- Color used throughout to enhance neuroanatomic pathways
- Color used to block in tables and highlight clinical correlations
- Cerebellar atrophies
- Localization of sensory disorders

To the Student
To make the most of this book, carefully study the illustrations, computed tomography scans, magnetic resonance images, and angiograms, as well as the figure legends; much of the board question information lies within the images and legends. **The answers to at least 30 common USMLE questions are outlined below;** refer to these tips as you review the chapters:

Chapter 1: The mini-atlas provides you with the essential examination structures labeled on computed tomography scans, magnetic resonance images, and gross stained sections.

Chapter 2: Meninges and cerebrospinal fluid (CSF). Three membranes envelop the brain and spinal cord. What is their function? CSF is produced by the **choroid plexus** and absorbed by the **arachnoid villi** that jut into the dural venous sinuses. Name a noninvasive tumor that arises from the arachnoid granulations. Distinguish between **normal-pressure hydrocephalus** and **pseudotumor cerebri (benign intracranial hypertension).**

Chapter 3: Blood supply of the central nervous system (CNS). The essential arteries and the functional areas that they irrigate are shown: The anterior spinal artery (ASA) perfuses the anterior two-thirds of the spinal cord including the corticospinal and spinothalamic tracts. In the medial medulla the ASA supplies the corticospinal tract and medial lemniscus. In the lateral medulla the posterior inferior cerebellar artery (PICA) irrigates the nucleus ambiguus, the inferior cerebellar peduncle, spinal trigeminal nucleus and tract, and the spinothalamic tract. In the posterolateral pons the PICA irrigates the nucleus of facial nerve, nucleus and tract of the trigeminal nerve. In the rostral midbrain the posterior cerebral artery (PCA) irrigates the intra-axial fibers of cranial nerve III and the corticospinal tracts. Know the **arterial circle of Willis!** What is the most common cause of nontraumatic intraparenchymal hemorrhage? Study the distribution of the anterior, medial, and posterior cerebral arteries!

Chapter 4: Development of the nervous system. The **neural tube** (neuroectoderm) gives rise to the CNS. Failure of the **neuropores** to close results in neural tube defects such as **anencephaly.** Name the derivatives of the **neural crest.** Know the following congenital malfunctions: **spina bifida, meningohydroencephalocele, Arnold-Chiari,** and **Dandy-Walker** malfunctions.

Chapter 5: Neurohistology. Where are **pseudounipolar** and **bipolar neurons found? What is Wallerian degeneration? What is Nissl substance? Hortega** cells arise from monocytes, which enter the CNS via abnormal blood vessels. Schwann cells are myelin-forming peripheral neuroglial cells. The **glioblastoma multiforme** is the most rapid-growing and fatal glioma.

Chapter 6: The adult **spinal cord terminates (conus terminalis)** at the lower border of the first lumbar vertebra. The newborn's spinal cord extends to the third lumbar vertebra. The adult **cauda equina** extends from vertebral levels L2 to Co.

Chapter 7: Tracts of the spinal cord are reduced to four: corticospinal tract, spinothalamic tract, dorsal column-medial lemniscus, and hypothalamospinal tract. Transection of this descending autonomic tract results in **Horner syndrome.**

Chapter 8: Lesions of the spinal cord. Review the eight classic national board lesions of the spinal cord: **poliomyelitis, multiple sclerosis, dorsal column disease** (syphilis, locomotor ataxia, tabes dorsalis), **amyotrophic lateral sclerosis** (ALS), **hemisection of spinal cord (Brown-Séquard syndrome), subacute combined degeneration** (vitamin B_{12} neuropathy), **syringomyelia,** and **anterior** (ventral) **spinal artery syndrome.**

Chapter 9: Brainstem. Study the transverse sections of the brainstem and localize the cranial nerve nuclei. Study the ventral surface of the brainstem and identify the exiting and entering cranial nerves. On the dorsal surface of the brainstem, identify the only exiting cranial nerve, the trochlear nerve.

Chapter 10: Trigeminal system. The trigeminal nerve (CN V) is the largest cranial nerve. Which is the smallest? Name the afferent and efferent limbs of the corneal and jaw jerk reflexes. Study the sensory pathway of the ventral trigeminothalamic tract. Where is the cave of Meckel? What is tic douloureux? Trigeminal neuralgia? Which trigeminal nerve branches pass through the cavernous sinus?

Chapter 11: Auditory system. Study the auditory pathway and its way stations: hair cells of the **organ of Corti** → cochlear nuclei → superior olivary nucleus → lateral lemniscus → nucleus of inferior colliculus → brachium of inferior colliculus → medial geniculate body → auditory radiations → auditory cortex, transverse gyrus of **Heschl, Brodmann areas 41 and 42.**

Chapter 12: Vestibular system. Study the vestibular pathways; recall the anatomy and function of the sensory hair cells found in the **utricle** and **saccule.** Lesions of the vestibular system result in nystagmus. **What is vestibular, postrotational, optokinetic and caloric nystagmus? What is Ménière disease? What is benign positional vertigo?**

Chapter 13: Cranial nerves and their major functions: CN I smells. CN II sees. CN III moves the eyeball and elevates the upper eye lid. CN IV depresses, intorts, and abducts the eyeball. CN V provides sensory innervation of the face and innervates the muscles of chewing. CN VI abducts the eyeball. CN VII moves the face, tastes, salivates, and cries. CN VIII hears and mediates balance. CN IX tastes, swallows, and mediates input from the **carotid sinus** that via **baroreceptors** regulate arterial blood pressure. It also mediates input from the **carotid body** that monitors the carbon dioxide and oxygen concentration of the blood. CN X phonates, swallows, and innervates the viscera of the neck and the thoracic and abdominal cavities. Understand the **carotid sinus reflex;** what is the **gag reflex**?

Chapter 14: Lesions of the brainstem. The seven most important lesions of the **brainstem are the anterior spinal artery syndrome (Figure 14-1), the anterior inferior cerebellar artery syndrome** (Figure 14-1), the **posterior inferior cerebellar artery syndrome** (Figure14-2), the **medial longitudinal fasciculus** (MLF) (Figures 9-6 and 9-7). The MLF syndrome is seen in **multiple sclerosis.** Three important midbrain lesions are **Parinaud, Benedikt,** and **Weber.** Name the cranial nerves involved in these syndromes!

Chapter 15: Cerebellum. Figure 15-4 shows the most important cerebellar circuit. The inhibitory gamma-aminobutyric acid (GABA) –ergic Purkinje axons give rise to the cerebellodentatothalamic tract. What are mossy and climbing fibers? What is **von Hippel-Lindau** syndrome? Review the cerebellar atrophies!

Chapter 16: Thalamus. Review the nuclei of the thalamus, the afferent and efferent connections. Study the blood supply to the thalamus, the basal ganglia, and the internal capsule. Understanding the thalamus will get you some points on the United States Medical Licensing Examination (USMLE).

Chapter 17: Visual system. Study the histology of the retina. Study the visual pathways and visual field defects (e.g. hemianopsias and quadrantanopias). Know the visual reflexes, such as the pupillary light reflex and pupillary dilation pathway; these connections are clinically important and appear on the boards. Don't forget **Horner syndrome;** it's on there!

Chapter 18: Autonomic nervous system. The important anatomy of the autonomic nervous system is clearly seen in **Figures 18-1** and **18-2.**

Chapter 19: Hypothalamus. Figures 19-2 and **19-5** show that the paraventricular and supraoptic nuclei synthesize and release antidiuretic hormone and oxytocin. The suprachiasmatic nucleus receives direct input from the retina and plays a role in the regulation of circadian rhythms. **Wernicke encephalopathy** results from the deficiency of thiamine (vitamin B_1); lesions are found in the mamillary bodies, thalamus, and midbrain tegmentum (**Figure 19-6**).

Chapter: 20: Olfactory, gustatory, and limbic systems. Bilateral lesions of the amygdala result in Klüver-Bucy syndrome. Recall the triad of hyperphagia, hypersexuality, and psychic blindness. Memory loss is associated with bilateral lesions of the hippocampus. Know the Papez circuit, a common board topic (**Figure 20-4**).

Chapter 21: Basal ganglia and the striatal motor system. Figure 21-4 shows the **circuitry of the basal ganglia and their associated neurotransmitters.** Parkinson disease is associated with depopulation of neurons in the substantia nigra. Huntington disease results in a loss of nerve cells in the caudate nucleus and putamen. Hemiballism results from infarction of the contralateral subthalamic nucleus.

Chapter 22: Neurotransmitters and their pathways. The **pathways of the major neurotransmitters** are shown in separate brain maps. Glutamate is the major excitatory transmitter of the brain; GABA is the major inhibitory transmitter. Purkinje cells in the cerebellum are GABA-ergic.

Chapter 23: Cerebral cortex. This chapter describes the cortical localization of functional areas of the brain. How does the dominant hemisphere differ from the nondominant hemisphere? **Figure 23-4** outlines the **effects of the various major hemispheric lesions.** What symptoms result from a lesion of the right inferior parietal lobe? What is Gerstmann syndrome?

Chapter 24: Apraxia, aphasia, and dysprosody. Be able to differentiate Broca aphasia from Wernicke aphasia. What is conduction aphasia? This is board-relevant material.

Review Tests and Comprehensive Examination: Take time to read the explanations given with the answers. Many confusing issues of neuroanatomy are settled in the explanations to the questions—for example, the difference between stria medullaris and stria terminalis or the important difference between a lower motor neuron and an upper motor neuron.

I wish you success,

James D. Fix

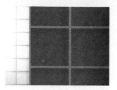

Acknowledgments

I thank my students and colleagues for their valuable comments, suggestions, and help. I also thank the Lippincott Williams & Wilkins staff and their associates for their contributions to this edition—Crystal Taylor, acquisitions editor, and Kelly Horvath, managing editor—and the student and faculty reviewers—in particular, Thomas A. Marino, Ph.D.—who were invited by the publisher to provide valuable feedback and suggestions.

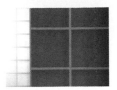

Contents

Gross Anatomy of the Brain

I. Introduction: The Brain

- is the part of the central nervous system (CNS) that lies within the cranial vault, the **encephalon.** Its hemispheric surface is convoluted (i.e., gyrencephalic) and has **gyri** and **sulci.**
- consists of the **cerebrum** (cerebral hemispheres and diencephalon), the **brainstem** (midbrain, pons, and medulla), and the **cerebellum.**
- weighs 350 g in the newborn and 1400 g in the adult.
- is covered by three connective tissue membranes, the **meninges.**
- is surrounded by **cerebrospinal fluid (CSF),** which supports it and protects it from trauma.

II. Divisions of the Brain

- The brain is classified into six postembryonic divisions: **telencephalon, diencephalon, mesencephalon, pons, medulla oblongata,** and **cerebellum.**

A. **Telencephalon**
   - consists of the **cerebral hemispheres** (which comprise both cerebral cortex and white matter) and the **basal ganglia.** The cerebral hemispheres contain the **lateral ventricles.**
   1. **Cerebral hemispheres** (Figures 1-1 through 1-5)
      - are separated by the longitudinal cerebral fissure and the falx cerebri.
      - are interconnected by the corpus callosum.
      - consist of six lobes and the olfactory structures:
         a. **Frontal lobe** (see Figures 1-3 and 1-4)
            - extends from the central sulcus to the frontal pole.
            - lies above the lateral sulcus and anterior to the central sulcus.
            - contains the following gyri:
               (1) **Precentral gyrus**
                  - consists of the motor area (area 4).
               (2) **Superior frontal gyrus**
                  - contains the supplementary motor cortex on the medial surface (area 6).
               (3) **Middle frontal gyrus**
                  - contains the frontal eye field (area 8).
               (4) **Inferior frontal gyrus**
                  - contains the Broca speech area in the dominant hemisphere (areas 44 and 45).

Some authorities classify the diencephalon as part of the brainstem, not as part of the cerebrum.

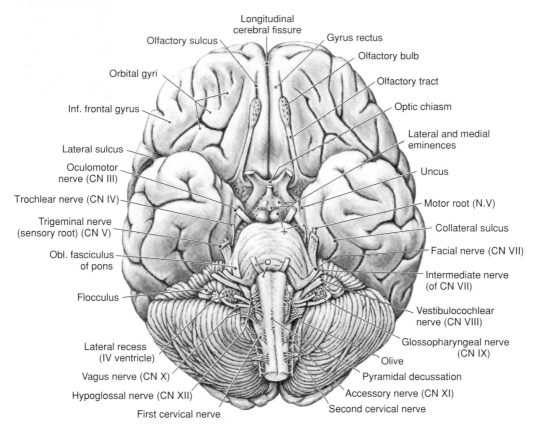

Longitudinal cerebral fissure — Olfactory sulcus — Gyrus rectus — Orbital gyri — Olfactory bulb — Olfactory tract — Inf. frontal gyrus — Optic chiasm — Lateral and medial eminences — Lateral sulcus — Oculomotor nerve (CN III) — Uncus — Trochlear nerve (CN IV) — Motor root (N.V) — Trigeminal nerve (sensory root) (CN V) — Collateral sulcus — Facial nerve (CN VII) — Obl. fasciculus of pons — Intermediate nerve (of CN VII) — Flocculus — Vestibulocochlear nerve (CN VIII) — Glossopharyngeal nerve (CN IX) — Lateral recess (IV ventricle) — Olive — Vagus nerve (CN X) — Pyramidal decussation — Hypoglossal nerve (CN XII) — Accessory nerve (CN XI) — First cervical nerve — Second cervical nerve

+ = Mamillary body; cerebral peduncle
o = Abducens nerve; pyramid of medulla

Figure 1-1. Base of the brain with the attached cranial nerves. (Reprinted with permission from Truex RC, Kellner CE: *Detailed Atlas of the Head and Neck*. New York, Oxford University Press, 1958, p 34.)

(5) **Gyrus rectus and orbital gyri**
- are separated by the olfactory sulcus.

(6) **Anterior paracentral lobule**
- is found on the medial surface between the superior frontal gyrus (paracentral sulcus) and the central sulcus.
- represents a continuation of the precentral gyrus on the medial hemispheric surface.

b. **Parietal lobe** (see Figures 1-3 through 1-5)
- extends from the central sulcus to the occipital lobe and lies superior to the temporal lobe.
- contains the following lobules and gyri:

(1) **Postcentral gyrus**
- is the primary somatosensory area of the cerebral cortex (areas 3, 1, and 2).

(2) **Superior parietal lobule**
- comprises association areas involved in somatosensory functions (areas 5 and 7).

(3) **Inferior parietal lobule**
(a) **Supramarginal gyrus**
- interrelates somatosensory, auditory, and visual input (area 40).
(b) **Angular gyrus** (area 39)
- receives impulses from primary visual cortex.

(4) **Precuneus**
- is located between the paracentral lobule and the cuneus.

(*text continues on page 5*)

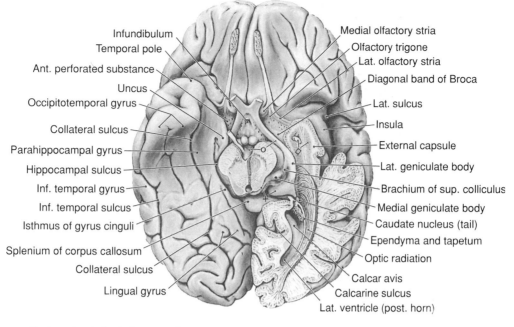

Infundibulum
Temporal pole
Ant. perforated substance
Uncus
Occipitotemporal gyrus
Collateral sulcus
Parahippocampal gyrus
Hippocampal sulcus
Inf. temporal gyrus
Inf. temporal sulcus
Isthmus of gyrus cinguli
Splenium of corpus callosum
Collateral sulcus
Lingual gyrus

Medial olfactory stria
Olfactory trigone
Lat. olfactory stria
Diagonal band of Broca
Lat. sulcus
Insula
External capsule
Lat. geniculate body
Brachium of sup. colliculus
Medial geniculate body
Caudate nucleus (tail)
Ependyma and tapetum
Optic radiation
Calcar avis
Calcarine sulcus
Lat. ventricle (post. horn)

o = Post. perforated substance; optic tract
◊ = Ant. commissure; lenticular nucleus
+ = Pulvinar of thalamus; brachium of inf. colliculus

Figure 1-2. Inferior surface of the brain showing the principal gyri and sulci. The left hemisphere has been dissected to show the visual pathways and relation of the optic radiation to the lateral ventricle. (Reprinted with permission from Truex RC, Kellner CE: *Detailed Atlas of the Head and Neck*. New York, Oxford University Press, 1958, p 46.)

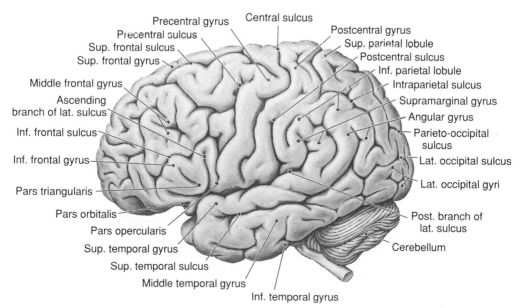

Precentral gyrus
Precentral sulcus
Sup. frontal sulcus
Sup. frontal gyrus
Middle frontal gyrus
Ascending branch of lat. sulcus
Inf. frontal sulcus
Inf. frontal gyrus
Pars triangularis
Pars orbitalis
Pars opercularis
Sup. temporal gyrus
Sup. temporal sulcus
Middle temporal gyrus
Inf. temporal gyrus

Central sulcus
Postcentral gyrus
Sup. parietal lobule
Postcentral sulcus
Inf. parietal lobule
Intraparietal sulcus
Supramarginal gyrus
Angular gyrus
Parieto-occipital sulcus
Lat. occipital sulcus
Lat. occipital gyri
Post. branch of lat. sulcus
Cerebellum

Figure 1-3. Lateral convex surface of the brain showing the principal gyri and sulci. The central sulcus separates the primary motor cortex (precentral gyrus) from the primary somatosensory cortex (postcentral gyrus). (Reprinted with permission from Truex RC, Kellner CE: *Detailed Atlas of the Head and Neck*. New York, Oxford University Press, 1958, p 47.)

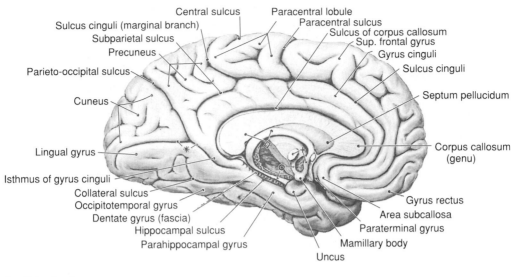

* = Calcarine fissure
◊ = Splenium of corpus callosum; body of fornix
+ = Interthalamic connection: ant. column of fornix
o = Fimbria of hippocampus; mamillothalamic tract

Figure 1-4. Medial surface of the brain showing the principal gyri and sulci. Parts of the thalamus and hypothalamus have been removed to show the fimbria and anterior column of the fornix and the mamillothalamic tract. (Reprinted with permission from Truex RC, Kellner CE: *Detailed Atlas of the Head and Neck*. New York, Oxford University Press, 1958, p 49.)

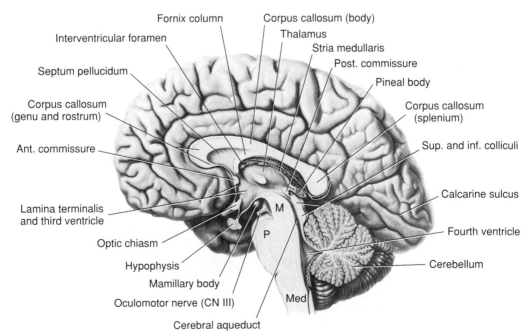

Figure 1-5. Midsagittal section of the brain and brainstem showing the structures surrounding the third and fourth ventricles. The brainstem includes the midbrain (*M*), pons (*P*), and medulla oblongata (*Med*). (Reprinted with permission from Wolf-Heidegger G: *Atlas der systematischen Anatomie des Menschen*, vol III, 3rd ed. Basel, S Karger AG, 1972.)

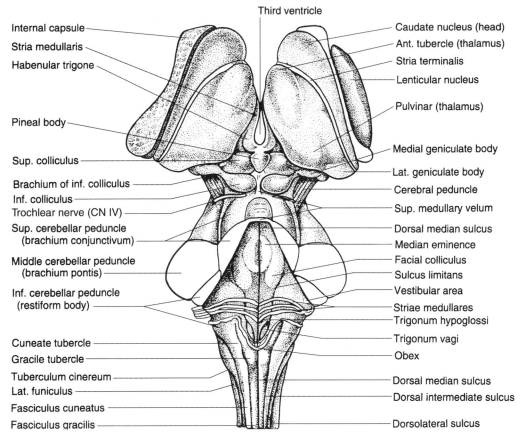

Figure 1-6. Surface anatomy of the brainstem and relationships of the attached cranial nerves (dorsal surface). The cerebellum has been removed to show the three cerebellar peduncles and the floor of the fourth ventricle (rhomboid fossa). (Reprinted with permission from Truex RC, Carpenter MB: *Human Neuroanatomy.* Baltimore, Williams & Wilkins, 1969, p 31.)

    (5) Posterior paracentral lobule
- is located on the medial surface between the central sulcus and the precuneus.
- represents a continuation of the postcentral gyrus on the medial hemispheric surface.

  c. Temporal lobe (see Figures 1-2 through 1-4)
- extends from the temporal pole to the occipital lobe, lying below the lateral sulcus.
- extends from the lateral sulcus to the collateral sulcus.
- contains the following gyri:

    (1) Transverse temporal gyri of Heschl
- lie buried within the lateral sulcus.
- extend from the superior temporal gyrus toward the medial geniculate body (Figure 1-6).
- are the primary auditory areas of the cerebral cortex (areas 41 and 42).

    (2) Superior temporal gyrus
- is associated with auditory functions.
- contains the **Wernicke speech area** in the dominant hemisphere (area 22).
- contains the planum temporale on its superior hidden surface.

    (3) Middle temporal gyrus

    (4) Inferior temporal gyrus

    (5) Lateral occipitotemporal gyrus (fusiform gyrus)
- lies between the inferior temporal sulcus and the collateral sulcus.

    d. Occipital lobe (see Figures 1-3 through 1-5)
- lies posterior to a line connecting the parieto-occipital sulcus and the preoccipital notch.
- contains two structures:
  - **(1) Cuneus**
    - lies between the parieto-occipital sulcus and the calcarine sulcus.
    - contains the visual cortex (areas 17, 18, and 19).
  - **(2) Lingual gyrus (medial occipitotemporal gyrus)**
    - lies below the calcarine sulcus.
    - contains the visual cortex (areas 17, 18, and 19).

    e. Insular lobe (insula) (see Figure 1-2)
- lies buried within the lateral sulcus.
- has short and long gyri.

    f. Limbic lobe (see Figures 1-4 and 23-1B)
- is a **C-shaped structure** of the medial hemispheric surface that encircles the corpus callosum and the lateral aspect of the midbrain.
- includes the following structures:
  - **(1) Paraterminal gyrus and subcallosal area** (see Figure 1-4)
    - are located anterior to the lamina terminalis and ventral to the rostrum of the corpus callosum.
  - **(2) Cingulate gyrus**
    - lies directly above the corpus callosum.
    - merges with the parahippocampal gyrus at the isthmus.
  - **(3) Parahippocampal gyrus**
    - lies between the hippocampal and collateral sulci and terminates in the **uncus**.
  - **(4) Hippocampal formation** (see Figures 1-2 and 1-4)
    - lies between the choroidal and hippocampal fissures.
    - is jelly-rolled into the parahippocampal gyrus.
    - is connected to the hypothalamus and septal area via the **fornix**.
    - includes the following three structures:
      - **(a) Dentate gyrus** (see Figure 1-4)
      - **(b) Hippocampus**
      - **(c) Subiculum** (see Figure 20-5)

    g. Olfactory structures (see Figure 1-2)
- are found on the orbital surface of the brain and include:
  - **(1) Olfactory bulb and tract**
    - are an outpouching of the telencephalon.
  - **(2) Olfactory bulb**
    - receives the olfactory nerve (cranial nerve [CN] I).
  - **(3) Olfactory trigone and striae**
  - **(4) Anterior perforated substance**
    - is created by penetrating striate arteries.
  - **(5) Diagonal band of Broca** (see Figure 1-2)
    - interconnects the amygdaloid nucleus and the septal area.

2. Basal ganglia (Figure 1-7; see Figures 1-6 and 21-1)
- are the subcortical nuclei of the telencephalon.
- include the following structures:
  - **a. Caudate nucleus**
    - is part of the striatum, together with the putamen.
  - **b. Putamen**
    - is part of the striatum, together with the caudate nucleus.
    - is part of the lentiform nucleus, together with the globus pallidus.

Some authorities include the parahippocampal gyrus as a temporal lobe structure.

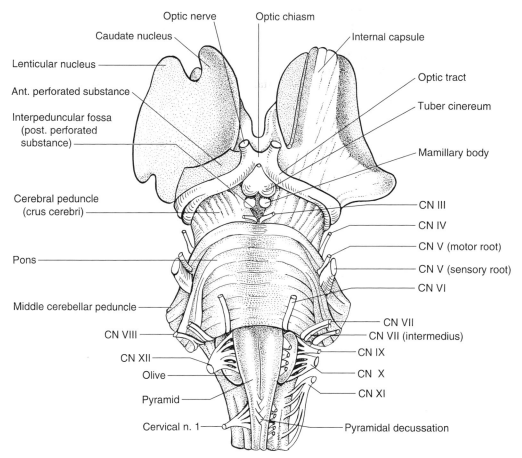

Figure 1-7.   Surface anatomy of the brainstem and relationships of the attached cranial nerves (ventral surface). (Reprinted with permission from Truex RC, Carpenter MB: *Human Neuroanatomy.* Baltimore, Williams & Wilkins, 1969, p 31.)

  c. **Globus pallidus**
    • is part of the lentiform nucleus, together with the putamen.
  d. **Amygdaloid nuclear complex (amygdala)**
  3. **Lateral ventricles** (see Figure 2-4)
    • are ependyma-lined cavities of the cerebral hemispheres.
    • contain **CSF** and **choroid plexus**.
    • communicate with the third ventricle via the two interventricular foramina of Monro (see Figure 2-3).
    • are separated from each other by the septa pellucida.
  4. **Cerebral cortex**
    • consists of a thin layer or mantle of gray substance.
    • covers the surface of each cerebral hemisphere.
    • is folded into gyri that are separated by sulci.
  5. **White matter**
    • includes the cerebral commissures and the internal capsule.
    a. **Cerebral commissures** (see Figures 1-4 and 1-5)
      • interconnect the cerebral hemispheres and include:
      (1) **Corpus callosum**
        • is the largest commissure of the brain.
        • interconnects the two hemispheres.
        • has four parts:

        (a) Rostrum

        (b) Genu

        (c) Body

        (d) Splenium

    (2) Anterior commissure

- is located in the midsagittal section between the lamina terminalis and the column of the fornix.
- interconnects the olfactory bulbs and the middle and inferior temporal lobes.

    (3) Hippocampal commissure (commissure of the fornix)

- is located between the fornices and ventral to the splenium of the corpus callosum.

  b. Internal capsule (see Figures 1-6, 1-7, and 16-3)

- consists of the white matter located between the basal ganglia and the thalamus.
- has three parts:

    (1) Anterior limb

- is located between the caudate nucleus and putamen.

    (2) Genu

- is located between the anterior and posterior limbs.
- contains corticobulbar fibers.

    (3) Posterior limb

- is located between the thalamus and lentiform nucleus (which is made up of the putamen and the globus pallidus).
- contains corticospinal fibers.

B. Diencephalon (see Figures 1-5 and 1-6)

- is located between the telencephalon and mesencephalon and between the interventricular foramen and the posterior commissure.
- receives the optic nerve (CN II).
- consists of the epithalamus, thalamus, hypothalamus, subthalamus, and the third ventricle and associated structures.

  1. Epithalamus (see Figures 1-5 and 1-6)

    a. Pineal body (epiphysis cerebri)

    b. Habenular trigone (see Figure 1-6)

    c. Medullary stria of the thalamus

    d. Posterior commissure

- mediates the consensual reaction of the pupillary light reflex.

    e. Tela choroidea and choroid plexus of the third ventricle

  2. Thalamus (see Figure 1-6)

- is separated from the hypothalamus by the **hypothalamic sulcus**.
- consists of the following surface structures:

    a. Pulvinar

    b. Metathalamus

      (1) Medial geniculate body (auditory system)

      (2) Lateral geniculate body (visual system)

    c. Anterior tubercle

    d. Interthalamic adhesion (massa intermedia)

  3. Hypothalamus (see Figures 1-1, 1-2, and 1-6)

    a. Optic chiasm

    b. Mamillary body

    c. Infundibulum

    d. Tuber cinereum

  4. Subthalamus (ventral thalamus)

- lies ventral to the thalamus and lateral to the hypothalamus.
- is not visible on midsagittal sections through the third ventricle.
- consists of:

    a. Subthalamic nucleus

    b. Zona incerta and fields of Forel (see Figure 21-3)

   5. **Third ventricle and associated structures** (see Figures 1-5 and 2-4)
      a. **Lamina terminalis**
         • results from closure of the anterior neuropore.
      b. **Tela choroidea**
      c. **Choroid plexus**
      d. **Interventricular foramen of Monro**
         • interconnects the lateral ventricle and the third ventricle.
      e. **Optic recess**
      f. **Infundibular recess**
      g. **Suprapineal recess**
      h. **Pineal recess**

C. **Mesencephalon (midbrain)** (see Figure 1-6)
   • is located between the diencephalon and the pons.
   • extends from the posterior commissure to the frenulum of the superior medullary velum.
   • contains the **cerebral aqueduct**, which interconnects the third and fourth ventricles.
   1. **Ventral surface**
      a. **Cerebral peduncle**
      b. **Interpeduncular fossa**
         (1) **Oculomotor nerve (CN III)**
         (2) **Posterior perforated substance**
            • is created by penetrating branches of the posterior cerebral and posterior communicating arteries.
   2. **Dorsal surface**
      a. **Superior colliculus (visual system)**
      b. **Brachium of the superior colliculus**
      c. **Inferior colliculus (auditory system)**
      d. **Brachium of the inferior colliculus**
      e. **Trochlear nerve (CN IV)**
         • is the only cranial nerve to exit the brainstem from the dorsal aspect.

D. **Pons** (see Figures 1-1 and 1-7)
   • is located between the midbrain and the medulla.
   • extends from the inferior pontine sulcus to the superior pontine sulcus.
   1. **Ventral surface**
      a. **Base of the pons**
      b. **Cranial nerves**
         (1) **Trigeminal nerve (CN V)**
         (2) **Abducent nerve (CN VI)**
         (3) **Facial nerve (CN VII)**
         (4) **Vestibulocochlear nerve (CN VIII)**
   2. **Dorsal surface (rhomboid fossa)**
      a. **Locus ceruleus**
         • contains the largest collection of norepinephrinergic neurons in the CNS.
      b. **Facial colliculus**
         • contains the abducent nucleus and internal genu of the facial nerve.
      c. **Sulcus limitans**
         • separates the alar plate from the basal plate.
      d. **Striae medullares of the rhomboid fossa**
         • divide the rhomboid fossa into the superior pontine portion and the inferior medullary portion.

E. **Medulla oblongata (myelencephalon)** (see Figures 1-1 and 1-7)
   • is located between the pons and the spinal cord.
   • extends from the first cervical nerve (C1) to the inferior pontine sulcus (also called the pontobulbar sulcus).

1. **Ventral surface**
   a. **Pyramid**
      • contains the corticospinal tract.
   b. **Olive**
      • contains the inferior olivary nucleus.
   c. **Cranial nerves**
      (1) **Glossopharyngeal nerve (CN IX)**
      (2) **Vagal nerve (CN X)**
      (3) **Accessory nerve (CN XI)**
      (4) **Hypoglossal nerve (CN XII)**
2. **Dorsal surface**
   a. **Gracile tubercle**
   b. **Cuneate tubercle**
   c. **Rhomboid fossa** (see Figure 1-6)
      (1) **Striae medullares of the rhomboid fossa**
      (2) **Vagal trigone**
      (3) **Hypoglossal trigone**
      (4) **Sulcus limitans**
      (5) **Area postrema (vomiting center)**

F. **Cerebellum** (see Figures 1-1 and 1-5)
   • is located in the posterior cranial fossa.
   • is attached to the brainstem by three cerebellar peduncles.
   • forms the roof of the fourth ventricle.
   • is separated from the occipital and temporal lobes by the **tentorium cerebelli**.
   • consists of **folia** and **fissures** on its surface.
   • contains the following surface structures:
      1. **Hemispheres**
         • are made up of two lateral lobes.
      2. **Vermis**
         • is a midline structure.
      3. **Flocculus and vermal nodulus**
         • form the flocculonodular lobule.
      4. **Tonsil**
         • is a rounded lobule on the inferior surface of each cerebellar hemisphere.
         • may herniate, with increased intracranial pressure, through the foramen magnum.
      5. **Superior cerebellar peduncle** (see Figure 1-6)
         • connects the cerebellum to the pons and midbrain.
      6. **Middle cerebellar peduncle** (see Figure 1-6)
         • connects the cerebellum to the pons.
      7. **Inferior cerebellar peduncle** (see Figure 1-6)
         • connects the cerebellum to the medulla.
      8. **Anterior lobe**
         • lies anterior to the primary fissure.
      9. **Posterior lobe**
         • is located between the primary and posterolateral fissures.
      10. **Flocculonodular lobe**
         • lies posterior to the posterolateral fissure.

III.   Atlas of the Brain and Brainstem (Figures 1-8 through 1-18)

• includes midsagittal, parasagittal, coronal, and axial sections of thick, stained brain slices.

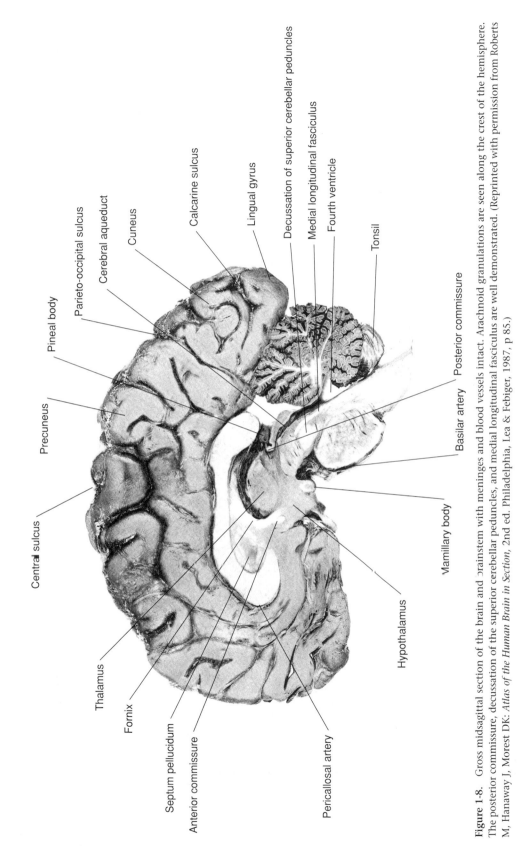

Figure 1-8. Gross midsagittal section of the brain and brainstem with meninges and blood vessels intact. Arachnoid granulations are seen along the crest of the hemisphere. The posterior commissure, decussation of the superior cerebellar peduncles, and medial longitudinal fasciculus are well demonstrated. (Reprinted with permission from Roberts M, Hanaway J, Morest DK: *Atlas of the Human Brain in Section,* 2nd ed. Philadelphia, Lea & Febiger, 1987, p 85.)

Central sulcus

Precuneus

Pineal body

Parieto-occipital sulcus

Cerebral aqueduct

Cuneus

Calcarine sulcus

Lingual gyrus

Decussation of superior cerebellar peduncles

Medial longitudinal fasciculus

Fourth ventricle

Tonsil

Basilar artery   Posterior commissure

Mamillary body

Hypothalamus

Pericallosal artery

Anterior commissure

Septum pellucidum

Fornix

Thalamus

11

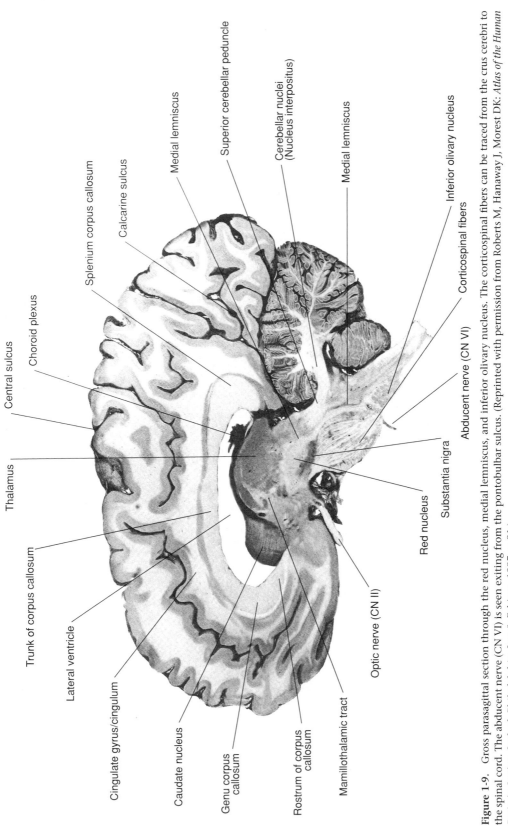

Figure 1-9. Gross parasagittal section through the red nucleus, medial lemniscus, and inferior olivary nucleus. The corticospinal fibers can be traced from the crus cerebri to the spinal cord. The abducent nerve (CN VI) is seen exiting from the pontobulbar sulcus. (Reprinted with permission from Roberts M, Hanaway J, Morest DK: *Atlas of the Human Brain in Section,* 2nd ed. Philadelphia, Lea & Febiger, 1987, p 81.)

Central sulcus

Choroid plexus

Thalamus

Splenium corpus callosum

Calcarine sulcus

Medial lemniscus

Superior cerebellar peduncle

Cerebellar nuclei
(Nucleus interpositus)

Medial lemniscus

Inferior olivary nucleus

Corticospinal fibers

Abducent nerve (CN VI)

Substantia nigra

Red nucleus

Optic nerve (CN II)

Mamillothalamic tract

Rostrum of corpus callosum

Genu corpus callosum

Caudate nucleus

Cingulate gyrus/cingulum

Lateral ventricle

Trunk of corpus callosum

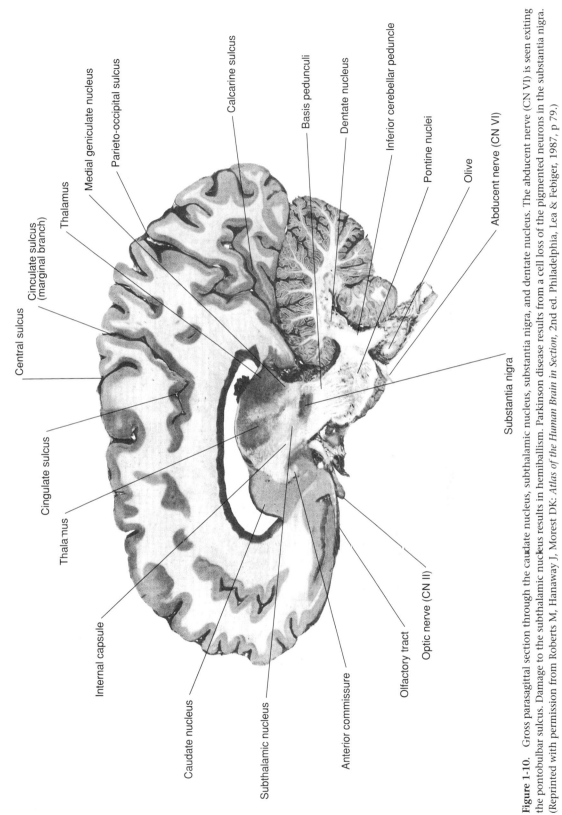

Figure 1-10. Gross parasagittal section through the caudate nucleus, subthalamic nucleus, substantia nigra, and dentate nucleus. The abducent nerve (CN VI) is seen exiting the pontobulbar sulcus. Damage to the subthalamic nucleus results in hemiballism. Parkinson disease results from a cell loss of the pigmented neurons in the substantia nigra. (Reprinted with permission from Roberts M, Hanaway J, Morest DK: *Atlas of the Human Brain in Section*, 2nd ed. Philadelphia, Lea & Febiger, 1987, p 79.)

13

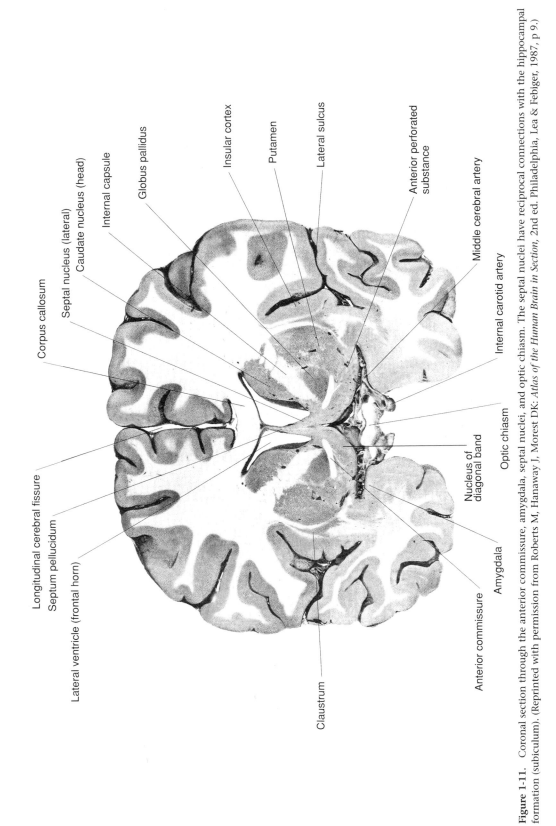

Figure 1-11. Coronal section through the anterior commissure, amygdala, septal nuclei, and optic chiasm. The septal nuclei have reciprocal connections with the hippocampal formation (subiculum). (Reprinted with permission from Roberts M, Hanaway J, Morest DK: *Atlas of the Human Brain in Section*, 2nd ed. Philadelphia, Lea & Febiger, 1987, p 9.)

Corpus callosum

Septal nucleus (lateral)
Caudate nucleus (head)
Internal capsule

Globus pallidus

Insular cortex

Putamen

Lateral sulcus

Anterior perforated
substance

Middle cerebral artery

Internal carotid artery

Longitudinal cerebral fissure
Septum pellucidum

Lateral ventricle (frontal horn)

Claustrum

Anterior commissure

Amygdala

Nucleus of
diagonal band

Optic chiasm

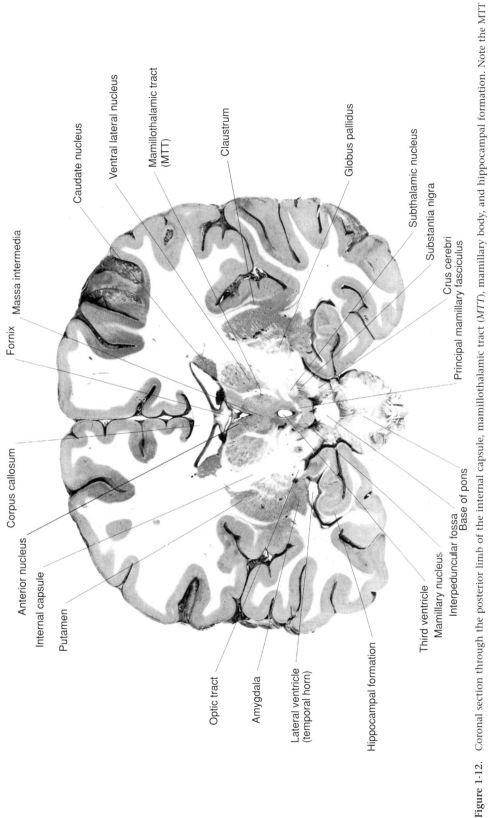

Figure 1-12. Coronal section through the posterior limb of the internal capsule, mamillothalamic tract (*MTT*), mamillary body, and hippocampal formation. Note the MTT entering the anterior ventral nucleus. The optic tracts are visible bilaterally. (Reprinted with permission from Roberts M, Hanaway J, Morest DK: *Atlas of the Human Brain in Section*, 2nd ed. Philadelphia, Lea & Febiger, 1987, p 19.

Caudate nucleus

Ventral lateral nucleus

Mamillothalamic tract (MTT)

Claustrum

Globus pallidus

Subthalamic nucleus

Substantia nigra

Crus cerebri

Principal mamillary fasciculus

Massa intermedia

Fornix

Corpus callosum

Anterior nucleus

Internal capsule

Putamen

Optic tract

Amygdala

Lateral ventricle (temporal horn)

Hippocampal formation

Third ventricle

Mamillary nucleus

Interpeduncular fossa

Base of pons

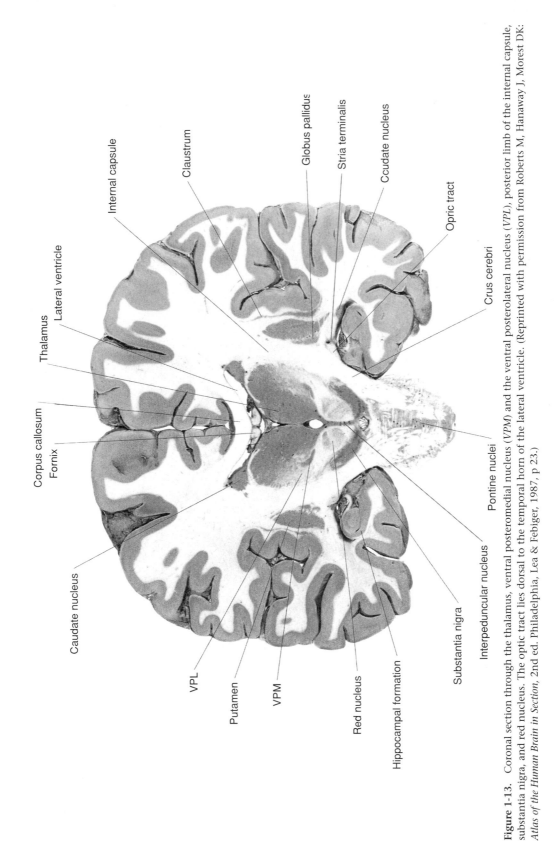

Figure 1-13. Coronal section through the thalamus, ventral posteromedial nucleus (*VPM*) and the ventral posterolateral nucleus (*VPL*), posterior limb of the internal capsule, substantia nigra, and red nucleus. The optic tract lies dorsal to the temporal horn of the lateral ventricle. (Reprinted with permission from Roberts M, Hanaway J, Morest DK: *Atlas of the Human Brain in Section*, 2nd ed. Philadelphia, Lea & Febiger, 1987, p 23.)

Labels on figure:
Internal capsule
Claustrum
Globus pallidus
Stria terminalis
Ccudate nucleus
Opric tract
Crus cerebri
Lateral ventricle
Thalamus
Corpus callosum
Fornix
Caudate nucleus
VPL
Putamen
VPM
Red nucleus
Hippocampal formation
Substantia nigra
Interpeduncular nucleus
Pontine nuclei

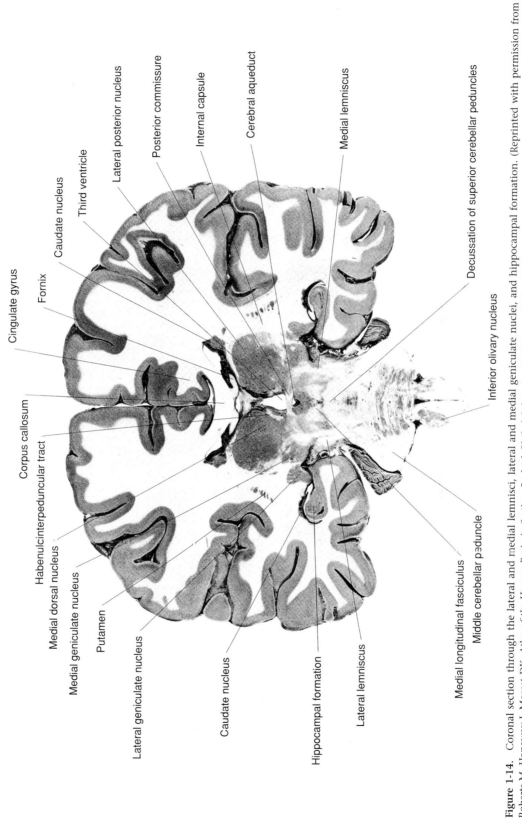

Figure 1-14. Coronal section through the lateral and medial lemnisci, lateral and medial geniculate nuclei, and hippocampal formation. (Reprinted with permission from Roberts M, Hanaway J, Morest DK: *Atlas of the Human Brain in Section*, 2nd ed. Philadelphia, Lea & Febiger, 1987, p 25.)

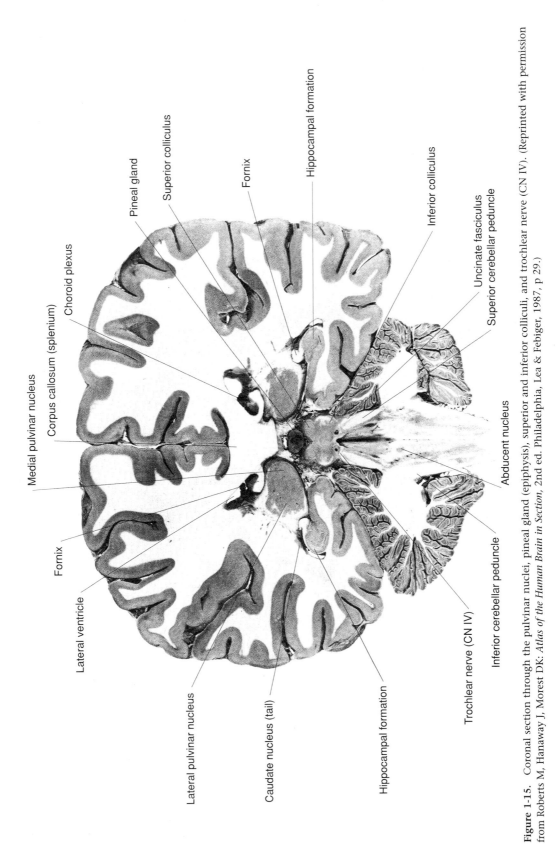

Figure 1-15. Coronal section through the pulvinar nuclei, pineal gland (epiphysis), superior and inferior colliculi, and trochlear nerve (CN IV). (Reprinted with permission from Roberts M, Hanaway J, Morest DK: *Atlas of the Human Brain in Section*, 2nd ed. Philadelphia, Lea & Febiger, 1987, p 29.)

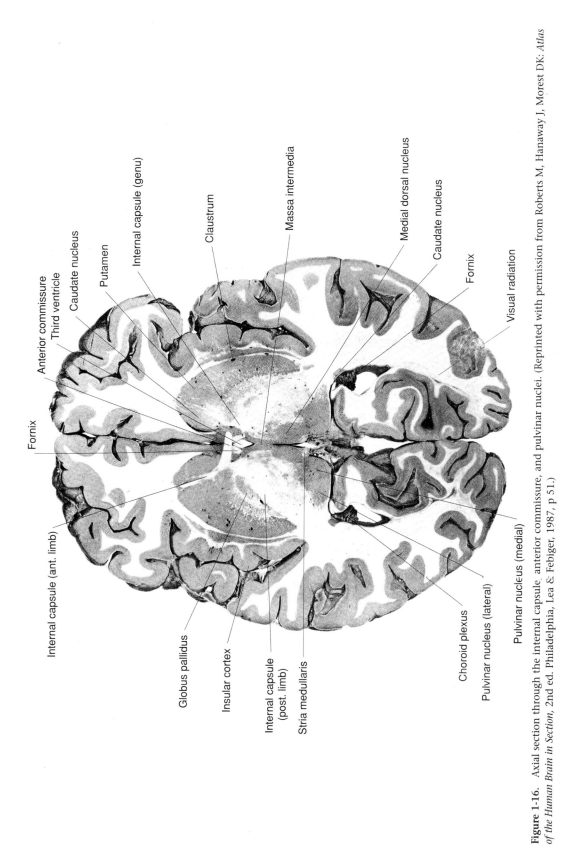

Figure 1-16. Axial section through the internal capsule, anterior commissure, and pulvinar nuclei. (Reprinted with permission from Roberts M, Hanaway J, Morest DK: *Atlas of the Human Brain in Section*, 2nd ed. Philadelphia, Lea & Febiger, 1987, p 51.)

Anterior commissure

Third ventricle

Caudate nucleus

Putamen

Internal capsule (genu)

Claustrum

Massa intermedia

Medial dorsal nucleus

Caudate nucleus

Fornix

Visual radiation

Fornix

Internal capsule (ant. limb)

Globus pallidus

Insular cortex

Internal capsule (post. limb)

Stria medullaris

Choroid plexus

Pulvinar nucleus (lateral)

Pulvinar nucleus (medial)

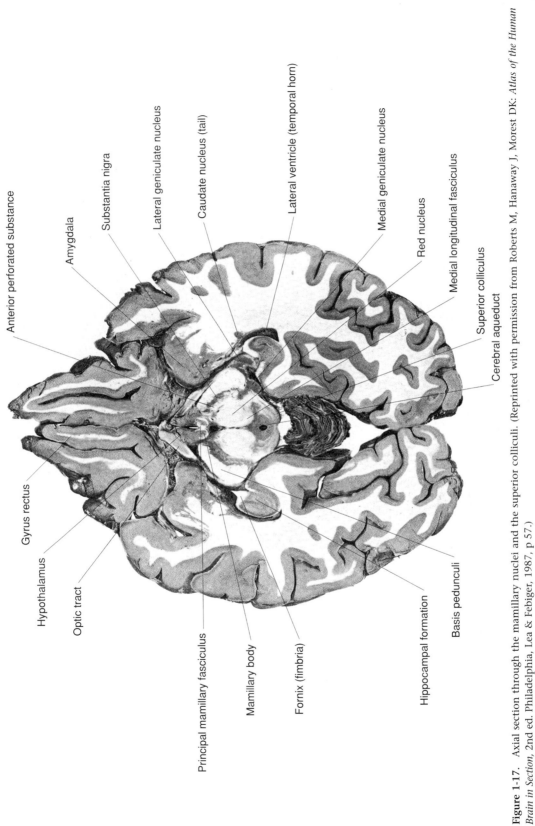

Anterior perforated substance

Amygdala

Substantia nigra

Lateral geniculate nucleus

Caudate nucleus (tail)

Lateral ventricle (temporal horn)

Medial geniculate nucleus

Red nucleus

Medial longitudinal fasciculus

Superior colliculus

Cerebral aqueduct

Gyrus rectus

Hypothalamus

Optic tract

Principal mamillary fasciculus

Mamillary body

Fornix (fimbria)

Hippocampal formation

Basis pedunculi

Figure 1-17. Axial section through the mamillary nuclei and the superior colliculi. (Reprinted with permission from Roberts M, Hanaway J, Morest DK: *Atlas of the Human Brain in Section*, 2nd ed. Philadelphia, Lea & Febiger, 1987, p 57.)

20

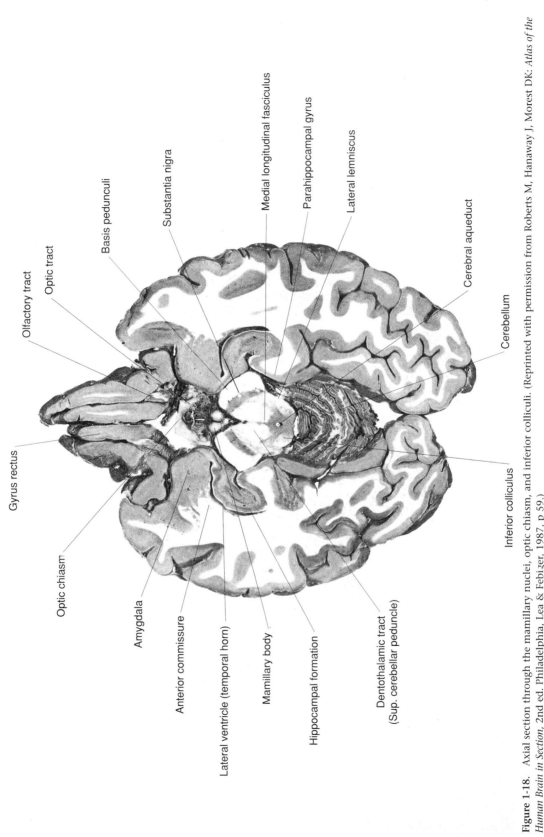

Figure 1-18. Axial section through the mamillary nuclei, optic chiasm, and inferior colliculi. (Reprinted with permission from Roberts M, Hanaway J, Morest DK: *Atlas of the Human Brain in Section*, 2nd ed. Philadelphia, Lea & Febiger, 1987, p 59.)

21

REVIEW TEST

1. Which one of the following structures is found in the diencephalon?

(A) thalamus
(B) cerebral hemispheres
(C) globus pallidus
(D) caudate nucleus
(E) internal capsule

2. The hippocampal formation is part of the

(A) frontal lobe
(B) parietal lobe
(C) insular lobe
(D) limbic lobe
(E) occipital lobe

3. Which one of the cranial nerves exits the brainstem from the dorsal aspect?

(A) CN I
(B) CN II
(C) CN III
(D) CN IV
(E) CN VI

4. Heschl's gyrus receives input from which of the following neural structures?

(A) angular gyrus
(B) medial geniculate nucleus
(C) primary auditory cortex
(D) sensory strip
(E) supramarginal gyrus

Questions 5 to 9

Match the descriptions in items 5 to 9 with the appropriate lettered structure shown in the T₁-weighted magnetic resonance image (MRI) of the coronal section of the brain.

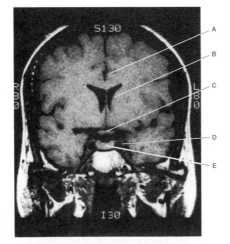

5. Lies within the cavernous sinus

6. Lies within the sella turcica

7. Is part of the striatum

8. Is part of the limbic lobe

9. Lies within a cistern

Questions 10 to 14

Match the structure or description in items 10 to 14 with the appropriate lettered structure shown in the stained thick section of the brain.

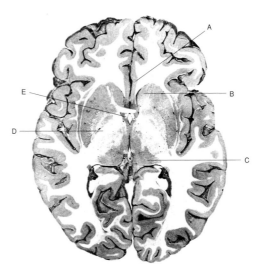

(From Roberts M, Hanaway J, Morest DK: *Atlas of the Human Brain in Section,* 2nd ed. Philadelphia, Lea & Febiger, 1987, p 51.)

10. Has reciprocal connections between the hippocampal formation and the septal nuclei

11. Largest nucleus of the diencephalon

12. Internal capsule

13. Cingulate gyrus

14. Caudate nucleus

ANSWERS AND EXPLANATIONS

1–A. The thalamus, along with the epithalamus, hypothalamus and the subthalamus comprise the diencephalon. The diencephalon lies deep to the prosencephalon and rostral to the midbrain.

2–D. The hippocampus is part of the limbic system and plays a role in memory. The name derives from Greek and is based on its jelly-roll shape, which resembles a sea horse. The hippocampus is one of the first regions damaged in Alzheimer's disease.

3–D. The trochlear nerve (CN IV) is the only cranial nerve to exit the brainstem from the dorsal aspect.

4–B. Primary auditory cortex (41, 42) is found in the Heschl gyrus, and receives input from the medial geniculate nucleus. The postcentral gyrus is the "sensory strip," the somatosensory cortex (3,1,2). The parietal lobe includes the angular gyrus, which receives visual impulses (39) and supramarginal gyrus, which interrelates somatosensory, auditory, and visual input (40). Destruction of the angular and supramarginal gyri on the dominant (usually left) side gives rise to the Gerstmann syndrome, whose symptoms include agraphia, acalculia, finger agnosia and left-right disorientation.

5–D. The carotid artery lies within the cavernous sinus, in company with CN III, CN IV, CN V-1, CN V-2, and CN VI; aneurysms of the internal carotid artery and tumors of the cavernous sinus may cause cranial nerve palsies.

6–E. The hypophysis (pituitary gland) lies within the hypophyseal fossa of the sella turcica; common tumors in this region are pituitary adenomas, craniopharyngiomas, and meningiomas.

7–B. The caudate nucleus and putamen are parts of the striatum. In Huntington disease there is a loss of neurons in the caudate nucleus; in Parkinson disease there is a loss of pigmented neurons in the substantia nigra.

8–A. The cingulate gyrus is part of the limbic lobe; lesions may result in akinesia, mutism, apathy, and indifference to pain.

9–C. The optic chiasm lies within the chiasmatic cistern.

10 E. The fornix contains fibers from the hippocampal formation and from the septal nuclei. The fornix projects massively to the mamillary nuclei of the hypothalamus.

11–C. The pulvinar nucleus is the largest nucleus of the thalamus. It has reciprocal connections with the association cortex of the occipital, parietal, and posterior lobes and is concerned with the integration of visual, auditory, and somesthetic input.

12–D. The posterior limb of the internal capsule lies between the lentiform nucleus and the thalamus. It contains the corticospinal tract and is perfused by the lateral striate arteries (branches of MCA) and the anterior choroidal artery.

13–A. The cingulate gyrus contains the cingulum, a fiber bundle that interconnects the hippocampal formation with the septal nucleus. Bilateral destruction of the cingulate gyrus causes loss of inhibition as well as dulling of the emotions. Memory is unaffected. Lesions of the anterior cingulate gyri cause placidity; cingulectomy is used to treat severe anxiety and depression.

14–B. The caudate nucleus and the putamen comprise the striatum, a basal ganglion. In Huntington disease, massive loss of neurons in the head of the caudate nucleus results in hydrocephalus ex vacuo. The globus pallidus and subthalamic nucleus are also basal ganglia.

Meninges and Cerebrospinal Fluid (CSF)

I. Meninges (Figure 2-1)

- are three connective tissue membranes that invest the spinal cord and brain.
- consist of the **pia mater** and the **arachnoid** (together known as the leptomeninges) and the **dura mater** (pachymeninx).

A. Pia mater
- is a delicate, highly vascular layer of connective tissue.
- closely covers the surface of the brain and spinal cord.
- is connected to the arachnoid by trabeculae.
  1. **Denticulate ligaments** (see Figure 2-1)
     - consist of two lateral flattened bands of pial tissue.
     - adhere to the spinal dura mater with 21 attachments.
  2. **Filum terminale** (Figure 2-2)
     - consists of a nonneural band of tissue that is a condensation of the pia mater.
     - extends from the conus medullaris to the end of the dural sac and fuses with it.

B. Arachnoid
- is a delicate, nonvascular connective tissue membrane between the dura mater and the pia mater.
  1. **Arachnoid granulations or arachnoid villi**
     - enter the venous dural sinuses and permit the one-way flow of **CSF** from the subarachnoid space into the venous circulation.
     - are found in large numbers along the **superior sagittal sinus** but are associated with all dural sinuses.
  2. **Subarachnoid space** (see I D 4)

C. Dura mater
- is the outer layer of the meninges and consists of dense connective tissue.
- The supratentorial dura is innervated by the trigeminal nerve; the posterior fossa is innervated by the vagal and upper spinal nerves.
- forms three major reflections and the walls of the dural venous sinuses:
  1. **Falx cerebri**
     - lies between the cerebral hemispheres in the longitudinal cerebral fissure.
     - contains the superior and inferior sagittal sinuses between its two layers.

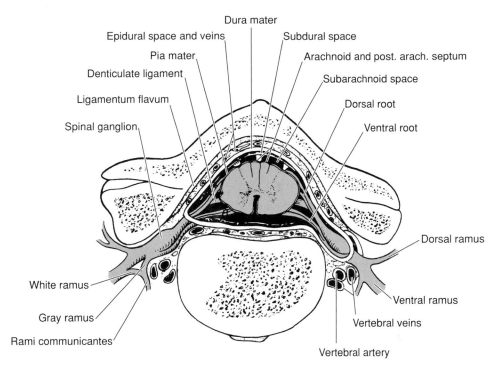

Figure 2-1.   Cross-section of the spinal cord and its meningeal investments. The subarachnoid, subdural, and epidural spaces are visible. The anterior and posterior longitudinal ligaments are seen but are not labeled. (Reprinted with permission from Carpenter MB, Sutin J: *Human Neuroanatomy,* 8th ed. Baltimore, Williams & Wilkins, 1983, p 9.)

    2. Tentorium cerebelli (Figure 2-3)
- separates the posterior cranial fossa from the middle cranial fossa.
- separates the temporal and occipital lobes from the cerebellum and infratentorial brainstem.
- contains the **tentorial incisure**, or notch, through which the brainstem passes.

    3. Diaphragma sellae
- forms the roof of the **hypophyseal fossa**.
- contains an aperture through which the **hypophyseal stalk** (infundibulum) passes.

    4. Dural sinuses (see Figure 2-3)
- are endothelium-lined, valveless venous blood channels.

D. Meningeal spaces (see Figures 2-1 through 2-3)
    1. Spinal epidural space
- is located between the dura and the vertebral periosteum.
- contains loose areolar tissue, venous plexuses, and lymphatics.
- may be injected with a local anesthetic to produce a paravertebral nerve block.

    2. Cranial epidural space
- is a *potential* space between the periosteal and meningeal layers of the dura.
- contains the meningeal arteries and veins.

    3. Subdural space
- is a *potential* space between the dura and the arachnoid.
- intracranially transmits the superior cerebral veins to the venous lacunae of the superior sagittal sinus. Laceration of these "bridging veins" results in **subdural hemorrhage** (hematoma).

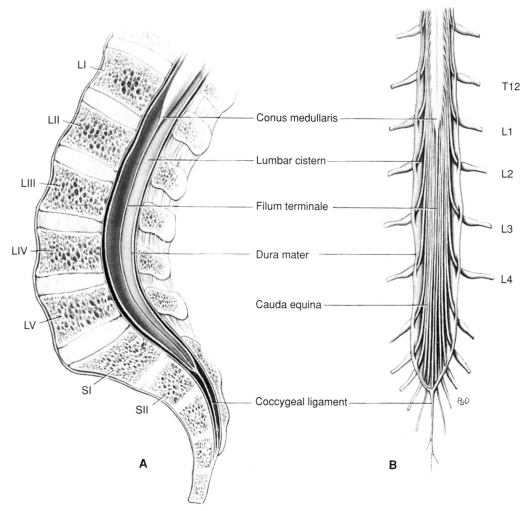

Figure 2-2. Diagrammatic representations of the caudal part of the spinal cord and lumbar cistern. **(A)** Longitudinal section through the caudal vertebral column and canal showing the conus medullaris and the lumbar cistern. Lumbar puncture is made between the spinous processes of L3 and L4 (or L4 and L5). **(B)** Dorsal view of the cauda equina and spinal nerves. The adult spinal cord terminates at the L1–L2 interspace. (Reprinted with permission from Carpenter MB, Sutin J: *Human Neuroanatomy,* 8th ed. Baltimore, Williams & Wilkins, 1983, p 8.)

4. Subarachnoid space
- is located between the pia mater and the arachnoid.
- contains **CSF.**
- surrounds the entire brain and spinal cord.
- extends, in the adult, below the conus medullaris to the level of the second sacral vertebra, the **lumbar cistern** (see Figure 2-2A).

5. Subarachnoid cisterns (see Figure 2-3)
- are dilations of the subarachnoid space, which contains CSF.
- are named after the structures over which they lie (e.g., pontine, chiasmatic, and interpeduncular cisterns).
  a. Cerebellopontine angle cistern
    - receives CSF from the fourth ventricle via the lateral foramina of Luschka.

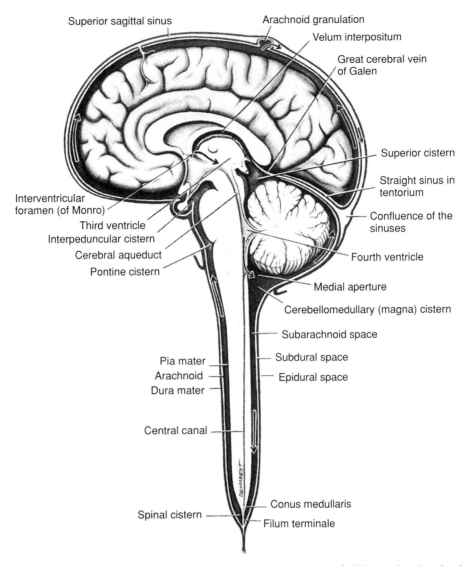

Figure 2-3. The subarachnoid spaces and cisterns of the brain and spinal cord. CSF is produced in the choroid plexuses of the ventricles, exits the fourth ventricle, circulates in the subarachnoid space, and enters the superior sagittal sinus via the arachnoid granulations. (Reprinted with permission from Noback CR, Strominger NL, Demarest RJ: *The Human Nervous System,* 4th ed. Baltimore, Williams & Wilkins, 1991, p 68.)

- contains the facial nerve (**cranial nerve [CN] VII**) and the vestibulocochlear nerve (**CN VIII**).
  b. **Cerebellomedullary cistern (cisterna magna)**
    - is located in the midline between the cerebellum and the medulla.
    - receives CSF from the fourth ventricle via the median foramen of Magendie.
    - can be tapped for CSF (suboccipital tap).
  c. **Ambient cistern**
    - interconnects the superior and interpeduncular cisterns; contains the trochlear nerve (**CN IV**).
  d. **Superior cistern**
    - overlies the midbrain tectum.

E. **Meningiomas**
- are benign, slow-growing, well-demarcated tumors that arise from meningotheal arachnoid cells.
- comprise 20% of primary intracranial tumors and 25% of spinal tumors.
- are found most frequently in the anterior cranial fossa (parasagittal 25%, convexity 20%, and basal 40%).
- are histologically characterized by a whorling pattern and calcified **psammoma bodies**.
- enlarge slowly and create a cavity in the adjacent brain.
- occur in adults between 20 and 60 years of age, most often in women (60%).

II.   Ventricles (Figure 2-4; see Figure 2-3)

- are lined with ependyma and contain CSF.
- contain choroid plexus, which produces CSF at a rate of 500 ml/day.
- communicate with the subarachnoid space via three foramina in the fourth ventricle.
- consist of four fluid-filled communicating cavities within the brain.

A. **Lateral ventricles**
- are the two ventricles located within the cerebral hemispheres.
- communicate with the third ventricle via the **interventricular foramina of Monro**.
- consist of five parts:
  1. **Frontal (anterior) horn**
     - is located in the frontal lobe; its lateral wall is formed by the head of the caudate nucleus.
     - lacks choroid plexus.
  2. **Body**
     - is located in the medial portion of the frontal and parietal lobes.
     - has choroid plexus.
     - communicates via the interventricular foramen of Monro with the third ventricle.
  3. **Temporal (inferior) horn**
     - is located in the medial part of the temporal lobe.
     - has choroid plexus.
  4. **Occipital (posterior) horn** (see Figure 1-2)
     - is located in the parietal and occipital lobes.
     - lacks choroid plexus.
  5. **Trigone (atrium)**
     - is found at the junction of the body, occipital horn, and temporal horn of the lateral ventricle.
     - contains the **glomus**, a large tuft of choroid plexus, which is calcified in adults and is visible on x-ray film and computed tomography (CT).

B. **Third ventricle** (see Figures 1-5, 2-3, and 2-4)
- is a slitlike vertical midline cavity of the diencephalon.
- communicates with the lateral ventricles via the interventricular foramina of Monro and with the fourth ventricle via the cerebral aqueduct.
- contains a pair of choroid plexuses in its roof.

C. **Cerebral aqueduct (aqueduct of Sylvius)**
- lies in the midbrain.
- connects the third ventricle with the fourth ventricle.
- lacks choroid plexus.
- Blockage leads to hydrocephalus (aqueductal stenosis).

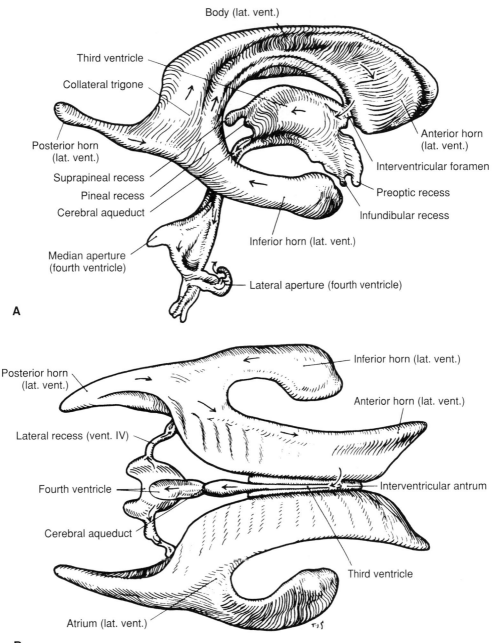

Figure 2-4. The ventricle system of the brain. **(A)** Lateral aspect. **(B)** Dorsal aspect. (Reprinted with permission from Carpenter MB, Sutin J: *Human Neuroanatomy*, 8th ed. Baltimore, Williams & Wilkins, 1983, p 44.)

D. **Fourth ventricle** (see Figures 1-5, 2-3, and 2-4)
   • lies between the cerebellum and the brainstem.
   • contains a pair of choroid plexuses in its caudal roof.
   • expresses CSF into the subarachnoid space via the two lateral foramina of Luschka and the single medial foramen of Magendie.

III. Cerebrospinal Fluid

- is a clear, colorless, acellular fluid found in the subarachnoid space and ventricles.
- has several **features**:

A. Formation
- is produced by the **choroid plexus** at a rate of 500 ml/day. The total CSF volume equals 140 ml (see Figures 1-5, 1-7, and 2-3).

B. Function
- supports and cushions the central nervous system (CNS) against concussive injury.
- transports hormones and hormone-releasing factors.
- removes metabolic waste products through absorption; the sites of greatest absorption are the **arachnoid villi** (see Figure 2-3).

C. Circulation (see Figure 2-3)
- flows from the ventricles via the three foramina of the fourth **ventricle** into the subarachnoid space and over the convexity of the hemisphere to the superior sagittal sinus, where it enters the venous circulation.

D. Composition
- contains no more than 5 lymphocytes/μl and usually is sterile.
- other **normal values** are:
  1. **pH:** 7.35
  2. **Specific gravity:** 1.007
  3. **Glucose:** 66% of plasma glucose
  4. **Total protein:** < 45 mg/dl in the lumbar cistern

E. Normal pressure
- is 80 to 180 mm of water (CSF) in the lumbar subarachnoid space when the patient is in a lateral recumbent (decubitus) position.

IV. Hydrocephalus

- is dilation of the cerebral ventricles caused by blockage of the CSF pathways.
- is characterized by excessive accumulation of CSF in the cerebral ventricles or subarachnoid space.

A. Noncommunicating hydrocephalus
- results from obstruction within the ventricles (e.g., congenital aqueductal stenosis).

B. Communicating hydrocephalus
- results from blockage within the subarachnoid space (e.g., adhesions after meningitis).

C. Normal-pressure hydrocephalus
- occurs when the CSF is not absorbed by the arachnoid villi, possibly secondary to post-traumatic meningeal hemorrhage.
- is characterized clinically by the triad of progressive dementia, ataxic gait, and urinary incontinence (**wacky, wobbly, and wet**).

D. Hydrocephalus ex vacuo
- results from a loss of cells in the caudate nucleus (e.g., Huntington disease).

E. **Pseudotumor cerebri (benign intracranial hypertension)**
- results from increased resistance to CSF outflow at the arachnoid villi.
- is characterized by papilledema without mass, elevated CSF pressure, and deteriorating vision. The ventricles may be slit-like.
- occurs in obese young women.

V.   Meningitis (pl. meningitides)

- is an inflammation of the pia–arachnoid of the brain, spinal cord, or both.

A. **Bacterial (pyogenic) meningitis**
- occurs most often in children under 5 years of age (>70% of all cases).
- is characterized clinically by fever, headache, and nuchal rigidity with Kernig sign.
- may result in cranial nerve palsies (CN III, CN IV, CN VI, and CN VIII) and hydrocephalus.
  1. **Common etiologic agents**
     a. In **newborns** (<1 month of age), it is most frequently caused by group B streptococci (*S. agalactiae*) and *Escherichia coli.*
     b. In **older infants and young children** (1 month–9 years of age), it is most frequently caused by *Haemophilus influenzae.*
     c. In **older children to middle-aged adults** (10–60 years of age), it is most frequently caused by *S. pneumoniae* and *Neisseria meningitidis.*
     d. In **older adults**, it is most frequently caused by *S. pneumoniae.*
     e. **In newborns**, immunization against *Haemophilus influenzae* has significantly reduced this type of meningitis.
  2. **CSF findings** (Table 2-1)
     a. **Numerous neutrophils**
     b. **Decreased glucose level**
     c. **Elevated protein level** — *bact stkproduct*

B. **Viral (lymphocytic) meningitis**
- is also called aseptic meningitis.
- is characterized by fever, headache, and nuchal rigidity with Kernig sign.

TABLE 2-1	*Properties of CSF in Subarachnoid Hemorrhage, Bacterial Meningitis, and Viral Encephalitis*			
CSF	Normal	Subarachnoid Hemorrhage	Bacterial Meningitis	Viral Encephalitis
Color	Clear	Bloody	Cloudy	Clear, cloudy
Cell count (per mm^3)	<5 lymphocytes	Red blood cells present (~5 × 10^6/mm^3)	>1000 PML	25–500 lymphocytes
Protein	<45 mg/dl	Normal to slightly elevated	Elevated (>100 mg/dl)	Slightly elevated (<100 mg/dl)
Glucose (~66% of blood [80–120 mg/dl])	>45 mg/dl	Normal	Reduced	Normal

PML = polymorphonuclear leukocytes.
In infants: cell counts <10 cells/mm^3; protein 20–170 mg/dl.

1. Viruses isolated include the following:
   a. Mumps virus
   b. Enteric cytopathic human orphan (ECHO) viruses
   c. Coxsackie virus
   d. Epstein-Barr virus
   e. Herpes simplex virus (type 2)
2. CSF findings
   a. Numerous lymphocytes
   b. Normal glucose
   c. Normal to slightly increased protein

VI. Herniation (Figures 2-5 through 2-8)

A. **Transtentorial (uncal) herniation**
   - is protrusion of the brain through the tentorial incisure.

B. **Transforaminal (tonsillar) herniation**
   - is protrusion of the brainstem and cerebellum through the foramen magnum.

C. **Subfalcial herniation**
   - is herniation below the falx cerebri.

VII. Circumventricular Organs

- are chemosensitive zones that monitor the varying concentrations of circulating hormones in blood and CSF.
- are located in the periphery of the third ventricle; the **area postrema** is found in the floor of the fourth ventricle.
- are highly vascularized with fenestrated capillaries and no blood–brain barrier (the subcommissural organ is an exception).
- include the following structures:

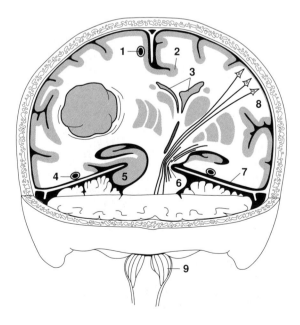

Figure 2-5 Coronal section of a tumor in the supratentorial compartment. **(1)** Anterior cerebral artery; **(2)** subfalcial herniation; **(3)** shifting of ventricles; **(4)** posterior cerebral artery (compression results in contralateral hemianopia); **(5)** uncal (transtentorial) herniation; **(6)** Kernohan notch, with damaged corticospinal and corticobulbar fibers; **(7)** tentorium cerebelli; **(8)** pyramidal cells that give rise to the corticospinal tract; **(9)** tonsillar (transforaminal) herniation, which damages vital medullary centers. (Adapted with permission from Leech RW, Shuman RM: *Neuropathology.* New York, Harper & Row, 1982, p 16.)

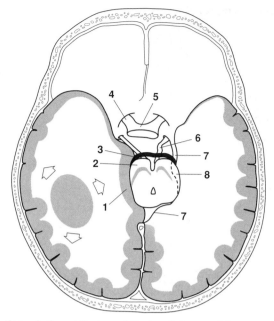

Figure 2-6   Axial section through the midbrain and the herniating parahippocampal gyrus (**arrows**). The left oculomotor nerve is being stretched (dilated pupil). The left posterior cerebral artery is compressed, resulting in a contralateral hemianopia. The right crus cerebri is damaged (Kernohan notch) by the free edge of the tentorial incisure, resulting in a contralateral hemiparesis; the Kernohan notch results in a false localizing sign. The caudal displacement of the brainstem causes rupture of the paramedian arteries of the basilar artery. Hemorrhage into the midbrain and rostral pontine tegmentum is usually fatal (Duret hemorrhages). The posterior cerebral arteries lie superior to the oculomotor nerves. (**1**) Parahippocampal gyrus; (**2**) crus cerebri; (**3**) posterior cerebral artery; (**4**) optic nerve; (**5**) optic chiasma; oculomotor nerve; (**6**) oculomotor nerve; (**7**) free edge of tentorium; (**8**) Kernohan notch. (Adapted with permission from Leech RW, Shuman RM: *Neuropathology.* New York, Harper & Row, 1982, p 19.)

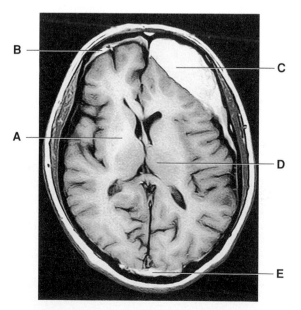

Figure 2-7   Magnetic resonance imaging scan (T_1-weighted image) showing brain trauma. Epidural hematomas may cross dural attachments. Subdural hematomas do not cross dural attachments. The hyperintense signals are caused by methemoglobin. (**A**) Internal capsule; (**B**) subdural hematoma; (**C**) subdural hematoma; (**D**) thalamus; (**E**) epidural hematoma. (Reprinted with permission from Fix JD: *High-Yield Neuroanatomy,* 3rd ed. Philadelphia, Lippincott Williams & Wilkins, 2005, p 27.)

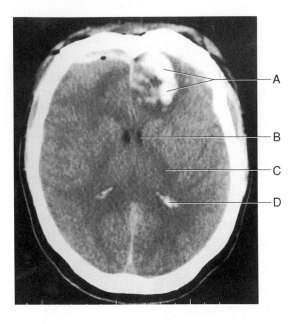

Figure 2-8 CT scan (axial section) showing an intraparenchymal hemorrhage in the left frontal lobe. **(A)** Intraparenchymal hemorrhage; **(B)** lateral ventricle; **(C)** internal capsule; **(D)** calcified glomus in the trigone region of the lateral ventricle. (Reprinted with permission from Fix JD: *High-Yield Neuroanatomy*, 3rd ed. Philadelphia, Lippincott Williams & Wilkins, 2005, p 27.)

OVLT

A. Organum vasculosum of the lamina terminalis
- is considered to be a vascular outlet for luteinizing hormone–releasing hormone and somatostatin.

B. Median eminence of the tuber cinereum (see Figure 1-1)
- contains neurons that elaborate releasing and inhibiting hormones into the hypophyseal portal system.

C. Subfornical organ
- is located on the inferior surface of the fornix at the level of the interventricular foramen of Monro.
- contains neurons that project to the supraoptic nuclei and the organum vasculosum.
- is a central receptor site for angiotensin II.

D. Subcommissural organ
- is located below the posterior commissure at the junction of the third ventricle and the cerebral aqueduct.
- is composed of specialized ependymal cells, glial elements, and a capillary bed containing nonfenestrated endothelial cells.

E. Pineal body (see Figures 1-5 and 1-6)
- contains **calcareous granules**, in **brain sand** or acervulus, which are seen on x-ray film and CT; calcification occurs after 16 years of age.
- contains **pinealocytes** (epiphyseal cells) and is highly vascular with fenestrated capillaries.
- is derived from the diencephalon.
- is innervated solely via postganglionic fibers from the superior cervical ganglion of the autonomic nervous system.
- synthesizes serotonin and melatonin. Clinical observation suggests an **antigonadotrophic function**.
- **Pinealomas** may result in dorsal midbrain syndrome (see Figure 14-3A).

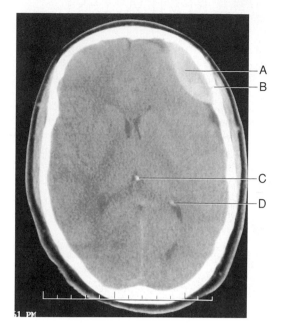

Figure 2-9 CT scan (axial section) showing an epidural hematoma and a skull fracture. The epidural hematoma has a classic biconvex, or lentiform, shape. **(A)** Epidural hematoma; **(B)** skull fracture; **(C)** calcified pineal gland; **(D)** calcified glomus in the trigone region of the lateral ventricle.

F. **Area postrema** (Figure 2-9)
   • consists of two small subependymal oval areas on either side of the fourth ventricle rostral to the obex.
   • contains modified neurons and astrocyte-like cells surrounded by fenestrated capillaries.
   • is considered to be a chemoreceptor zone that triggers vomiting in response to circulating emetic substances.
   • plays a role in food intake and cardiovascular regulation.

1. A 25-year-old housewife complains of headaches of 4 months' duration. She is obese and has bilateral papilledema, and her vision is deteriorating. Her opening CSF pressure is elevated; other CSF findings are normal. CT and magnetic resonance imaging (MRI) scans are normal. These signs are due to impairment of CSF egress. Obstruction at which of the following loci is most likely?

(A) Arachnoid villi
(B) Cerebral aqueduct
(C) Foramen of Luschka
(D) Foramen of Magendie
(E) Foramen of Monro

2. The total volume of CSF found in the sub-arachnoid space and cerebral ventricles is

(A) 110 ml
(B) 140 ml
(C) 160 ml
(D) 170 ml
(E) 190 ml

3. Which of the following pathogens would most likely be seen in bacterial meningitis of the newborn?

(A) *Streptococcus agalactiae*
(B) *Haemophilus influenzae*
(C) *Neisseria meningitides*
(D) *Streptococcus pneumoniae*
(E) Herpes simplex type 2

4. Which part of the ventricular system contains choroid plexus?

(A) Frontal horn
(B) Occipital horn
(C) Cerebral aqueduct
(D) Third ventricle
(E) Terminal ventricle

5. Which one of the following circumventricular organs is solely innervated by postganglionic fibers from the superior cervical ganglion of the ANS?

(A) Area postrema
(B) Pineal body
(C) Organum vasculosum of the lamina terminalis
(D) Subfornical organ
(E) Subcommissural organ

6. Choose the normal quantity of CSF daily production.

(A) 300 ml
(B) 400 ml
(C) 500 ml
(D) 600 ml
(E) 700 ml

7. Which one of the following tumors contains cellular whorls and psammoma bodies?

(A) Astrocytoma
(B) Acoustic schwannoma
(C) Glioblastoma multiforme
(D) Oligodendroglioma
(E) Meningioma

Questions 8 to12

Match each structure or description in items 8 to 12 with the appropriate lettered structure shown in the T$_1$-weighted magnetic resonance image of a coronal section of the brain.

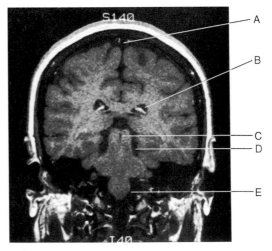

8. Olive

9. It contains the trochlear nerve (CN IV)

10. Its stenosis results in hydrocephalus

11. Contains a calcified glomus

12. Receives CSF from the arachnoid villi

Questions 13 to 17

Match each structure or description in items 13 to 17 with the appropriate lettered structure shown on the T_1-weighted magnetic resonance image of a midsagittal section of the brain.

13. Superior cistern

14. Blockage resulting in hydrocephalus

15. Lateral ventricle

16. Contains the two foramina of Luschka

17. Receives CSF via the foramen of Magendie

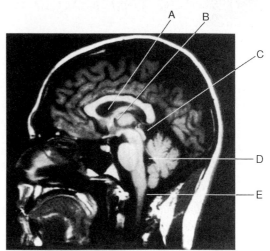

ANSWERS AND EXPLANATIONS

1–A. This condition, called pseudotumor cerebri (benign intracranial hypertension), is seen primarily in young obese women. Impaired absorptive function of the arachnoid villi is thought to be the cause.

2–B. The total volume of CSF found in the subarachnoid space and ventricles is 140 ml.

3–A. *Streptococcus agalactiae* is seen frequently in newborns. *Haemophilus influenzae* immunization has greatly reduced this type of meningitis. *S. pneumoniae* is frequently the cause of meningitis in older adults. *Neisseria meningitides* is seen in older children to middle-aged adults. Herpes simplex type 2 is a virus.

4–D. The third ventricle has a choroid plexus; the frontal lobe, the occipital lobe, and the cerebral aqueduct all are devoid of a choroid plexus; a terminal ventricle is a localized dilation of the caudal end of the central canal with no choroid plexus.

5–B. The pineal body (epiphysis) is innervated solely via postganglionic fibers from the superior ganglion of the autonomic nervous system; it synthesizes melatonin; it has antigonadotrophic function; the area postrema is a chemoreceptor zone that triggers vomiting in response to circulating emetic substances; the organum vasculosum of the lamina terminalis is a vascular outlet for luteinizing hormone–releasing hormone and somatostatin; the subfornical organ is a central receptor for angiotensin II; the subcommissural organ has a capillary bed with nonfenestrated endothelial cell and a blood–brain barrier.

6–C. The choroid plexus produces CSF at a rate of 500 ml/day.

7–E. Meningiomas contain cellular whorls and calcified psammoma bodies; are associated with neurofibromatosis-2; gender females> males; astrocytomas type II have near normal cellularity, little nuclear pleomorphism, no endothelial proliferation, and no necrosis; acoustic schwannomas are benign tumors arising from Schwann cells—histopathology shows Antoni A and Antoni B tissue and Verocay bodies; oligodendrogliomas show calcification in 50% of cases—cells look like fried eggs (perinuclear halos); glioblastoma multiforme represents 55% of gliomas, is malignant and rapidly fatal; most common primary brain tumor; contains pseudopalisades, perivascular pseudorosettes, and microvascular proliferation.

8–E. The olive is a prominent surface structure of the medulla.

9–D. The ambient cistern contains the trochlear nerve (CN IV).

10–C. Stenosis of the cerebral aqueduct prevents CSF from entering the fourth ventricle; this results in a noncommunicating hydrocephalus.

11–B. The trigone of the lateral ventricle contains a large tuft of choroid plexus called the glomus. It is usually calcified and highly visible in CT images.

12–A. The superior sagittal sinus receives CSF via the arachnoid villi.

13–C. The superior (quadrigeminal) cistern overlies the dorsal aspect of the midbrain.

14–B. Blockage of the interventricular foramen of Monro (e.g., due to a colloid cyst of the third ventricle) results in hydrocephalus involving the lateral ventricle.

15–A. The lateral ventricle is seen between the corpus callosum and the fornix.

16–D. The fourth ventricle contains the two foramina of Luschka, which drain into the two cerebellopontine angle cisterns.

17–E. The cerebellomedullary cistern receives CSF via the foramen of Magendie.

CHAPTER

3

Blood Supply of the Central Nervous System (CNS)

I. Arteries of the Spinal Cord

- arise from the vertebral and segmental arteries.

A. **Vertebral artery** (Figure 3-1)
  - is a branch of the subclavian artery.
  - gives rise to the anterior spinal artery and may give rise to the posterior spinal artery.
  1. **Anterior spinal artery**
     - supplies the anterior two-thirds of the spinal cord, including the anterior and lateral horns.
     - supplies the pyramids, medial lemniscus, and intra-axial fibers of the hypoglossal nerve (cranial nerve [CN] XII) in the medulla.
  2. **Posterior spinal arteries**
     - supply the posterior third of the spinal cord, including the posterior horns and columns.
     - supply the gracile and cuneate fasciculi and nuclei in the medulla.

B. **Segmental arteries**
  - arise from the aorta, vertebral arteries, and common iliac arteries as medullary arteries, which supply the anterior and posterior spinal arteries.
  - provide the main blood supply to the spinal cord at thoracic and lumbar levels. The second lumbar artery gives rise to a large anterior medullary artery, the **artery of Adamkiewicz**. Its origin varies from T12 to L4, and it usually arises on the left side.

C. **Segmental vulnerability**
  - is due to inadequate blood supply after injury (e.g., dissecting aneurysms, atherosclerosis, arterial thrombosis). Segments T1 to T4 and L1 are poorly vascularized and are at risk.
  - may explain the etiology of the anterior spinal artery syndrome.

II. Venous Drainage of the Spinal Cord

- follows, in general, the arterial pattern.
- passes from spinal veins within the subarachnoid space to the epidural internal venous plexus before draining into intracranial, cervical, thoracic, intercostal, or abdominal veins.
- is conducted by valveless veins that permit bidirectional flow, depending on the existing pressure gradients.
- is a pathway for transmission of infectious agents and tumor cells.

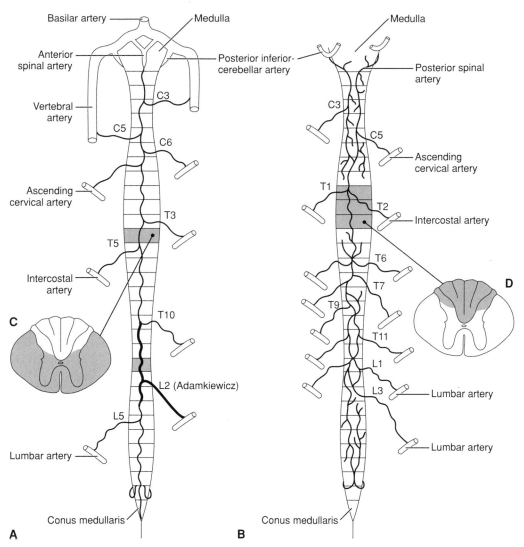

Figure 3-1. Arterial blood supply of the spinal cord. (A) Anterior surface, (B) posterior surface, (C) occlusion of the anterior spinal artery resulting in infarction of the anterior two-thirds of the spinal cord, (D) occlusion of the posterior spinal arteries resulting in infarction of the posterior columns. Note the large lumbar feeder artery of Adamkiewicz, whose origin varies from segments T12 to L4. Stippled areas show spinal cord segments that are vulnerable to hypoperfusion. (Adapted from Parent A: *Carpenter's Human Neuroanatomy*, 9th ed. Baltimore, Williams & Wilkins, 1995, p 94.)

III.   Arteries of the Brain (Figures 3-2 through 3-6)

- supply 15% of the cardiac output to the brain.
- provide the brain with 20% of the oxygen used by the body.
- have a normal blood flow of 50 ml/100 g of brain tissue per minute.
- consist of two pairs of vessels, the **internal carotid arteries** and the **vertebral arteries**, and their divisions. At the junction between the medulla and the pons, the two vertebral arteries fuse to form the **basilar artery**.

A.   Internal carotid artery
- enters the cranium via the carotid canal of the temporal bone.
- lies within the cavernous sinus as the carotid siphon.

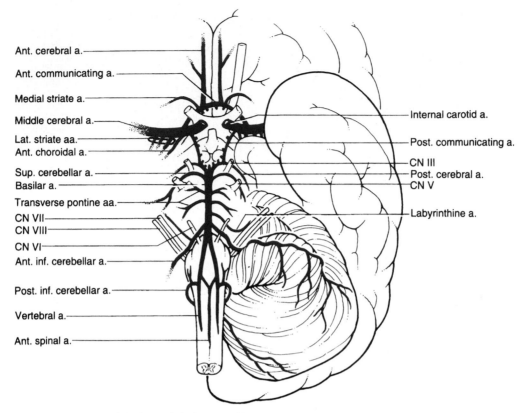

Figure 3-2. Arteries of the base of the brain and brainstem, including the arterial circle of Willis. The medial and lateral striate arteries and the anterior choroidal artery supply the basal ganglia and internal capsule.

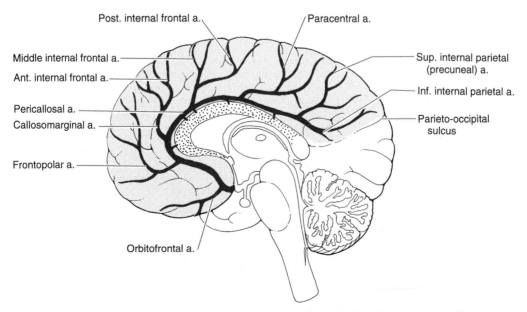

Figure 3-3. Cortical branches of the anterior cerebral artery on the medial hemispheric surface. The temporal pole is supplied by the middle cerebral artery; the occipital lobe is supplied by the posterior cerebral artery.

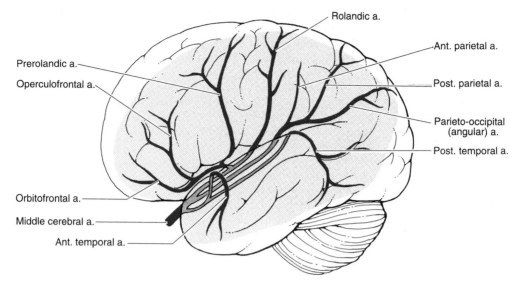

Figure 3-4. Cortical branches of the middle cerebral artery. The *unshaded* area represents the terminal territories of the anterior and posterior cerebral arteries.

- supplies tributaries to the dura, hypophysis, tympanic cavity, and trigeminal ganglion.
- provides direct branches to the optic nerve, optic chiasm, hypothalamus, and genu of the internal capsule.
- divides into the following branches:
  1. **Ophthalmic artery**
     - enters the orbit via the optic canal with the optic nerve.
  2. **Central artery of the retina**
     - is a branch of the **ophthalmic artery.**
     - provides the only blood supply to the inner five layers of the retina.
     - is an end artery; its **occlusion results in blindness.**
  3. **Posterior communicating artery** (see Figures 3-2 and 3-6)
     - arises from the carotid siphon and joins the posterior cerebral artery.

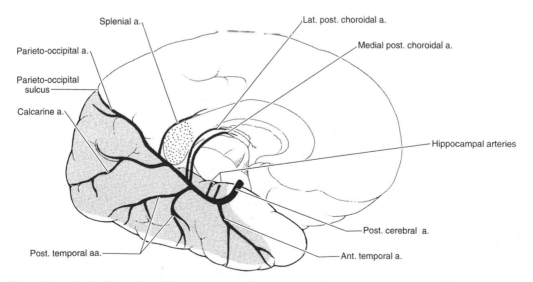

Figure 3-5. Cortical branches of the posterior cerebral artery seen from the ventral and medial surfaces. The splenium of the corpus callosum is supplied by the callosal branch of the posterior cerebral artery.

- supplies the optic chiasm and tract, hypothalamus, subthalamus, and anterior half of the ventral portion of the thalamus.
- is a common site of berry aneurysms.

4. **Anterior choroidal artery** (see Figures 3-2 and 3-6)
   - arises from the internal carotid artery.
   - supplies the choroid plexus of the temporal horn of the lateral ventricle, hippocampus, amygdala, optic tract, lateral geniculate body, globus pallidus, and ventral part of the posterior limb of the internal capsule.
   - supplies the proximal portion of optic radiations as they leave the lateral geniculate body to form Meyer loop.

5. **Anterior cerebral artery** (see Figure 3-3)
   - originates at the terminal bifurcation of the internal carotid artery.
   - gives direct branches to the optic chiasm.
   - supplies the medial surface of the frontal and parietal lobes and corpus callosum.
   - supplies part of the caudate nucleus and putamen and anterior limb of the internal capsule via the **medial striate artery of Heubner** (see Figure 3-2).
   - supplies the leg and foot area of the motor and sensory cortices (paracentral lobule) (see Figure 23-1).

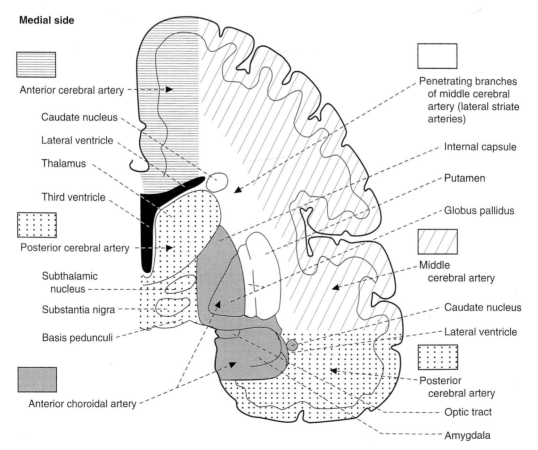

Figure 3-6.   Schematic drawing of a coronal (frontal) section through the cerebral hemisphere at the level of the internal capsule and thalamus, showing the major vascular territories. (Modified with permission from Fix JD: *High-Yield Neuroanatomy,* 3rd ed. Philadelphia, Lippincott Williams & Wilkins, 2005, p 31.)

   6. **Anterior communicating artery**
      - connects the two anterior cerebral arteries.
      - is the most common site of berry aneurysms.
   7. **Middle cerebral artery** (see Figures 3-3 and 3-5)
      - begins at the bifurcation of the internal carotid artery.
      - supplies the lateral convexity of the hemisphere and underlying insula.
      - supplies the trunk, arm, and face areas of the motor and sensory cortices.
      - supplies the Broca and Wernicke speech areas.
      - supplies the caudate nucleus, putamen, globus pallidus, and anterior and posterior limbs of the internal capsule via the **lateral striate arteries**.

B. **Vertebral artery** (see Figure 3-1)
   - is a branch of the subclavian artery.
   - joins its opposite partner to form the basilar artery.
   - gives rise to:
      1. **Anterior spinal artery**
      2. **Posterior spinal artery**
         - is occasionally a branch of the vertebral artery.
      3. **Posterior inferior cerebellar artery**
         - gives rise to the posterior spinal artery.
         - supplies the dorsolateral zone of the medulla.
         - supplies the inferior surface of the cerebellum and the choroid plexus of the fourth ventricle.
         - supplies the medial and inferior vestibular nuclei, inferior cerebellar peduncle, nucleus ambiguus, intra-axial fibers of the glossopharyngeal nerve (CN IX) and the vagal nerve (CN X), spinothalamic tract, and spinal trigeminal nucleus and tract.
         - supplies the hypothalamospinal tract to the ciliospinal center of Budge at T1–T2 (Horner syndrome).

C. **Basilar artery** (see Figure 3-1)
   - is formed by the two vertebral arteries.
   - gives rise to:
      1. **Pontine arteries**
         - include penetrating and short circumferential branches.
         - supply corticospinal tracts and the intra-axial exiting fibers of the abducent nerve (CN VI).
      2. **Labyrinthine artery**
         - arises from the basilar artery in 15% of the population.
         - perfuses the cochlea and the vestibular apparatus.
      3. **Anterior inferior cerebellar artery**
         - supplies the inferior surface of the cerebellum.
         - supplies the facial nucleus and intra-axial fibers, spinal trigeminal nucleus and tract, vestibular nuclei, cochlear nuclei, intra-axial fibers of the vestibulocochlear nerve, spinothalamic tract, and inferior and middle cerebellar peduncles.
         - gives rise to the labyrinthine artery in 85% of the population.
         - supplies the hypothalamospinal tract (Horner syndrome).
      4. **Superior cerebellar artery**
         - supplies the superior surface of the cerebellum and the cerebellar nuclei (dentate nucleus).
         - supplies the rostral and lateral pons, including the superior cerebellar peduncle and spinothalamic tract.
      5. **Posterior cerebral artery** (see Figure 3-5)
         - originates from the internal carotid (fetal origin) in 20% of the population.
         - is formed by bifurcation of the basilar artery.
         - provides the major blood supply to the midbrain.

- supplies the posterior half of the thalamus and the medial and lateral geniculate bodies.
- supplies the occipital lobe, visual cortex, and inferior surface of the temporal lobe, including the hippocampal formation.
- gives rise to the lateral and medial **posterior choroidal arteries,** which supply the dorsal thalamus, pineal body, and choroid plexus of the third and lateral ventricles.

IV. Arterial Circle of Willis (see Figure 3-2)

- is formed by the anterior communicating, anterior cerebral, internal carotid, posterior communicating, and posterior cerebral arteries.
- gives off penetrating arteries to supply the ventral diencephalon (hypothalamus, subthalamus, and thalamus) and the midbrain.

V. Meningeal Arteries

- supply the intracranial dura.
- usually arise from branches of the external carotid artery.

A. Anterior meningeal arteries
- arise from the anterior and posterior ethmoidal arteries.
- supply the dura of the anterior cranial fossa.

B. Middle meningeal artery
- is a branch of the **maxillary artery.**
- enters the cranium via the **foramen spinosum.**
- lies between the periosteal and meningeal dura, below the temporal and parietal bones.
- supplies most of the dura and almost its entire calvarial portion.
- Laceration results in **epidural hemorrhage** (hematoma).

C. Posterior meningeal arteries
- are branches of the ascending pharyngeal, vertebral, and occipital arteries.
- supply the dura of the posterior cranial fossa.

VI. Veins of the Brain

- are devoid of valves and lie along surface sulci.
- arise from the cortex and subcortical medullary substance and terminate in the dural sinuses.

A. Superficial cerebral veins
- drain into the superior sagittal sinus (bridging veins).
- Laceration of these vessels results in subdural hemorrhage (hematoma).

B. Deep cerebral veins (see Figures 3-8 and 3-13)
- drain the deep subcortical structures of the cerebral hemispheres: **septal area, thalamus, and basal ganglia.**
  1. **Internal cerebral veins**
     - drain the following:
       a. **Septal vein**
       b. **Thalamostriate vein**

      c. **Terminal vein**

      d. **Venous angle**
- is the point where the septal vein and the thalamostriate vein meet.
- marks the interventricular foramen of Monro.

  2. **Great vein of Galen**
- receives blood from the internal cerebral veins and drains into the straight sinus.

VII.   Venous Dural Sinuses (Figure 3-7)

- are endothelium-lined valveless channels whose walls are formed by two layers of dura mater.
- collect blood from the superficial and deep cerebral veins and the calvarium and represent the major drainage pathway of the cranial cavity.
- receive arachnoid granulations and absorb cerebrospinal fluid (CSF).

A. Superior sagittal sinus (see Figure 2-3)
- extends from the foramen cecum to the internal occipital protuberance and usually terminates in the right transverse sinus.
- receives blood from the superficial cerebral veins, diploic veins, and parietal emissary veins.
- receives arachnoid granulations and drains CSF from the subarachnoid space.

B. Inferior sagittal sinus
- courses in the inferior edge of the falx cerebri.
- joins the great cerebral vein to form the straight sinus.

C. Straight sinus
- is formed by the great cerebral vein and the inferior sagittal sinus.
- terminates at the internal occipital protuberance and usually drains into the left transverse sinus.
- drains the superior surface of the cerebellum.

D. Left and right transverse sinuses
- originate at the confluence of the sinuses and course anterolaterally along the edge of the tentorium cerebelli to become the sigmoid sinus.
- receive venous blood from the temporal and occipital lobes.

E. Confluence of the sinuses
- lies at the internal occipital protuberance.
- is formed by the union of the superior sagittal, straight, and transverse sinuses.

F. Sigmoid sinus
- is a continuation of the transverse sinus.
- passes inferiorly and medially into the jugular foramen.

G. Sphenoparietal sinus
- lies along the curve of the lesser wing of the sphenoid bone and drains into the cavernous sinus.

H. Superior petrosal sinus
- extends from the cavernous sinus to the sigmoid sinus.
- receives tributaries from the pons, medulla, cerebellum, and inner ear.

I. Inferior petrosal sinus
- passes between the glossopharyngeal (CN IX) and vagal (CN X) nerves and drains into the jugular bulb.
- receives major venous drainage from the inferior portion of the cerebellum.
- drains the cavernous sinus and clival plexus into the internal jugular vein.

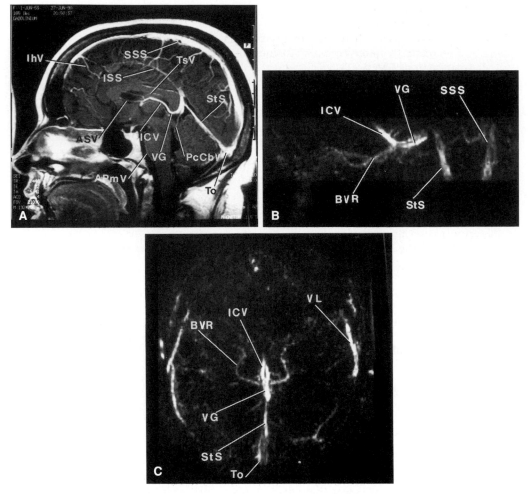

Figure 3-7. Venous anatomy of an MR section; midsagittal **(A)**, lateral **(B)**, submental-vertex **(C)**. IhV = inter-hemispheric veins; SSS = straight sinus; PcCbV = precentral cerebellar vein; To = torcula; VG = vein of anteri-or pontomesencephalic veins. (Reprinted with permission from Grossman CB: *Magnetic Resonance Imaging and Computed Tomography of the Head and Spine,* 2nd ed. Philadelphia, Williams & Wilkins, 1996, p 124.)

J. Cavernous sinus (see Figure 10-4)
- surrounds the sella turcica and the body of the sphenoid bone.
- contains, *within the sinus,* the internal carotid artery, sympathetic plexus, and abducent nerve (CN VI).
- contains, *within the lateral wall of the sinus,* the oculomotor nerve (CN III), the trochlear nerve (CN IV), the ophthalmic nerve (CN V-1), and the maxillary branches (CN V-2) of the trigeminal nerve.
- receives blood from the superior and the inferior ophthalmic veins.

VIII. Angiography

A. Carotid angiography (Figures 3-8A and B through 3-11) shows the following arteries:
1. Internal carotid artery
2. Anterior cerebral artery
3. Middle cerebral artery

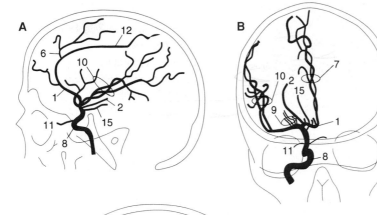

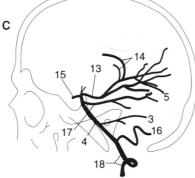

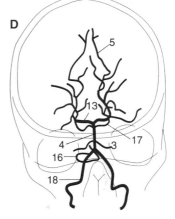

List of structures:

1. Anterior cerebral artery
2. Anterior choroidal artery
3. Anterior inferior cerebellar artery
4. Basilar artery
5. Calcarine artery (of posterior cerebral artery)
6. Callosomarginal artery (of anterior cerebral artery)
7. Callosomarginal and pericallosal arteries
   (of anterior cerebral artery)
8. Internal carotid artery
9. Lateral striate arteries (of middle cerebral artery)

10. Middle cerebral artery
11. Ophthalmic artery
12. Pericallosal artery (of anterior cerebral artery)
13. Posterior cerebral artery
14. Posterior choroidal arteries
    (of posteior cerebral artery)
15. Posterior communicating artery
16. Posterior inferior cerebellar artery
17. Superior cerebellar artery
18. Vertebral artery

Figure 3-8. (A) Carotid angiogram, lateral projection; (B) carotid angiogram, anteroposterior projection; (C) vertebral angiogram, lateral projection; (D) vertebral angiogram, anteroposterior projection. (Modified with permission from Fix JD: *High-Yield Neuroanatomy,* 3rd ed. Philadelphia, Lippincott Williams & Wilkins, 2005, p 33.)

B. **Vertebral angiography** (see Figure 3-8C and D; Figures 3-12 and 3-13) shows the following arteries:
1. Vertebral artery
2. Posterior inferior cerebellar artery
3. Basilar artery
4. Anterior inferior cerebellar artery
5. Superior cerebellar artery
6. Posterior cerebral artery

C. **Cerebral veins and dural sinuses** (Figure 3-14)

(text continues on page 53)

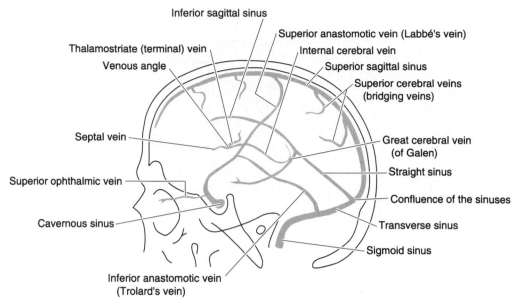

Figure 3-9. Carotid angiogram, venous phase, lateral projection showing cerebral veins and venous sinuses. (Modified with permission from Fix JD: *High-Yield Neuroanatomy,* 3rd ed. Philadelphia, Lippincott Williams & Wilkins, 2005, p 36.)

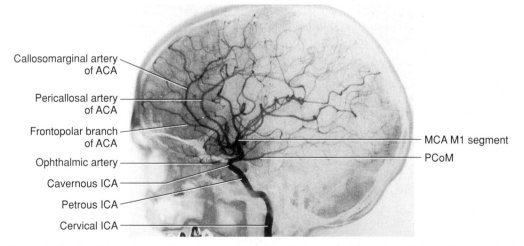

Figure 3-10. Carotid angiogram, lateral projection. Identify the cortical branches of the anterior cerebral artery (ACA) and middle cerebral artery (MCA). Follow the course of the internal carotid artery (ICA). Remember that aneurysms of the posterior communicating artery may result in third nerve palsy. The paracentral lobule is irrigated by the callosomarginal artery. Cortical branches of the MCA are designated with dots. *PCoM* = posterior communicating artery. (Reprinted with permission from Fix JD: *High-Yield Neuroanatomy,* 3rd ed. Philadelphia, Lippincott Williams & Wilkins, 2005, p 36.)

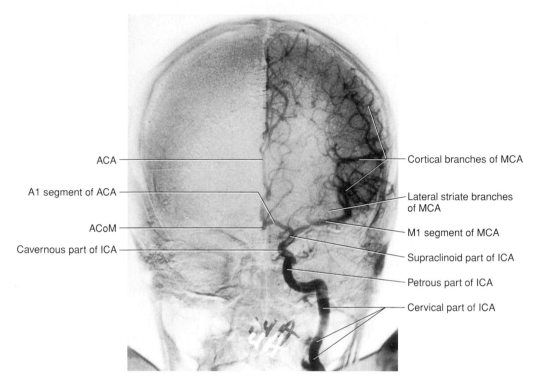

Figure 3-11. Carotid angiogram, anteroposterior projection. Identify the anterior cerebral artery (ACA), middle cerebral artery (MCA), and internal carotid artery (ICA). The horizontal branches of the MCA perfuse the basal ganglia and internal capsule. *ACoM* = anterior communicating artery. (Reprinted with permission from Fix JD: *High-Yield Neuroanatomy,* 3rd ed. Philadelphia, Lippincott Williams & Wilkins, 2005, p 37.)

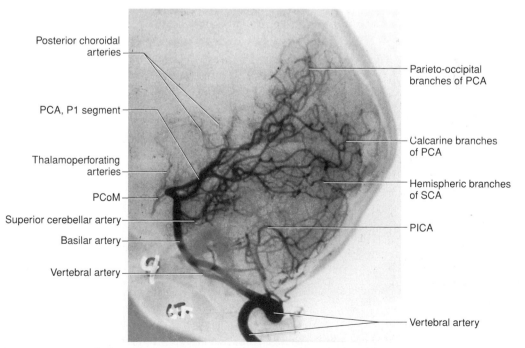

Figure 3-12. Vertebral angiogram, lateral projection. Two structures are found between the posterior cerebral artery (*PCA*) and the superior cerebellar artery: the tentorium and the third cranial nerve. *PCoM* = posterior communicating artery; *PICA* = posterior inferior cerebellar artery; *SCA* = superior cerebellar artery. (Reprinted with permission from Fix JD: *High-Yield Neuroanatomy,* 3rd ed. Philadelphia, Lippincott Williams & Wilkins, 2005, p 37.)

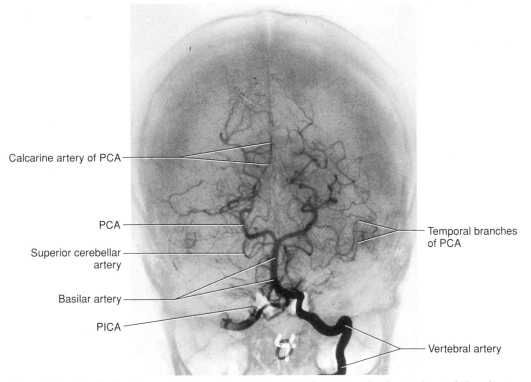

Calcarine artery of PCA

PCA

Superior cerebellar artery

Basilar artery

PICA

Temporal branches of PCA

Vertebral artery

Figure 3-13. Vertebral angiogram, anteroposterior projection. Which artery supplies the visual cortex? The calcarine artery, a branch of the posterior cerebral artery (*PCA*). Occlusion of the PCA (calcarine artery) results in a contralateral homonymous hemianopia, with macular sparing. *PICA* = posterior inferior cerebellar artery. (Reprinted with permission from Fix JD: *High-Yield Neuroanatomy,* 3rd ed. Philadelphia, Lippincott Williams & Wilkins, 2005, p 38.)

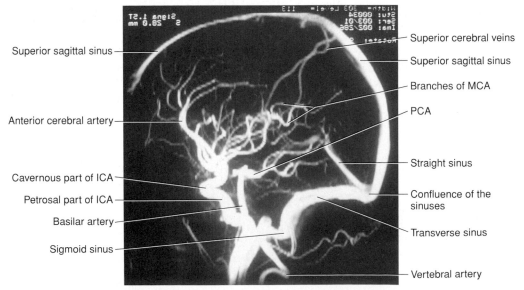

Superior sagittal sinus

Anterior cerebral artery

Cavernous part of ICA

Petrosal part of ICA

Basilar artery

Sigmoid sinus

Superior cerebral veins

Superior sagittal sinus

Branches of MCA

PCA

Straight sinus

Confluence of the sinuses

Transverse sinus

Vertebral artery

Figure 3-14. Magnetic resonance angiogram, lateral projection, showing the major venous sinuses and arteries. Note the bridging veins entering the superior sagittal sinus. *ICA* = internal carotid artery; *MCA* = middle cerebral artery; *PCA* = posterior cerebral artery. (Reprinted with permission from Fix JD: *High-Yield Neuroanatomy,* 3rd ed. Philadelphia, Lippincott Williams & Wilkins, 2005, p 32.)

IX.   Intracranial Hemorrhage

A. **Aneurysms**
- are circumscribed **dilations (ectasias) of an artery**.
  1. **Berry (saccular) aneurysms** (Figure 3-15)
     - develop at arterial bifurcations. The **arterial circle of Willis** contains 60%; 30% arise from the middle cerebral artery; and the remaining 10% are found in the vertebrobasilar system.
     - of the anterior communicating artery frequently pressure the optic chiasm and cause a **bitemporal lower quadrantanopia**.
     - of the posterior communicating artery frequently cause a **third nerve palsy**.
     - Rupture is the most common cause of nontraumatic **subarachnoid hemorrhage**.
  2. **Microaneurysms (Charcot-Bouchard aneurysms)**
     - are found in small arteries, most frequently within the territory of the middle cerebral artery (the lenticulostriate arteries).
     - Rupture occurs most frequently in the basal ganglia and is the most common cause of nontraumatic **intraparenchymal hemorrhage**.

B. **Subdural hemorrhage (hematoma)** (Figure 3-16)
- results from **rupture of the superior cerebral veins**, the "bridging" veins that drain into the superior sagittal sinus.

C. **Epidural hemorrhage (hematoma)** (Figure 3-17)
- results from **rupture of the middle meningeal artery**, which lies between the dura and the inner table of the skull.

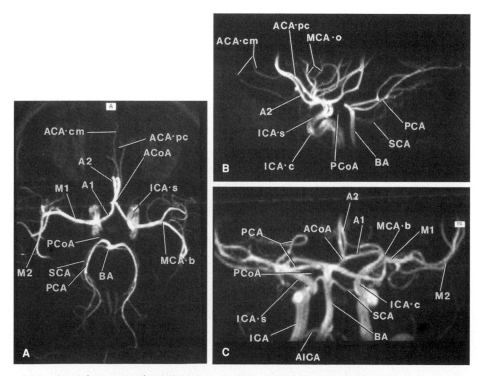

Figure 3-15.   Arterial anatomy of an MR section: axial (**A**), sagittal (**B, C**), coronal (**C**). ACAcm = anterior cerebral artery, callosal marginal branch; A2 and A1 are branches of the anterior cerebral artery: ACApc = pericallosal branch of the anterior cerebral artery; ACoA = anterior communicating artery; M1 and M2 are segments of the middle cerebral artery (MCA); MCAb = bifurcation; ICAs = internal carotid artery siphon; PAC = posterior cerebral artery; PCoA = posterior communicating artery; BA = basilar artery; SCA = superior cerebellar artery. (Reprinted with permission from Grossman CB: *Magnetic Resonance Imaging and Computed Tomography of the Head and Spine,* 2nd ed. Philadelphia, Williams & Wilkins, 1996, p 124.)

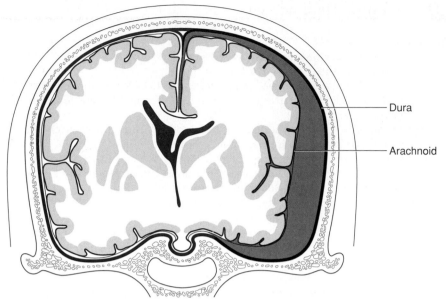

Figure 3-16. Subdural hematomas result from lacerated bridging veins. Subdural hematomas are frequently accompanied by traumatic subarachnoid hemorrhages and cortical contusions. Sudden deceleration of the head causes tearing of the superior cerebral veins. The hematoma extends over the crest of the convexity into the interhemispheric fissure but does not cross the dural attachment of the falx cerebri; the clot can be crescent-shaped, biconvex, or multiloculated. Subdural hematomas, which are more common than epidural hematomas, always cause brain damage. (Modified with permission from Osburn AG, Tong KA: *Handbook of Neuroradiology: Brain and Skull.* St Louis, Mosby, 1996, p 192.)

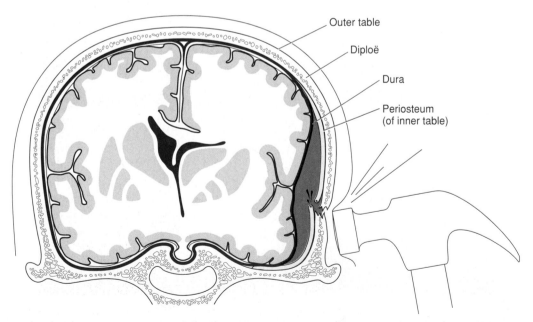

Figure 3-17. Epidural hematomas result from laceration of the middle meningeal artery. Arterial bleeding into the epidural space forms a biconvex clot. The classic lucid interval is seen in 50% of cases. Skull fractures are usually found. Epidural hematomas rarely cross sutural lines. (Modified with permission from Osburn AG, Tong KA: *Handbook of Neuroradiology: Brain and Skull.* St Louis, Mosby, 1996, p 191.)

Q REVIEW TEST

1. A 50-year-old hypertensive woman complains of numbness and weakness in her left leg and foot. Occlusion of which of the following vessels may account for this complaint?

(A) Anterior choroidal artery
(B) Anterior cerebral artery
(C) Interior carotid artery
(D) Middle cerebral artery
(E) Posterior artery

2. A 15-year-old boy is hit on the temple with a baseball and becomes unconscious. After about 10 minutes, he regains consciousness, but he soon becomes lethargic, and over the next 2 hours, he becomes stuporous. His pupils are unequal. Intracranial hemorrhage is suspected. Which of the following vessels is most likely to be the source of the hemorrhage?

(A) Anterior cerebral artery
(B) Anterior communicating artery
(C) Basilar artery
(D) Middle cerebral artery
(E) Middle meningeal artery

3. Which artery supplies the caudate and putamen and anterior limb of the internal capsule via the medial striate artery of Heubner?

(A) Middle cerebral
(B) Anterior communicating
(C) Anterior cerebral
(D) Anterior choroidal
(E) Posterior communicating

4. Which artery supplies the cochlea?

(A) Pontine
(B) Labyrinthine
(C) Superior cerebellar
(D) Posterior cerebral
(E) Anterior inferior cerebellar

5. Which sinus drains the superior surface of the cerebellum?

(A) Straight
(B) Inferior sagittal
(C) Inferior petrosal
(D) Sigmoid
(E) Sphenoparietal

6. A 40-year-old female graduate student had an excruciating headache. When she looked in the mirror, she noticed that her eyelid was drooping; when she lifted the eyelid, she saw that her eyeball was looking down and out and her pupil was huge. She complained of both blurred and double vision. An MRA scan showed an aneurysm of the circle of Willis. Which artery gives rise to the offending aneurysm?

(A) Heubner's
(B) anterior communicating
(C) posterior communicating
(D) Charcot-Bouchard's
(E) anterior choroidal

Questions 7 to 11

The response options for items 7 to 11 are the same. Select one answer for each item in the set.

(A) Posterior cerebral artery
(B) Superior cerebellar artery
(C) Anterior inferior cerebellar artery
(D) Posterior inferior cerebellar artery
(E) Anterior spinal artery

Match each of the following descriptions with the most appropriate artery.

7. Usually gives rise to the artery that supplies the inner ear

8. Supplies the facial nucleus and the spinal trigeminal nucleus and tract

9. Is the terminal branch of the basilar artery

10. Supplies the deep cerebellar nuclei

11. Supplies the nucleus ambiguus

Questions 12 to 16

Match the statements in items 12 to 16 with the appropriate lettered artery shown in the figure.

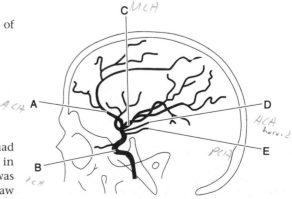

12. An aneurysm of this artery may cause a third nerve palsy *E*

13. Irrigates the posterior limb of the internal capsule   *D*

14. Occlusion of this artery results in a fluent receptive aphasia *C*

15. An aneurysm of this artery may result in Horner syndrome   *B*

16. Occlusion of this artery results in infarction of the paracentral lobule with Babinski sign *A*

Questions 17 to 23

Match the statements in items 17 to 23 with the appropriate lettered artery shown in the figure.

17. Thrombosis may result in an abducent palsy *A*

18. Drains the deep cerebral veins *E*

19. Marks the site of the foramen of Monro *B*

20. Receives the arachnoid granulations *C*

21. Receives blood from the ophthalmic veins *A*

22. Laceration results in subdural hemorrhage *D*

23. Receives blood from the straight, sagittal, superior, and transverse sinuses *F*

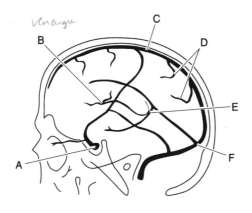

ANSWERS AND EXPLANATIONS

1–B. The anterior cerebral artery perfuses the paracentral lobule, which represents the motor and sensory strips of the leg and foot areas.

2–E. Laceration of the middle meningeal artery gives rise to an epidural hematoma. Classic signs of an epidural hematoma are skull trauma, usually with fracture, and sequential progression from unconsciousness to lucidity to progressive coma to death due to transtentorial herniation with ipsilateral third palsy.

3–C. The anterior cerebral artery supplies part of the caudate nucleus and putamen and anterior limb of the internal capsule via the medial striate artery of Heubner (see Figure 3-2).

4–B. The labyrinthine artery supplies the cochlea and the vestibular apparatus. In 15% of the population, it arises from the basilar artery; in the other 85% of the population, it arises from the anterior inferior cerebellar artery.

5–A. The straight sinus drains the superior surface of the cerebellum. It is formed by the great cerebral vein and the inferior sagittal sinus.

6–C. The posterior communicating artery may give rise to a berry aneurysm, which compresses the third cranial nerve and results incomplete third nerve palsy (see Figure 3-14). Heubner's artery is a branch of the anterior cerebral artery. A communicating artery may harbor berry aneurysms that impinge on the optic chiasm, causing a bitemporal lower quadrantanopia. Charcot-Bouchard microaneurysms are found in the territory of the lateral striate arteries and are the most common cause of nontraumatic intraparenchymal hemorrhage. Rupture occurs most frequently in the basal ganglia. The anterior choroidal artery is a branch of the internal carotid artery and irrigates the globus pallidus and posterior limb of the internal capsule.

7–C. The anterior inferior cerebellar artery usually gives rise to the labyrinthine artery, which supplies the structures of the inner ear (i.e., the cochlea and vestibular apparatus).

8–C. The facial nucleus and the spinal trigeminal nucleus and tract are supplied by the anterior inferior cerebellar artery.

9–A. The posterior cerebral artery is the terminal branch of the basilar artery.

10–B. The superior cerebellar artery supplies the superior surface of the cerebellum and the cerebellar nuclei (dentate nucleus).

11–D. The posterior inferior cerebellar artery supplies the dorsolateral medullary field, including the nucleus ambiguus.

12–E. An aneurysm of the posterior communicating artery may cause a third nerve palsy.

13–D. The anterior choroidal artery irrigates the posterior limb of the internal capsule.

14–C. Occlusion of the proximal stem of the left middle cerebral artery results in Wernicke aphasia, a fluent receptive aphasia.

15–B. An aneurysm of the internal carotid artery within the cavernous sinus can interrupt postganglionic sympathetic fibers, resulting in Horner syndrome.

16–A. The anterior cerebral artery perfuses the mesial aspect of the hemisphere from the frontal pole to the parieto-occipital sulcus, including the paracentral lobule. The paracentral lobule gives rise to corticospinal fibers to the contralateral foot and leg. Destruction of these fibers results in the Babinski sign.

17–A. Cavernous sinus thrombosis may result in cranial nerve palsies, including CN III, IV, VI, V-1, and V-2.

18–E. The great cerebral vein of Galen drains the deep cerebral veins that drain the thalamus and basal ganglia. The vein of Galen empties into the straight sinus.

19–B. The venous angle marks the site of the interventricular foramen of Monro; it is the point where the septal and thalamostriate veins meet.

20–C. The superior sagittal sinus receives cerebrospinal fluid (CSF) via the arachnoid granulations.

21–A. The inferior and superior ophthalmic veins drain into the cavernous sinus.

22–D. Laceration of the superior cerebral veins (bridging veins) results in subdural hemorrhage (hematoma).

23–F. The confluence of the sinuses (torcular Herophili) receives blood from the straight, sagittal, superior, and transverse sinuses.

CHAPTER

4

Development of the Nervous System

I. **Overview**

A. **Central nervous system (CNS)**
   - begins to form in the third week of embryonic development as the **neural plate**. The neural plate becomes the **neural tube**, which gives rise to the brain and spinal cord.

B. **Peripheral nervous system (PNS)**
   - consists of spinal, cranial, and visceral nerves and spinal, cranial, and autonomic ganglia.
   - is derived from three sources:
      1. **Neural crest cells**
         - give rise to peripheral ganglia, Schwann cells, and afferent nerve fibers.
      2. **Neural tube**
         - gives rise to all preganglionic autonomic fibers and all fibers that innervate skeletal muscles.
      3. **Mesoderm**
         - gives rise to the dura mater and to connective tissue investments of peripheral nerve fibers (endoneurium, perineurium, and epineurium).

II. Development of the Neural Tube (Figures 4-1 and 4-2)

- begins in the third week and is complete in the fourth week.

A. **Neural plate**
   - is a thickened pear-shaped region of embryonic ectoderm between the primitive knot and the oropharyngeal membrane.

B. **Neural groove**
   - forms as the neural plate begins to fold inward.
   - is flanked by neural folds, which are parallel.
   - deepens as the neural folds begin to close over it.

C. **Neural folds**
   - fuse in the midline to form the neural tube.
   - edges are the sites of neural crest cell differentiation.

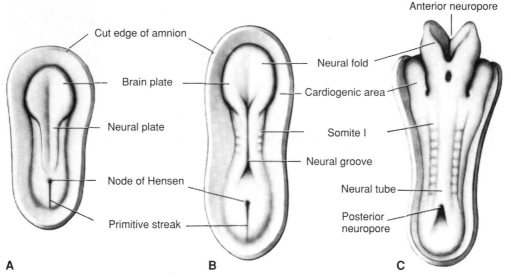

Figure 4-1.   Diagrams illustrating the dorsal aspect of the human embryo. **(A)** Late presomite and early neural plate stage. **(B)** Early somite stage and neural groove stage. **(C)** Eight-somite stage and early neural tube stage. The anterior and posterior neuropores provide transitory communication between the neural canal and the amniotic cavity. (Reprinted with permission from Carpenter MB, Sutin J: *Human Neuroanatomy,* 8th ed. Baltimore, Williams & Wilkins, 1983, p 63.)

D. **Neural tube**
   - forms as the neural folds fuse in the midline and separate from the surface ectoderm.
   - lies between the surface ectoderm and the notochord.
   - gives rise to the CNS:
     1. The **cranial part** becomes the brain.
     2. The **caudal part** becomes the spinal cord.
     3. The **cavity** gives rise to the central canal of the spinal cord and ventricles of the brain.
     4. The **two openings in the neural tube** connect the central canal with the amniotic cavity:
        a. **Anterior neuropore**
           - closes in the fourth week (day 25) and becomes the **lamina terminalis.**
        b. **Posterior neuropore**
           - closes in the fourth week (day 27).

III.   Neural Crest (see Figure 4-2)

- gives rise to:

A. **Pseudounipolar ganglion cells of the spinal and cranial nerve ganglia**

B. **Schwann cells** (neurolemmal sheath cells that form myelin in the PNS)

C. **Multipolar ganglion cells of the autonomic ganglia**

D. **Leptomeninges** (pia–arachnoid cells)

E. **Chromaffin cells of the suprarenal medulla**

F. **Pigment cells** (melanocytes)

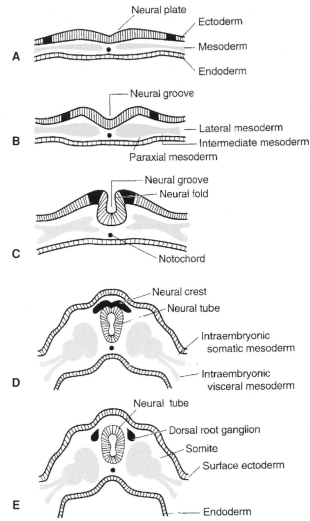

Figure 4-2. Schematic diagrams of transverse sections of embryos at various stages. (A) Neural plate stage. (B) Early neural groove stage. (C) Late neural groove stage. (D) Early neural tube and neural crest stage. (E) Neural tube and dorsal root ganglion stage. (Reprinted with permission from Truex RC, Carpenter MB: *Human Neuroanatomy*. Baltimore, Williams & Wilkins, 1969, p 91.)

G. **Odontoblasts** (dentin-forming cells), **dental papilla, and the dental follicle**

H. **Aorticopulmonary septum of the heart**

I. **Parafollicular cells** (calcitonin-producing C-cells)

J. **Skeletal and connective components of the pharyngeal arches**

IV.   Placodes

- are localized thickenings of the cephalic surface ectoderm.
- give rise to cells that migrate into the underlying mesoderm and develop into the sensory receptive organs of the olfactory nerve (cranial nerve [CN] I) and the vestibulocochlear nerve (CN VIII).

A. **Olfactory placodes**
   - differentiate into neurosensory cells that give rise to the **olfactory nerve (CN I).**
   - induce formation of the **olfactory bulbs.**

B. **Otic placodes**
   • give rise to the following statoacoustic organs:
   1. **Organ of Corti and spiral ganglion**
   2. **Cristae ampullares, maculae utriculi and sacculi, and vestibular ganglion**
   3. **Vestibulocochlear nerve (CN VIII)**

V.   Stages of Neural Tube Development

A. **Vesicle development**
   1. **The three primary brain vesicles and associated flexures** (Figure 4-3)
      • develop during the fourth week.
      • give rise to dilations of the primary brain vesicles and two curvatures.
      a. **Prosencephalon (forebrain)**
         • is associated with the appearance of the **optic vesicles.**
         • gives rise to:
            (1) **Telencephalon (endbrain)**
            (2) **Diencephalon (between-brain)**
      b. **Mesencephalon (midbrain)**
         • remains as the mesencephalon.
      c. **Rhombencephalon (hindbrain)**
         • gives rise to:
            (1) **Metencephalon (afterbrain)**
               • forms the pons and cerebellum.
            (2) **Myelencephalon (medulla oblongata)**
      d. **Cephalic flexure (midbrain flexure)**
         • is located between the prosencephalon and the rhombencephalon.
      e. **Cervical flexure**
         • is located between the rhombencephalon and the future spinal cord.

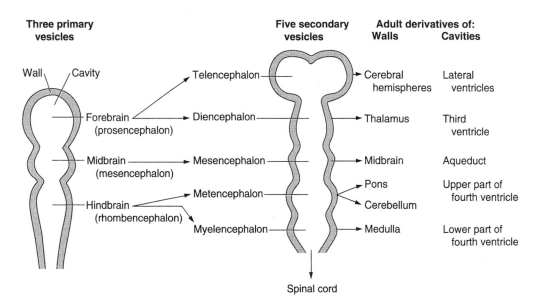

Figure 4-3. Diagrammatic sketches of the brain vesicles indicating the adult derivatives of their walls and cavities. (Reprinted with permission from Moore KL: *The Developing Human: Clinically Oriented Embryology,* 4th ed. Philadelphia, WB Saunders, 1988, p 380.)

2. **The five secondary brain vesicles (with four ventricles)** (see Figure 4-3)
   - become visible in the sixth week; the brain vesicles are visible as the primordia of the five major brain divisions.
   a. **Telencephalon**
      - has lateral outpocketings that form the **cerebral hemispheres.**
      - has ventral outpocketings that form the **olfactory bulbs.**
      - has visible lateral ventricles.
   b. **Diencephalon**
      - The third ventricle, optic chiasm and optic nerves, infundibulum, and mamillary eminences become visible.
   c. **Mesencephalon**
      - contains a large cavity that will become the **cerebral aqueduct.**
   d. **Metencephalon**
      - is separated from the mesencephalon by the rhombencephalic isthmus.
      - is separated from the myelencephalon by the pontine flexure.
      - contains **rhombic lips** on the dorsal surface, which give rise to the cerebellum.
      - becomes the **pons** and the **cerebellum.**
      - contains the **rostral half of the fourth ventricle.**
   e. **Myelencephalon (medulla oblongata)**
      - lies between the pontine and cervical flexures.
      - becomes the medulla.
      - contains the **caudal half of the fourth ventricle.**

B. **Histogenesis**
   1. **Cells of the neural tube wall**
      - are neuroepithelial cells that give rise to:
      a. **Neuroblasts**
         - form all neurons found in the CNS.
      b. **Glioblasts (spongioblasts)**
         - for the most part form after cessation of neuroblast formation (except for radial glial cells, which develop before neurogenesis is complete).
         - form the supporting cells of the CNS.
         (1) **Macroglia**
            (a) **Astroglia (astrocytes)**
               - contain glial fibrillary acidic protein (**GFAP**), a marker for astroblasts.
               - surround blood capillaries with their perivascular feet.
            (b) **Radial glial cells**
               - are of astrocytic lineage and are **GFAP**-positive.
               - provide guidance for migrating neuroblasts.
            (c) **Oligodendroglia (oligodendrocytes)**
               - produce the myelin of the CNS.
         (2) **Ependymal cells**
            - are ciliated.
            (a) **Ependymocytes**
               - line the ventricles and the central canal.
            (b) **Tanycytes**
               - are located in the wall of the third ventricle.
               - transport substances from the cerebrospinal fluid (**CSF**) to the hypophyseal portal system.
            (c) **Choroid plexus cells**
               - produce CSF.
               - are bound together by tight junctions (**zonulae occludentes**) that represent the blood–CSF barrier.
      c. **Microglia (gitter cells)**
         - are the scavenger cells of the CNS.
         - arise from monocytes, not from glioblasts.

- invade the developing nervous system in the third week with the developing blood vessels.

2. **Layers of the neural tube wall**
   - are formed within the wall of the primitive neural tube.
   a. **Neuroepithelial (ventricular) layer**
      - is the innermost layer.
      - is a monocellular layer of ependymal cells that lines the central canal and future brain ventricles.
   b. **Mantle (intermediate) layer**
      - is the middle layer.
      - consists of neurons and glial cells, the central **gray matter of the spinal cord.**
      - contains the developing **alar** and **basal plates.**
   c. **Marginal layer**
      - is the outermost layer.
      - contains nerve fibers of neuroblasts of the mantle layer and glial cells.
      - produces the **white matter of the spinal cord** through the myelination of axons growing into this layer.

VI. Spinal Cord (Medulla Spinalis) (Figure 4-4)

- develops from the neural tube caudal to the fourth pair of somites.

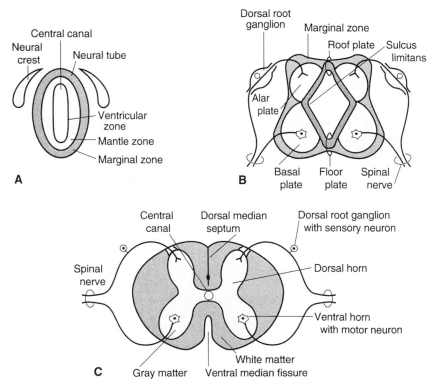

Figure 4-4. Schematic illustration of three successive stages in the development of the spinal cord. The neural crest gives rise to the dorsal root ganglion and the alar and basal plates give rise to the dorsal and ventral horns, respectively. (Modified with permission from Fix JD, Dudek RW: *BRS Embryology,* 3rd ed. Baltimore, Williams & Wilkins, 2005, p 67.)

A. Alar and basal plates, sulcus limitans, and roof and floor plates
  1. Alar plate
    • is a dorsolateral thickening of the mantle layer of the neural tube.
    • gives rise to second order **sensory neuroblasts** of the dorsal horn (general somatic afferent [GSA] and general visceral afferent [GVA] cell regions).
    • receives axons, which become the dorsal roots, from the dorsal root ganglion.
    • becomes the **dorsal horn** of the spinal cord.
  2. Basal plate
    • is a ventrolateral thickening of the mantle layer of the neural tube.
    • gives rise to the **motor neuroblasts** of the ventral and lateral horns (general somatic efferent [GSE] and general visceral efferent [GVE] cell regions). Axons from motor neuroblasts exit the spinal cord and form the ventral roots.
    • becomes the **ventral horn** of the spinal cord.
  3. Sulcus limitans
    • is a longitudinal groove in the lateral wall of the neural tube that appears during the fourth week.
    • separates the alar (sensory) and the basal (motor) plates.
    • disappears in the adult spinal cord but is retained in the rhomboid fossa of the brainstem.
    • extends from the spinal cord to the rostral midbrain.
  4. Roof plate
    • is the nonneural roof of the central canal.
  5. Floor plate
    • is the nonneural floor of the central canal.
    • contains the **ventral white commissure**.

B. Myelination
  • commences in the fourth fetal month in the spinal cord motor roots.
  1. Oligodendrocytes accomplish myelination of the CNS.
  2. Schwann cells accomplish myelination of the PNS.
  3. Myelination of the corticospinal tracts is not complete until the **end of the second postnatal year** (i.e., when the corticospinal tracts become myelinated and functional).
  4. Myelination of the association neocortex extends into the **third decade**.

C. Positional changes of the spinal cord
  • Disparate growth results in formation of the **cauda equina**, consisting of dorsal and ventral roots (L3–Co) that descend below the level of the conus medullaris, and in formation of the **nonneural filum terminale**, which anchors the spinal cord to the coccyx.
  1. At **8 weeks**, the spinal cord extends the entire length of the vertebral canal.
  2. At **birth**, the **conus medullaris** extends to the level of the third lumbar vertebra (VL3).
  3. In **adults**, the conus medullaris terminates at the VL1–VL2 interspace.

VII. Medulla Oblongata (Myelencephalon) (Figure 4-5)

• develops from the **caudal rhombencephalon**.
• contains the medullary pyramids (corticospinal tracts) in its base.

A. Alar (sensory) and basal (motor) plates
  1. Closed (caudal) medulla
    a. Alar plate sensory neuroblasts give rise to:
      (1) Dorsal column nuclei, which consist of the gracile and cuneate nuclei
      (2) Inferior olivary nuclei, which are cerebellar relay nuclei
      (3) Solitary nucleus, which forms the GVA (taste) and special visceral afferent (SVA) column

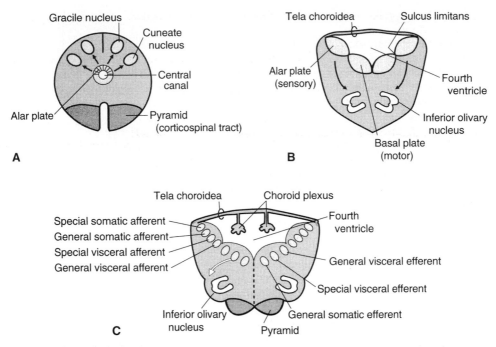

Figure 4-5. Schematic illustrations of the development of the medulla. **(A)** Transverse section of the caudal medulla showing the development of the gracile and cuneate nuclei from the alar plates. **(B)** Schematic sketch through the rostral (open) medulla showing the relationships of the alar and basal plates; the inferior olivary nucleus is derived from the alar plate. **(C)** A later stage of B shows the four sensory modalities of the alar plate and the three motor modalities of the basal plate; the *white arrow* indicates the lateral migration of the SVE column (CN IX, CN X, and CN XI); pyramids consist of motor fibers, the corticospinal tracts. (Adapted with permission from Fix JD, Dudek RW: *BRS Embryology,* 3rd ed. Baltimore, Williams & Wilkins, 2005, p 69.)

   (4) **Spinal trigeminal nucleus,** which forms the GSA column
   (5) **Cochlear and vestibular nuclei**
      • form the special somatic afferent (SSA) column.
      • lie in the medullopontine junction.
   b. **Basal plate motor neuroblasts give rise to:**
      (1) **Hypoglossal nucleus,** which forms the GSE column
      (2) **Nucleus ambiguus,** which forms the special visceral efferent (SVE) column (CN IX, CN X, and CN XI)
      (3) **Dorsal motor nucleus of the vagal nerve (CN X) and the inferior salivatory nucleus of the glossopharyngeal nerve (CN IX),** which form the GVE column
2. **Open (rostral) medulla** (Figure 4-6; see Figure 4-5)
   • extends from the **obex** to the **striae medullares** of the rhomboid fossa (see Figure 1-6:)
   • Formation of the pontine flexure causes the lateral walls of the rostral medulla to open like a book and form the rhomboid fossa (the floor of the fourth ventricle).
   a. **Alar plate**
      • lies lateral to the sulcus limitans.
      • its sensory neuroblasts give rise to:
      (1) **Solitary nucleus**
         • forms the GVA and SVA columns.
      (2) **Cochlear and vestibular nuclei**
         • form the special SSA column.
      (3) **Spinal trigeminal nucleus**
         • forms the GSA column.

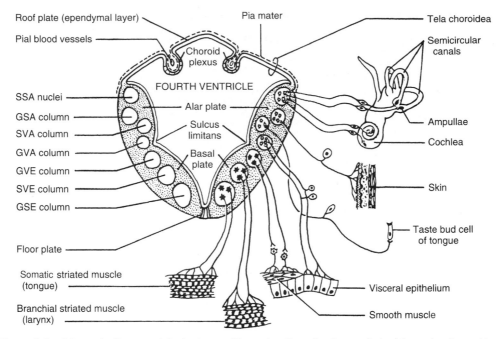

Figure 4-6. Schematic diagram of the brainstem illustrating the cell columns derived from the alar and basal plates. The seven cranial nerve modalities are shown. *GSA* = general somatic afferent, *GVA* = general visceral afferent, *GVE* = general visceral efferent; *SSA* = special somatic afferent, *SSE* = special somatic efferent; *SVA* = special visceral afferent, *SVE* = special visceral efferent. (Adapted with permission from Fix JD, Dudek RW: *BRS Embryology,* 3rd ed. Baltimore, Williams & Wilkins, 2005, p 69.)

> **b. Basal plate**
>> • lies medial to the sulcus limitans.
>> • its motor neuroblasts give rise to:
>>> **(1) Hypoglossal nucleus**
>>>> • forms the GSE column.
>>> **(2) Nucleus ambiguus**
>>>> • forms the SVE column.
>>> **(3) Dorsal motor nucleus of the vagal nerve and the inferior salivatory nucleus of CN IX**
>>>> • form the GVE column.

B. Roof plate
> • forms the caudal roof of the fourth ventricle.
> • is the **tela choroidea**, a monolayer of ependymal cells covered with pia mater.
> • is invaginated by pial vessels to form the **choroid plexus of the fourth ventricle.**

VIII. Metencephalon (Figure 4-7; see Figure 4-3)

> • develops from the **rostral division of the rhombencephalon.**
> • gives rise to the **pons and the cerebellum.**

A. Pons
> **1. Alar plate sensory neuroblasts** give rise to:
>> **a. Solitary nucleus,** which forms the GVA and the SVA (taste) columns of CN VII
>> **b. Cochlear and vestibular nuclei,** which form the SSA column of CN VIII

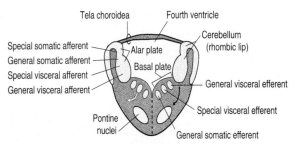

Figure 4-7. Schematic illustration (transverse section) of the development of the pons and cerebellum. The alar plate (rhombic lip) gives rise to the cerebellum, the four sensory cell columns, and the pontine nuclei. The basal plate gives rise to the three motor columns. The base of the pons contains the descending corticospinal tracts, which originate from the motor and sensory strips of the cerebral cortex. The *white arrow* indicates the lateral migration of the SVE column (V and CN VII). (Modified with permission from Fix JD, Dudek RW: *BRS Embryology,* 3rd ed. Baltimore, Williams & Wilkins, 2005, p 71.)

      c. Spinal and principal trigeminal nuclei, which form the GSA column of CN V

      d. Pontine nuclei, which consist of cerebellar relay nuclei (pontine gray)

  2. Basal plate motor neuroblasts give rise to:

      a. Abducent nucleus of CN VI, which forms the GSE column

      b. Facial and trigeminal motor nuclei of CN VII and CN V, which form the SVE column

      c. Superior salivatory nucleus, which forms the GVE column of CN VII

  3. Base of the pons

    • contains pontine nuclei from the alar plate.

    • contains corticobulbar, corticospinal, and corticopontine fibers with cell bodies located in the cerebral cortex.

    • contains pontocerebellar fibers, which are axons of neurons found in the pontine nuclei.

B. Cerebellum

  • is formed by the **rhombic lips,** which are the thickened alar plates of the mantle layer. The **rostral** part of the cerebellum is derived from the **caudal mesencephalon**.

  • The **cerebellar anlage (primordium)** gives rise to:

    1. Vermis, by midline growth

    2. Cerebellar hemispheres, by lateral growth

    3. Three-layered cerebellar cortex (molecular layer, Purkinje cell layer, and **granular [internal] cell layer) and four pairs of cerebellar nuclei,** by cell migration from the ventricular zone into the marginal layer

    4. External granular layer (EGL)

      • is a germinal (proliferative) layer on the surface of the cerebellum, present from week 8 of development to the end of the second postnatal year.

      • New evidence indicates that the EGL gives rise *only* to granule cells and not to basket (inner stellate) or stellate (outer stellate) neurons.

      • Persistent cell nests may give rise to a neoplasm, **medulloblastoma** (see Chapter 15 VI E 2).

      • is sensitive to antiviral agents, which block the synthesis of DNA.

    5. Folia and fissures, by cortical growth

IX.   Mesencephalon (Midbrain) (Figure 4-8; see Figure 4-3)

• develops from the walls of the mesencephalic vesicle.

• contains the **cerebral aqueduct,** which develops from the mesencephalic cavity.

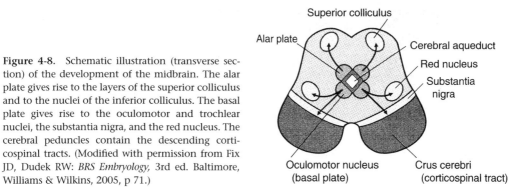

Figure 4-8. Schematic illustration (transverse section) of the development of the midbrain. The alar plate gives rise to the layers of the superior colliculus and to the nuclei of the inferior colliculus. The basal plate gives rise to the oculomotor and trochlear nuclei, the substantia nigra, and the red nucleus. The cerebral peduncles contain the descending corticospinal tracts. (Modified with permission from Fix JD, Dudek RW: *BRS Embryology,* 3rd ed. Baltimore, Williams & Wilkins, 2005, p 71.)

A. **Alar plate sensory neuroblasts**
   - form the cell layers of the superior colliculi and the nuclei of the inferior colliculi.

B. **Basal plate motor neuroblasts**
   - give rise to the:
     1. **Trochlear and oculomotor nuclei of CN IV and III**, which form the GSE column
     2. **Edinger-Westphal nucleus of CN III**, which forms the most rostral cell group of the GVE column
     3. **Red nucleus and substantia nigra**

C. **Basis pedunculi** (crus cerebri)
   - contains corticobulbar, corticospinal, and corticopontine fibers, derived from the cerebral cortex of the telencephalon.

X. Development of the Diencephalon, Optic Structures, and Hypophysis

A. **Diencephalon** (see Figure 4-3)
   - develops from the **caudal part of the prosencephalon,** within the walls of the primitive third ventricle.
     1. **Epithalamus**
        - develops from the embryonic roof plate and dorsal parts of the alar plates.
        - gives rise to the **pineal body** (epiphysis) and the habenular nuclei.
        - gives rise to the habenular and posterior commissures.
        - gives rise, from the roof plate and the pia mater, to the **tela choroidea** and **choroid plexus of the third ventricle.**
     2. **Thalamus (dorsal thalamus)**
        - is an alar plate derivative that gives rise to thalamic nuclei.
        - includes the **metathalamus,** which includes the lateral geniculate body (relays visual impulses) and the medial geniculate body (relays auditory impulses).
     3. **Hypothalamus**
        - develops ventral to the hypothalamic sulcus from the alar plate and floor plate.
        - gives rise to hypothalamic nuclei, including the **mamillary bodies,** and to the **neurohypophysis.**
     4. **Subthalamus (ventral thalamus)**
        - is an alar plate derivative located ventral to the thalamus and lateral to the hypothalamus.
        - includes the **subthalamic nucleus, zona incerta,** and **lenticular and thalamic fasciculi (fields of Forel).**
        - contains subthalamic neuroblasts that migrate into the telencephalon and form the **globus pallidus** (pallidum), a basal ganglion.

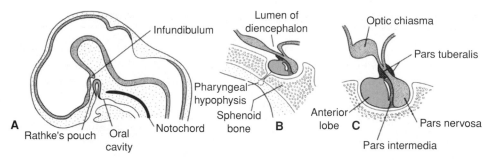

Figure 4-9. Schematic drawings illustrating the development of the hypophysis (pituitary gland). **(A)** Midsagittal section through the 6-week old embryo showing Rathke's pouch as a dorsal outpocketing of the oral cavity and the infundibulum as a thickening in the floor of the hypothalamus. **(B and C)** Development at 11 weeks and 16 weeks, respectively. The anterior lobe, the pars tuberalis, and the pars intermedia are derived from Rathke pouch. (Adapted with permission from Sadler TW: *Langman's Medical Embryology,* 10th ed. Baltimore, Lippincott Williams & Wilkins, 2006, p 301.)

B. **Optic vesicles, cups, and stalks** (see Figure 4-3)
- • are derivatives of diencephalic vesicle walls.
- • give rise to the retina, optic nerve, optic chiasm, and optic tract.

C. **Hypophysis (pituitary gland)** (Figure 4-9)
1. **Anterior lobe (adenohypophysis)**
   - • develops from the **Rathke pouch**, an ectodermal diverticulum of the primitive oral cavity (**stomodeum**). Remnants of the Rathke pouch may give rise to a congenital cystic tumor, a **craniopharyngioma** (Figure 4-10; see Chapter 19 VII A:).
   - • includes the **pars tuberalis, pars intermedia,** and **pars distalis.**
2. **Posterior lobe (neurohypophysis)**
   - • develops from a ventral evagination of the hypothalamus.
   - • includes the median eminence, infundibular stem, and pars nervosa.

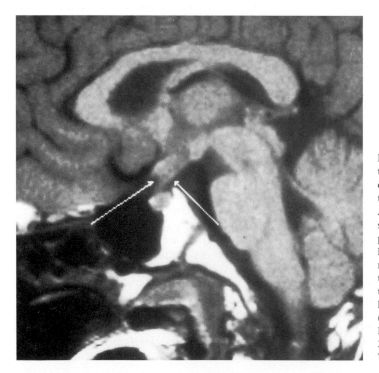

Figure 4-10. Midsagittal section of T_1-weighted magnetic resonance imaging scan through the brainstem and diencephalon. A craniopharyngioma (*arrow*) lies suprasellar in the midline, compressing the optic chiasm and hypothalamus. This tumor, the most common supratentorial tumor occurring in childhood, is the most common cause of hypopituitarism in children. (Reprinted with permission from Fix JD: *High-Yield Neuroanatomy,* 3rd ed. Philadelphia, Lippincott Williams & Wilkins, 2005, p 45.)

XI. Development of the Telencephalon

A. **Cerebral hemispheres** (Figure 4-11; see Figure 4-3)
   - develop as **bilateral evaginations** of the lateral walls of the **prosencephalic vesicle.**
   - contain the **cerebral cortex, cerebral white matter, basal ganglia,** and **lateral ventricles**.
   - are interconnected by three commissures: the **corpus callosum, anterior commissure, and hippocampal (fornix) commissure.**
   - continuous hemispheric growth gives rise to frontal, parietal, occipital, and temporal lobes, which overlie the insula and dorsal brainstem.

B. **Cerebral cortex (pallium)**
   - is formed by prosencephalic neuroblasts that migrate in waves from the mantle layer into the marginal layer and give rise to cortical cell layers.
   - is classified phylogenetically into:
     1. **Neocortex** (isocortex), a six-layered cortex
        - is separated from the paleocortex by the **rhinal sulcus**, a continuation of the collateral sulcus.
        - represents 90% of the cortical mantle.
     2. **Allocortex**, a three-layered cortex, including:
        a. **Paleocortex** (olfactory cortex)
        b. **Archicortex** (hippocampal cortex)

C. **Corpus striatum** (see Figure 4-11)
   - appears in the fifth week as a bulging striatal eminence in the ventral floor of the lateral telencephalic vesicle.
   - gives rise to the **basal ganglia**: the caudate nucleus, putamen, amygdaloid nucleus, and claustrum. The neurons of the **globus pallidus**, a basal ganglion, originate in the subthalamus; they migrate into the telencephalic white matter and become the medial segments of the lentiform nucleus.
   - is divided into the caudate nucleus and the lentiform nucleus by corticofugal and corticopetal fibers; these fibers make up the **internal capsule.**

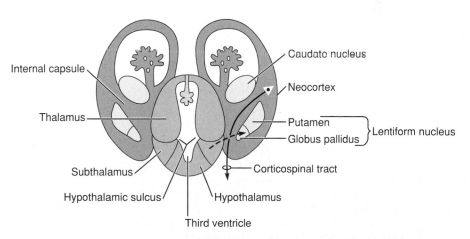

Figure 4-11. Schematic illustration (transverse section) of the development of the forebrain. The cerebral cortex and basal ganglia are shown. The internal capsule divides the corpus striatum into the caudate nucleus and the lentiform nucleus. The alar plate of the diencephalon gives rise to the thalamus and the hypothalamus. Cells from the subthalamus give rise to the globus pallidus. (Adapted with permission from Fix JD, Dudek RW: *BRS Embryology,* 2nd ed. Baltimore, Williams & Wilkins, 1998, p 90.)

D. Commissures
- are fiber bundles that interconnect the two cerebral hemispheres.
- cross the midline via the **lamina terminalis**.
  1. **Anterior commissure**
     - is the first commissure to appear.
     - interconnects the olfactory structures and the middle and inferior temporal gyri.
  2. **Hippocampal commissure (fornical commissure)**
     - is the second commissure to appear.
     - interconnects the two hippocampi.
  3. **Corpus callosum**
     - appears between weeks 12 and 22 of development.
     - is the third commissure to appear.
     - is the largest commissure of the brain and interconnects the corresponding neocortical areas of the two cerebral hemispheres.
     - does *not* project commissural fibers from the visual cortex (area 17) or the hand area of the motor or sensory strips (areas 1, 2, 3, and 4).

E. Gyri and sulci (fissures)
- In the fourth month, no gyri or sulci are present; the brain is smooth or **lissencephalic**.
- At the eighth month, all major gyri and sulci are present; the brain is convoluted or **gyrencephalic**.

XII. Congenital Malformations of the Central Nervous System (CNS)

- result from failure of the neural tube to close or separate from the surface ectoderm (e.g., spina bifida).
- result from failure of the vertebral arches to fuse.
- result from failure of midline cleavage of the embryonic forebrain (e.g., holoprosencephaly).

A. Neural tube defects (e.g., spina bifida and anencephaly)
- may be detected prenatally by screening for **high alpha-fetoprotein levels** in the amniotic fluid or in the maternal serum (**low alpha-fetoprotein levels** are found in **Down syndrome**) and subsequently confirmed through ultrasound.
  1. **Spina bifida** (Figure 4-12)
     - usually occurs in the sacrolumbar region.
     - results from failure of the **posterior neuropore** to close.
     - includes the following variations:
       a. **Spina bifida occulta**
          - is a defect in the vertebral arches.
          - is the least severe type of spina bifida.
          - occurs in 10% of the population.
       b. **Spina bifida cystica**
          - is the major form of **dysraphism**.
          - is most often localized in lumbar and lumbosacral regions.
          (1) **Spina bifida with meningocele**
              - occurs when the meninges project through a vertebral defect, forming a sac filled with CSF.
              - exists with the spinal cord remaining in its normal position.
          (2) **Spina bifida with meningomyelocele**
              - occurs when the meninges and spinal cord project through a vertebral defect, forming a sac.
              - is the most common variation of spina bifida cystica (80%–90%).
              - is usually present in Arnold-Chiari malformation.

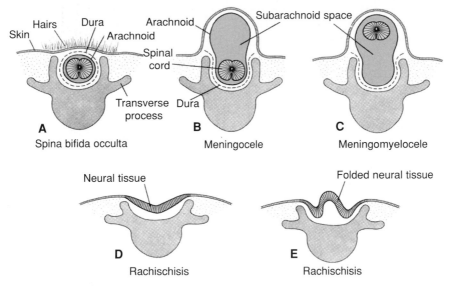

Figure 4-12.   Schematic drawings illustrating a variety of neural tube defects involving the spinal cord. The term *spina bifida* applies to all of the defects because the bony arch of one or more vertebrae has failed to fuse dorsal to the spinal cord. (Modified with permission from Sadler TW: *Langman's Medical Embryology,* 10th ed. Baltimore, Lippincott Williams & Wilkins, 2006, p 294.)

      (3) Spina bifida with myeloschisis
- is the most severe type of spina bifida.
- results in an open neural tube that lies on the surface of the back.

  2. Anencephaly (meroanencephaly)
- results from failure of the **anterior neuropore** to close.
- occurs when the brain fails to develop; a rudimentary brainstem is usually present, and no cranial vault is formed.
- is the most common serious birth defect in stillborn fetuses.
- occurs once in every 1000 births.

B. Ossification defects of the occipital bone (Figure 4-13)
- are also called **cranium bifidum**.
- occur once in every 2000 births.
- **Encephaloceles** occur in the occiput (75%) and in the sinciput (25%).
- include the following variations:

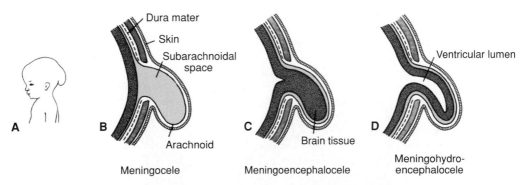

Figure 4-13.   Schematic drawings illustrating the various types of occipital encephaloceles (cranium bifidum). (Adapted with permission from Sadler TW: *Langman's Medical Embryology,* 10th ed. Baltimore, Lippincott Williams & Wilkins, 2006, p 308.)

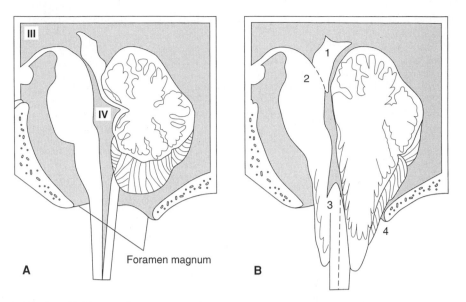

Figure 4-14. Arnold-Chiari malformation, midsagittal section. **(A)** Normal cerebellum, fourth ventricle, and brainstem. **(B)** Abnormal cerebellum, fourth ventricle, and brainstem showing the common congenital anomalies: (*1*) breaking of the tectal plate, (*2*) aqueductal stenosis, (*3*) kinking and transforaminal herniation of the medulla into the vertebral canal, and (*4*) herniation and unrolling of the cerebellar vermis into the vertebral canal. An accompanying meningomyelocele is common. (Modified with permission from Fix JD: *High-Yield Neuroanatomy,* 3rd ed. Philadelphia, Lippincott Williams & Wilkins, 2005, p 46.)

1. **Cranial meningocele**
2. **Meningoencephalocele**
3. **Meningohydroencephalocele**

C. **Arnold-Chiari malformation** (Figures 4-14 and 4-15)
   - is a cerebellomedullary malformation in which the caudal vermis, cerebellar tonsils, and medulla herniate through the foramen magnum, resulting in an obstructive hydrocephalus.
   - is frequently associated with spina bifida (meningomyelocele) and platybasia, with malformation of the occipitovertebral joint.

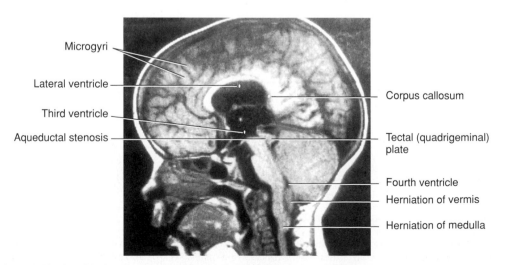

Figure 4-15 Arnold-Chiari malformation, midsagittal section, T_2-weighted magnetic resonance imaging scan.

- Affected children may have dysphonia, laryngeal stridor, and respiratory arrest (involvement of CN X).
- occurs once in every 1000 births.

D. **Dandy-Walker syndrome** (Figure 4-16)
- consists of a huge **cyst of the posterior fossa** associated with atresia of the outlet foramina of Luschka and Magendie.
- is associated with dilation of the fourth ventricle, **agenesis of the cerebellar vermis,** occipital meningocele, and frequently agenesis of the splenium of the corpus callosum.

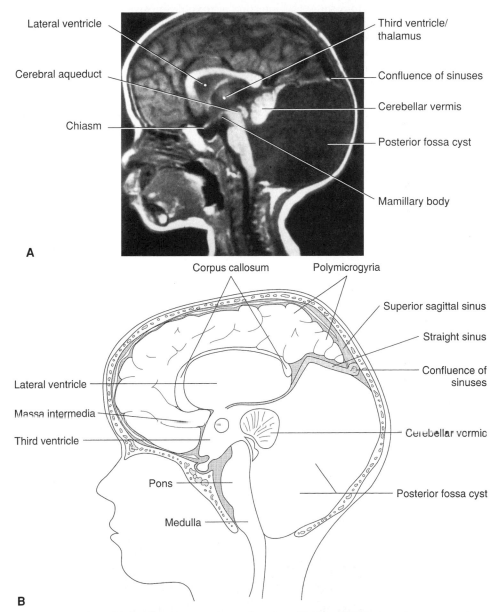

Figure 4-16. Dandy-Walker malformation, midsagittal section. (A) T_2-weighted magnetic resonance imaging scan. (B) Diagram. An enormous dilation of the fourth ventricle results from failure of the foramina of Luschka and Magendie to open. This condition is associated with occipital meningocele, elevation of the confluence of the sinuses (torcular Herophili), agenesis of the cerebellar vermis, and splenium of the corpus callosum. (Reprinted with permission from Fix JD: *High-Yield Embryology,* 3rd ed. Baltimore, Williams & Wilkins, 2005, p 46.)

E. Fetal alcohol syndrome
- includes growth retardation, microcephaly, and congenital heart anomalies.
- is considered the most common cause of mild mental retardation.
- occurs once in every 500 live births.

F. Hydrocephalus (Figure 4-17)
- is a dilation of the ventricles due to an excess of CSF.
- may result from blockage of CSF circulation (e.g., aqueductal stenosis) or overproduction of CSF (e.g., choroid plexus papilloma of lateral ventricle). **Aqueductal stenosis** is the most common cause of congenital hydrocephalus; it may be transmitted by an X-linked trait or may be caused by **cytomegalovirus** infection or **toxoplasmosis**.
  1. **Communicating hydrocephalus** results from obstruction distal to the ventricles (e.g., **subarachnoid hemorrhage** or **meningitis**).
  2. **Noncommunicating hydrocephalus** results from obstruction within the ventricle system (e.g., **aqueductal stenosis** or **ependymitis**).

G. Holoprosencephaly (Figure 4-18)
- results from failure of midline cleavage (diverticularization) of the embryonic forebrain. The telencephalon contains a single ventricular cavity.
- is characterized by the absence of olfactory bulbs and tracts (**arhinencephaly**).
- is seen in trisomy 13 (**Patau syndrome**).
- may result from alcohol abuse during pregnancy, especially in the first 4 weeks.
- is the most severe manifestation of **fetal alcohol syndrome**.
- in extreme forms (alobar and semilobar), it results in the absence of corpus callosum and septum pellucidum.

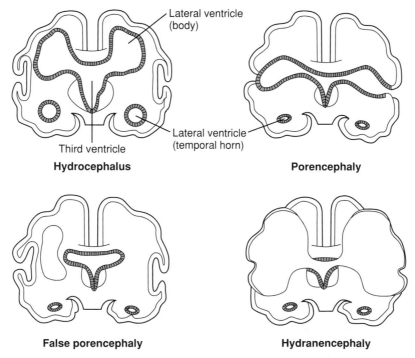

Figure 4-17. Cystic malformations of the prosencephalon (forebrain). Note the ependymal lining of these cysts. In hydranencephaly, the cyst is lined by glia and leptomeninges. In false porencephaly, the cyst is lined by glia. (Modified with permission from Dudek RW, Fix JD: *BRS Embryology,* 2nd ed. Baltimore, Williams & Wilkins, 1998, p 98.)

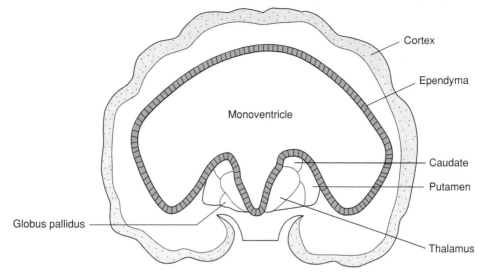

Figure 4-18. Holoprosencephaly results from failure of midline cleavage of the embryonic prosencephalon. The telencephalon contains a single ventricular cavity. It may result from alcohol abuse, especially during the first 4 weeks of pregnancy. (Modified with permission from Dudek RW, Fix JD: *BRS Embryology,* 2nd ed. Baltimore, Williams & Wilkins, 1998, p 99.)

H. Polyhydramnios
- is an excess of amniotic fluid, resulting from the inability of the fetus to swallow amniotic fluid.
- may result from esophageal atresia.

I. Hydranencephaly (see Figure 4-17)
- is a congenital absence of cerebral hemispheres, which are replaced by hugely dilated ventricles.
- results from bilateral hemispheral infarction secondary to occlusion of the carotid arteries in utero.
- also results from severe necrotizing encephalitis in utero from Toxoplasma, Rubella, Cytomegalovirus, or Herpesvirus (TORCH).

J. Porencephaly (see Figure 4-17)
- is cystic cavitation of the prosencephalon due to agenesis of the cortical mantle. The cavity is lined with ependyma and communicates with the lateral ventricle.
- is called schizencephaly when the condition is bilateral.

K. False porencephaly (see Figure 4-17)
- is a malformation consisting of cystic cavities that are lined with glia and do not communicate with the lateral ventricle.

L. Tethered spinal cord (filum terminale syndrome)
- results from a thick, short filum terminale.
- leads to weakness and sensory deficits in the lower extremity and a neurogenic bladder. Deficits usually improve after transection.

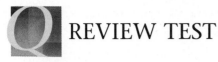

REVIEW TEST

1. The neural retina is derived from the

(A) alar plate
(B) choroid
(C) neural crest
(D) neural tube
(E) telencephalic vesicle wall

2. At birth, the conus medullaris is found at which vertebral level?

(A) VT12
(B) VL1
(C) VL3
(D) VS1
(E) VS4

3. Caudal herniation of the cerebellar tonsils and medulla through the foramen magnum is called

(A) Dandy-Walker syndrome
(B) Down syndrome
(C) Arnold-Chiari syndrome
(D) cranium bifidum
(E) myeloschisis

4. A newborn has multiple congenital defects due to dysgenesis of the neural crest. Which of the following cells is most likely to be spared?

(A) Dorsal root ganglion cells
(B) Geniculate ganglion cells
(C) Melanocytes
(D) Motor neurons
(E) Parafollicular cells

Questions 5 to 9

Match the statements in items 5 to 9 with the appropriate lettered structure shown in the figure.

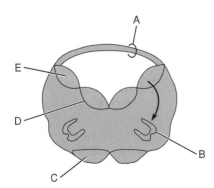

5. Is derived from the telencephalon

6. Gives rise to the choroid plexus

7. Is derived from the alar plate

8. Gives rise to motor neurons that innervate the tongue

9. Gives rise to the solitary nucleus

Questions 10 to 14

Match the statements in items 10 to 14 with the appropriate lettered structure shown in the figure.

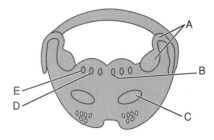

10. Innervates the lateral rectus muscle

11. Gives rise to a parasympathetic nucleus

12. Gives rise to the cerebellum

13. Is derived from the alar plate

14. Gives rise to motor neurons that migrate into the lateral pontine tegmentum

ANSWERS AND EXPLANATIONS

1–D. The retina is derived from the neural tube, which gives rise to the entire CNS.

2–C. At birth, the conus medullaris extends to VL3, and in the adult it extends to the VL1–VL2 interspace. At 8 weeks, the spinal cord extends the entire length of the vertebral canal.

3–C. Arnold-Chiari syndrome is a cerebellomedullary malformation in which the inferior vermis and medulla herniate through the foramen magnum, resulting in communicating hydrocephalus. Arnold-Chiari syndrome is frequently associated with spina bifida.

4–D. Motor neurons develop from the neural tube, more specifically from the basal plate. The other options are derivatives of the neural crest.

5–C. The corticospinal tract (pyramid) has its origin in the neocortex of the telencephalon.

6–A. The tela choroidea gives rise to the choroid plexus.

7–B. The inferior olivary nucleus is derived from the alar plate of the developing medulla.

8–D. The basal plate gives rise to the hypoglossal nucleus.

9–E. The alar plate gives rise to the solitary nucleus.

10–B. The GSE column innervates the lateral rectus muscle.

11–E. The GVE column gives rise to the superior salivatory nucleus of CN VII. This parasympathetic nucleus innervates the lacrimal, the sublingual, and the submandibular glands and also the palatine and nasal glands.

12–A. The cerebellum is derived from the alar plate. The alar plate gives rise to the rhombic lip, which becomes the cerebellum.

13–C. The pontine nuclei are derived from the alar plate.

14–D. The SVE column gives rise to motor neurons that migrate into the lateral pontine tegmentum and become the facial nucleus, CN VII.

Neurohistology

I. Overview: Nervous Tissue

- develops from ectoderm (neural tube and neural crest).
- consists of neurons and glial cells.

II. Neurons

- constitute the genetic, anatomic, trophic, and functional units of the nervous system (known as the neuron doctrine).
- have lost the capacity to undergo cell division.
- have the capacity to *receive* impulses from receptor organs or other neurons.
- have the capacity to *transmit* impulses to other neurons or effector organs.
- consist of the **cell body** and its processes, **dendrites**, and a single **axon**.

A. **Classification of neurons** (Figure 5-1)
- is according to **number of processes** (unipolar, bipolar, or multipolar), **axonal length, function**, and **neurotransmitter**.
    1. Processes
        a. **Unipolar or pseudounipolar neurons**
            - are sensory neurons in the dorsal root and cranial nerve ganglia and in the mesencephalic nucleus of the trigeminal nerve (cranial nerve [CN] V) of the brainstem.
        b. **Bipolar neurons**
            - are located in the vestibular and cochlear ganglia of the vestibulocochlear nerve (CN VIII), the retina, and the olfactory epithelium (CN I).
        c. **Multipolar neurons**
            - possess one axon and more than one dendrite.
            - are the largest population of nerve cells in the nervous system.
            - include motor neurons, interneurons, pyramidal cells of the cerebral cortex, and Purkinje cells of the cerebellar cortex.
    2. **Axonal length**
        a. **Golgi type I neurons**
            - have long axons (e.g., giant pyramidal cells of Betz of the motor cortex).
        b. **Golgi type II neurons**
            - have short axons (e.g., interneurons).
    3. **Function**
        a. **Motor neurons**
            - conduct impulses to muscles, glands, and blood vessels (e.g., ventral horn cells).

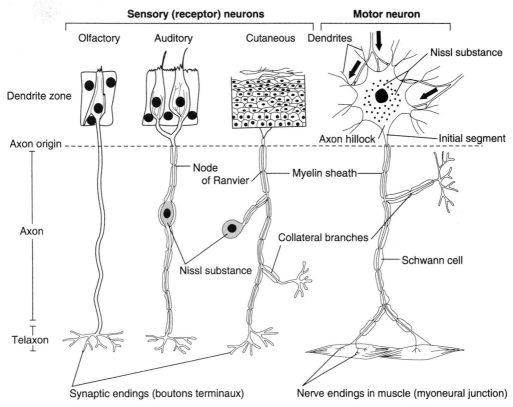

Figure 5-1. Types of nerve cells. Olfactory neurons are bipolar and unmyelinated. Auditory neurons are bipolar and myelinated. Dorsal root ganglion cells (cutaneous) are pseudounipolar and myelinated. Motor neurons are multipolar and myelinated. *Arrows* indicate input via axons of other neurons. Nerve cells are characterized by the presence of Nissl substance, rough endoplasmic reticulum. (Modified with permission from Carpenter MB, Sutin J: *Human Neuroanatomy,* 8th ed. Baltimore, Williams & Wilkins, 1983, p 92.)

    b. Sensory neurons
- receive stimuli from the external and internal environment (e.g., dorsal root ganglion cells).

    c. Interneurons
- are intercalated or internuncial neurons that interconnect motor or sensory neurons.

  4. Neurotransmitter (cholinergic neurons)
- elaborates acetylcholine as a neurotransmitter (e.g., ventral horn motor neurons).

B. Nerve cell body
- is also called the **soma** or **perikaryon**.
- contains the organelles found in other cells, including a large nucleus and a prominent nucleolus.
- has receptor molecules on its plasmalemmal surface that confer sensitivity to various neurotransmitters.
- incorporates or gives rise to the following structures:
    1. Nissl substance
- is characteristic of nerve cells and consists of rosettes of polysomes and rough endoplasmic reticulum.
- plays a role in **protein synthesis**.
- is abundant throughout cytoplasm and dendrites but is *not* found in the axon hillock or in the axon.

2. **Lysosomes**
   - are membrane-bound dense bodies that contain hydrolytic enzymes and are involved in the process of **intracellular digestion**.
   - A genetic defect in the synthesis of lysosomal enzymes results in a storage disease (e.g., Tay-Sachs disease [GM_2 gangliosidosis]).
3. **Filamentous protein structures**
   - form an internal supportive network, the **cytoskeleton**, consisting of:
     a. **Microtubules** (25 nm in diameter)
        - are found in the cell body, dendrites, and axons.
        - play a role in the **development** and **maintenance** of **cell shape**.
        - play a role in the **intracellular transport** of **peptide vesicles** and **organelles**.
     b. **Neurofilaments** (10 nm in diameter)
        - consist of spiral protein threads that play a role in **developing** and **regenerating nerve fibers**.
        - degenerate in Alzheimer disease to form **neurofibrillary tangles**.
        - contain neurofilament protein, which is exclusive to neurons and their precursors.
     c. **Microfilaments** (5 nm in diameter)
        - are composed of **actin**.
        - are found in the tips of growing axons.
        - facilitate **movement of plasma membrane** and **growth of nerve cell processes**.
4. **Inclusion bodies**
   - include pigment granules:
     a. **Lipofuscin (lipochrome) granules**
        - are common pigmented inclusions of cytoplasm that accumulate with aging.
        - are considered to be residual bodies derived from lysosomes.
     b. **Neuromelanin (melanin)**
        - is a blackish pigment in the neurons of the substantia nigra and locus ceruleus.
        - disappears from the substantia nigra and the locus ceruleus in Parkinson disease.
     c. **Lewy bodies**
        - are eosinophilic intracytoplasmic inclusion bodies found in the substantia nigra in patients with Parkinson disease.
     d. **Hirano bodies**
        - are intracytoplasmic inclusion bodies found in the hippocampus in patients with Alzheimer disease.
     e. **Negri and lyssa bodies**
        - are intracytoplasmic inclusion bodies found in people with rabies.
5. **Dendrites**
   - are processes that extend from the cell body.
   - contain cytoplasm similar in composition to that of the cell body; however, no Golgi apparatus is present.
   - conduct in a decremental fashion but may be capable of generating action potentials.
   - **receive synaptic input and transmit it toward the cell body.**
6. **Axons**
   - arise from either the cell body or a dendrite.
   - originate from the axon hillock, which lacks Nissl substance.
   - give rise to collateral branches.
   - may be myelinated or unmyelinated.
   - **generate, propagate, and transmit action potentials.**
   - end distally in terminal boutons in synapses with neurons, muscle cells, and glands.
7. **Nerve fibers** (Table 5-1)
   - consist of axons and their glial investments.
   - are classified by function, fiber size, and conduction velocity.
8. **Myelin sheath**
   - is produced in the peripheral nervous system (PNS) by Schwann cells.
   - is produced in the central nervous system (CNS) by oligodendrocytes.

TABLE 5-1	*Classification of Nerve Fibers*		
Fibers	Diameter (μm)*	Conduction Velocity (m/sec)	Function
Sensory axons			
Ia (A-α)	12–20	70–120	Proprioception, muscle spindles
Ib (A-α)	12–20	70–120	Proprioception, Golgi tendon organs
II (A-β)	5–12	30–70	Touch, pressure, and vibration
III (A-β)	2–5	12–30	Touch, pressure, fast pain, and temperature
IV (C)	0.5–1	0.5–2	Slow pain and temperature, unmyelinated fibers
Motor axons			
Alpha (A-α)	12–20	15–120	Alpha motor neurons of ventral horn (innervate extrafusal muscle fibers)
Gamma (A-γ)	2–10	10–45	Gamma motor neurons of ventral horn (innervate intrafusal muscle fibers)
Preganglionic autonomic fibers (B)	<3	3–15	Myelinated preganglionic autonomic fibers
Postganglionic autonomic fibers (C)	1	2	Unmyelinated postganglionic autonomic fibers

*Myelin sheath included if present.

- is interrupted by the nodes of Ranvier.
- consists of a spirally wrapped plasma membrane.

9. **Synapses**
   - are the **sites of functional contact** of a nerve cell with another nerve cell, an effector cell, or a sensory receptor cell.
   - consist of presynaptic membrane, synaptic cleft, and postsynaptic membrane.
   - are classified by the site of contact (e.g., axosomatic, axodendritic, or axoaxonic).
   - are also classified as chemical or electrical:
     a. **Chemical synapses**
        - use neurotransmitters.
     b. **Electrical synapses (ephapses)**
        - consist of gap junctions.
        - allow ions to pass from cell to cell.

III. Neuroglia

- are nonneuronal cells of the CNS and the PNS.
- arise from the neural tube and neural crest.
- are capable of mitotic cell division throughout adult life, especially in response to trauma or disease.
- are best revealed with gold and silver impregnation stains.
- are classified as **macroglia (astrocytes** and **oligodendrocytes), microglia,** and **ependyma.** Schwann cells are classified as peripheral neuroglia.

A. Astrocytes
- are the largest glial cells.
- consist of **fibrous astrocytes**, which are found mainly in white matter, and **protoplasmic astrocytes**, which are found mainly in gray matter.
- play a role in the metabolism of certain neurotransmitters (gamma-aminobutyric acid [GABA], serotonin, and glutamate).
- buffer the potassium concentration of the extracellular space.
- contain glial filaments and glycogen granules as their most characteristic cytoplasmic components.
- in damaged areas of the brain, form glial scars, a condition called **gliosis**.
- contain or give rise to the following structures:
  1. **Astrocytic end feet**
     - are the processes that form the external glial limiting membrane (interface between the pia mater and the CNS) and the internal glial limiting membrane (interface between the ependyma and the CNS).
     a. **Perivascular end feet**
        - surround capillaries.
     b. **Perineuronal end feet**
        - surround neurons.
  2. **Glial filaments**
     - contain **glial fibrillary acidic protein** (GFAP), a marker for astrocytes.
  3. **Glycogen granules**

B. Oligodendrocytes
- are small glial cells with few short processes.
- lack glial filaments and glycogen granules.
- are the myelin-forming cells of the CNS; one oligodendrocyte can myelinate numerous (up to 30) axons.
- consist of:
  1. **Interfascicular oligodendrocytes**
     - are found in white matter.
  2. **Satellite cells**
     - are found in gray matter.

C. Microglia (Hortega cells)
- arise from monocytes, which enter the CNS via abnormal blood vessels.
- are activated by inflammatory and degenerative processes.
- are macrophages, which are migratory and phagocytize debris of nerve tissue.

D. Ependymal cells
- line the central canal of the spinal cord and ventricles of the brain.
- possess cilia only in embryologic stages in man that originate from **blepharoplasts** (basal bodies), which can be stained by phosphotungstic acid–hematoxylin (PTAH).
- include choroid epithelial cells of the choroid plexus and tanycytes of the third ventricle; the choroid plexus cells produce cerebrospinal fluid (CSF) and are interconnected by tight junctions that constitute the **blood–CSF barrier**.

E. Schwann cells (neurolemmal cells)
- are derivatives of the neural crest.
- are myelin-forming cells of the PNS; a Schwann cell myelinates only one internode (only one peripheral axon).
- invest all unmyelinated axons of the PNS.
- function in regeneration and remyelination of severed axons in the PNS (Figure 5-2).
- are separated from each other by the **node of Ranvier**.

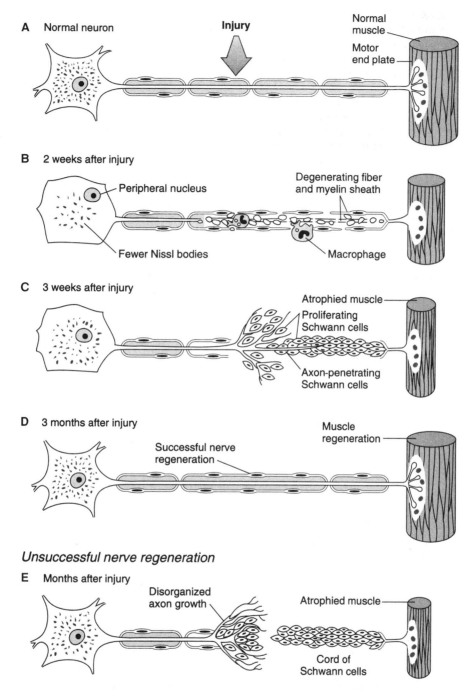

Figure 5-2. Wallerian (anterograde) degeneration and regeneration of a nerve fiber.

F. Tumors of neuroglial cells (gliomas) (Figure 5-3)
- are derived from the three glial cell types: astrocytes, oligodendrocytes, and ependymocytes.
- result from proliferation of glioblasts, embryonic precursors.
- represent 50% of primary intracranial tumors.

1. **Astrocytomas** (see Figure 5-3)
   - are most commonly found in the white matter of the cerebral hemisphere in middle and late life.
   - Astrocytomas of the cerebellum are the most common intracranial tumor in children.
   a. **Benign astrocytomas**
      - are slow-growing neoplasms of infiltrative character.
      - arise from **astroblasts**, embryonic precursors.
      - represent 25% of primary intracranial tumors.
      - frequently become malignant (**anaplastic astrocytomas**).
   b. **Malignant astrocytomas (glioblastoma multiforme)**
      - are rapid-growing, fatal astrocytic tumors; fewer than 20% of patients survive 1 year.
      - occur twice as frequently in men as in women.
      - arise from **astroblasts**.
      - represent 50% of gliomas.
      - are the most common primary brain tumors.
2. **Oligodendrogliomas** (see Figure 5-3)
   - are slow-growing, benign tumors that account for approximately 5% of primary intracranial gliomas.
   - occur mainly in adults.
   - are most frequently found in the cerebral hemisphere.
   - may arise from **oligodendroblasts**, embryonic precursors.
   - are usually well circumscribed and are frequently calcified.
   - may change and become glioblastomas.
3. **Ependymomas** (see Figure 5-3)
   - are slow-growing, benign circumscribed neoplasms typically found within the ventricles.
   - account for approximately 5% of primary intracranial gliomas.
   - are the most common gliomas found in the spinal cord, most frequently in the lumbosacral segments (filum terminale and cauda equina).
   - arise from **ependymal cells**.
4. **Schwannomas** (see Figure 5-3)
   - are benign tumors of peripheral nerves (e.g., acoustic neuromas of CN VIII).
   - account for 6% of primary intracranial tumors.
   - occur twice as frequently in females as in males.
   - arise from **Schwann cells**.
5. **Meningiomas** (see Figure 5-3)
   - are slow-growing tumors of mesenchymal origin.
   - account for 15% of primary intracranial tumors.
   - are supratentorial in 90% of cases.
   - have a female-to-male ratio of 3 : 2.
6. **Medulloblastomas** (see Figure 5-3)
   - arise exclusively in the cerebellum and are thought to arise from the external granular layer of the cerebellar cortex.
   - represent 20% of the primary intracranial tumors found in children.

IV.   Nerve Cell Degeneration and Regeneration (see Figure 5-2)

A. **Retrograde degeneration**
   - occurs toward the proximal end of an axon, including the cell body.
   - takes place in both the CNS and the PNS.
   - Reaction begins 2 days or sooner after insult and reaches a maximum in about 20 days.
   - involves the following:
     1. Disappearance of Nissl substance (chromatolysis)
     2. Swelling of the cell body
     3. Flattening and displacement of the nucleus to the periphery

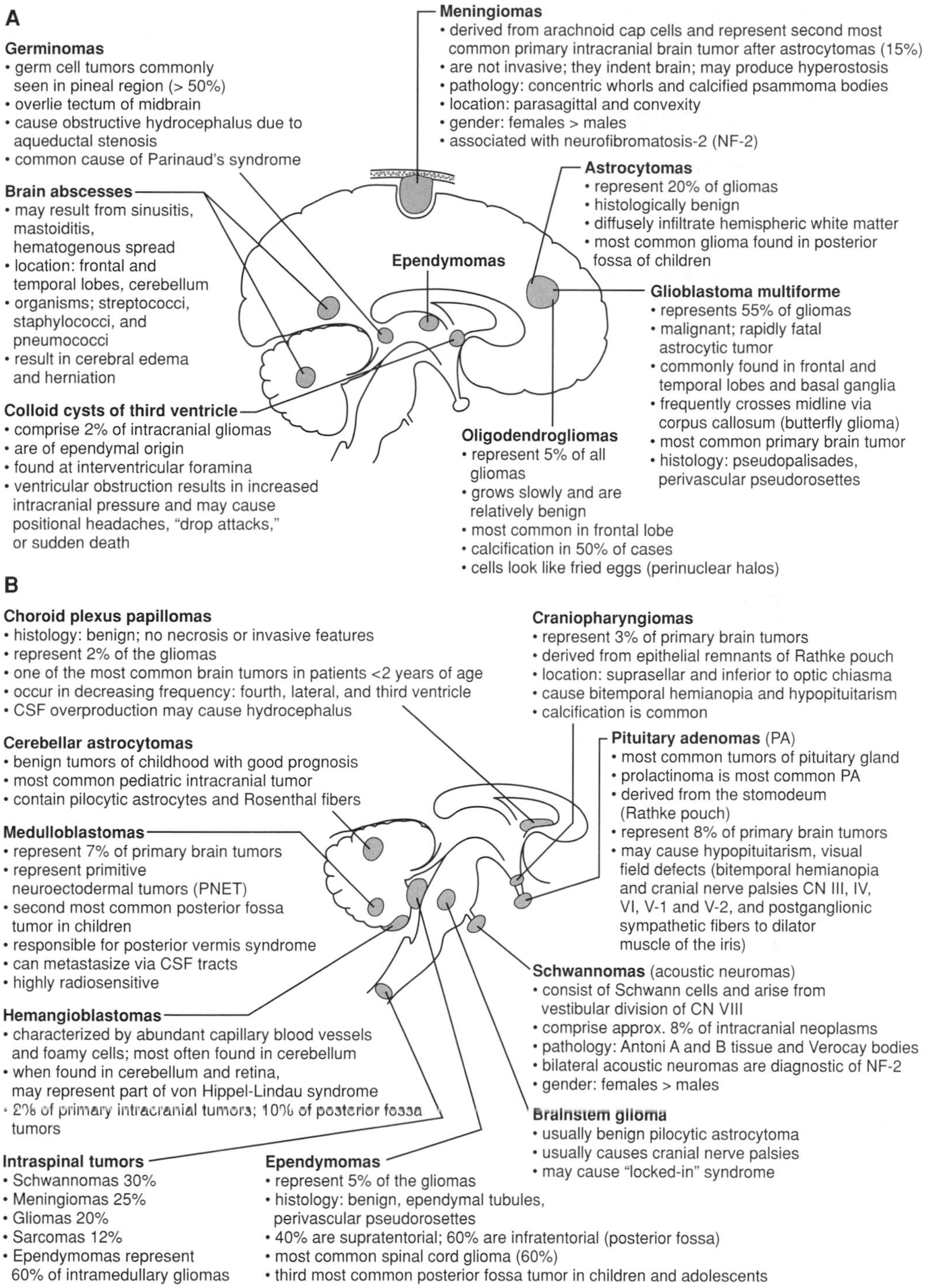

A

Germinomas
- germ cell tumors commonly seen in pineal region (> 50%)
- overlie tectum of midbrain
- cause obstructive hydrocephalus due to aqueductal stenosis
- common cause of Parinaud's syndrome

Brain abscesses
- may result from sinusitis, mastoiditis, hematogenous spread
- location: frontal and temporal lobes, cerebellum
- organisms; streptococci, staphylococci, and pneumococci
- result in cerebral edema and herniation

Colloid cysts of third ventricle
- comprise 2% of intracranial gliomas
- are of ependymal origin
- found at interventricular foramina
- ventricular obstruction results in increased intracranial pressure and may cause positional headaches, "drop attacks," or sudden death

Meningiomas
- derived from arachnoid cap cells and represent second most common primary intracranial brain tumor after astrocytomas (15%)
- are not invasive; they indent brain; may produce hyperostosis
- pathology: concentric whorls and calcified psammoma bodies
- location: parasagittal and convexity
- gender: females > males
- associated with neurofibromatosis-2 (NF-2)

Ependymomas

Astrocytomas
- represent 20% of gliomas
- histologically benign
- diffusely infiltrate hemispheric white matter
- most common glioma found in posterior fossa of children

Glioblastoma multiforme
- represents 55% of gliomas
- malignant; rapidly fatal astrocytic tumor
- commonly found in frontal and temporal lobes and basal ganglia
- frequently crosses midline via corpus callosum (butterfly glioma)
- most common primary brain tumor
- histology: pseudopalisades, perivascular pseudorosettes

Oligodendrogliomas
- represent 5% of all gliomas
- grows slowly and are relatively benign
- most common in frontal lobe
- calcification in 50% of cases
- cells look like fried eggs (perinuclear halos)

B

Choroid plexus papillomas
- histology: benign; no necrosis or invasive features
- represent 2% of the gliomas
- one of the most common brain tumors in patients <2 years of age
- occur in decreasing frequency: fourth, lateral, and third ventricle
- CSF overproduction may cause hydrocephalus

Cerebellar astrocytomas
- benign tumors of childhood with good prognosis
- most common pediatric intracranial tumor
- contain pilocytic astrocytes and Rosenthal fibers

Medulloblastomas
- represent 7% of primary brain tumors
- represent primitive neuroectodermal tumors (PNET)
- second most common posterior fossa tumor in children
- responsible for posterior vermis syndrome
- can metastasize via CSF tracts
- highly radiosensitive

Hemangioblastomas
- characterized by abundant capillary blood vessels and foamy cells; most often found in cerebellum
- when found in cerebellum and retina, may represent part of von Hippel-Lindau syndrome
- 2% of primary intracranial tumors; 10% of posterior fossa tumors

Intraspinal tumors
- Schwannomas 30%
- Meningiomas 25%
- Gliomas 20%
- Sarcomas 12%
- Ependymomas represent 60% of intramedullary gliomas

Ependymomas
- represent 5% of the gliomas
- histology: benign, ependymal tubules, perivascular pseudorosettes
- 40% are supratentorial; 60% are infratentorial (posterior fossa)
- most common spinal cord glioma (60%)
- third most common posterior fossa tumor in children and adolescents

Craniopharyngiomas
- represent 3% of primary brain tumors
- derived from epithelial remnants of Rathke pouch
- location: suprasellar and inferior to optic chiasma
- cause bitemporal hemianopia and hypopituitarism
- calcification is common

Pituitary adenomas (PA)
- most common tumors of pituitary gland
- prolactinoma is most common PA
- derived from the stomodeum (Rathke pouch)
- represent 8% of primary brain tumors
- may cause hypopituitarism, visual field defects (bitemporal hemianopia and cranial nerve palsies CN III, IV, VI, V-1 and V-2, and postganglionic sympathetic fibers to dilator muscle of the iris)

Schwannomas (acoustic neuromas)
- consist of Schwann cells and arise from vestibular division of CN VIII
- comprise approx. 8% of intracranial neoplasms
- pathology: Antoni A and B tissue and Verocay bodies
- bilateral acoustic neuromas are diagnostic of NF-2
- gender: females > males

Brainstem glioma
- usually benign pilocytic astrocytoma
- usually causes cranial nerve palsies
- may cause "locked-in" syndrome

Figure 5-3. Tumors of the CNS and PNS. (*A*) Supratentorial tumors. (*B*) Infratentorial tumors (posterior fossa) and intraspinal tumors. In children, 70% of tumors are infratentorial. In adults, 70% of tumors are supratentorial. CN = cranial nerve; CSF = cerebrospinal fluid. (Modified from Fix JD: *High-Yield Neuroanatomy,* 3rd ed. Philadelphia, Lippincott Williams & Wilkins, 2005, p 52.)

B. **Anterograde (wallerian) degeneration** (see Figure 5-2)
- occurs toward the distal end of the axon.
- takes place in both the PNS and the CNS.
- is characterized by successive fragmentation and disappearance of axons and myelin sheaths and by secondary proliferation of Schwann cells.

C. **Regeneration of the peripheral nerve fiber** (see Figure 5-2)
- A myelinated peripheral nerve fiber consists of an axon, a myelin sheath with its basement membrane, and a delicate connective sheath, the endoneurium.
- The severed distal nerve fiber maintains its integrity and provides a tube of basement membrane and endoneurium into which an axon sprout grows.
- Schwann cells proliferate along a degenerating axon and myelinate a new axon sprout, which grows at the rate of 3 mm/day (corresponds to slow axonal transport of 1–5 mm/day).
- If the path of regenerating axons is blocked, a traumatic neuroma forms at the site of obstruction (amputation neuroma). A neuroma consists of a proliferative mass of axons and Schwann cells.

D. **Regeneration of axons in the CNS**
- No Schwann cell basement membranes or endoneurial investments surround axons of the CNS.
- Effective regeneration does not occur in the CNS.

E. **Transsynaptic (transneuronal) degeneration**
- Interruption of certain CNS pathways results in degeneration of denervated neurons.
- Transection of the optic nerve results in degeneration of neurons in the lateral geniculate body.

V.   Axonal Transport

- mediates the intracellular distribution of secretory proteins, organelles, and cytoskeletal elements.
- is inhibited by colchicine, which depolymerizes microtubules.

A. **Fast anterograde transport**
- is responsible for transporting all newly synthesized membranous organelles (vesicles) and precursors of neurotransmitters at 200 to 400 mm/day.
- is mediated by microtubules and **kinesin** (fast transport is microtubule dependent).

B. **Fast mitochondrial transport**
- occurs at the rate of 50 to 100 mm/day.

C. **Slow anterograde transport**
- is responsible for transporting cytoskeletal and cytoplasmic elements at 1 to 5 mm/day.
- moves unidirectionally away from the cell body.
- transports neurofilaments and microtubules.

D. **Fast retrograde transport**
- returns used materials from the axon terminal to the cell body for degradation and recycling at the rate of 100–200 mm/day.
- transports nerve growth factor and neurotropic viruses and toxins (herpes simplex, rabies, polioviruses, and tetanus toxin).
- is mediated by microtubules and **dynein**.

E. **Tracing neuroanatomic pathways by axonal transport** (Figure 5-4)
  1. **Horseradish peroxidase (HRP) method**
     - is used primarily to study retrograde transport.
       a. HRP is injected into a region (nucleus) of the nervous system.

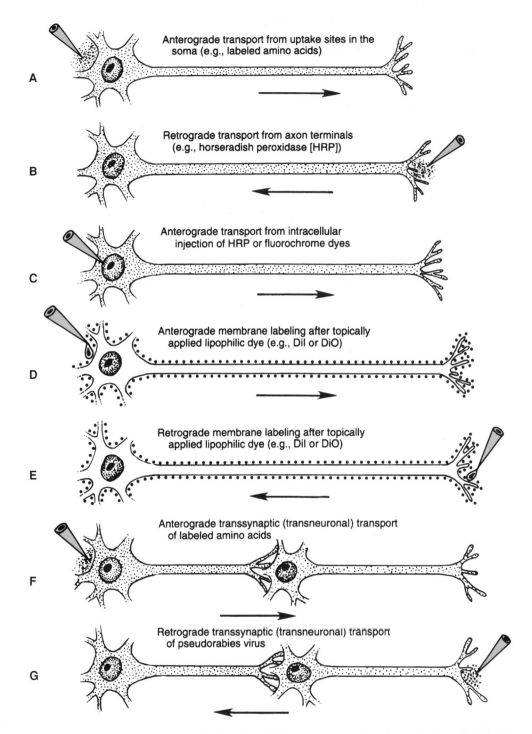

Figure 5-4. Some common tracing methods used to elucidate neuroanatomic pathways by intracellular labeling.

    b. It is taken up by the cell body and transported in an anterograde direction to the axon terminal.

    c. It is taken up by the axon terminal and transported in a retrograde direction to the cell body.

2. Autoradiographic method (see Figure 5-4)

    • is used to trace the axonal pathway in serial autoradiographs.

    a. Radioactive-labeled amino acids are injected into a region (nucleus) of the CNS.

    b. The radioactive substance is taken up by the cell body and transported to the axon terminal. (Only nerve cell bodies take up the label.)

3. Membrane labeling by externally applied carbocyanine dyes (see Figure 5-4)

    • traces neuronal pathways in fixed (dead) tissue.

    a. Commonly used **fluorescent dyes** are DiI, DiO, and DiS.

    b. These **lipophilic dyes** are used to trace neuronal pathways in fixed tissue by diffusion through the plasma membrane of the neuron.

    c. Labeling may be anterograde or retrograde.

VI. Capillaries of the Central Nervous System (Figure 5-5)

• have a higher density in gray matter than in white matter and consist of two types:

A. Nonfenestrated capillaries

• are ubiquitous in white and gray matter.

• have endothelial cells with tight junctions surrounded by a continuous basement membrane and an outer investment of astrocytic foot processes; the endothelial cells and their tight junctions constitute the **blood–brain barrier.**

B. Fenestrated capillaries

• consist of endothelial cells with fenestrations that permit the free passage of blood-borne substances into the extracellular spaces of the CNS.

• are located in specialized areas of the brain that lack a blood–brain barrier (e.g., circum-ventricular organs).

VII. Sensory Receptors

A. Pain and temperature receptors

• are free (nonencapsulated) nerve endings.

• are ubiquitous (e.g., are in the epidermis, dermis, cornea).

• are associated with A delta (group III) and C (group IV) fibers.

• project via the spinothalamic tracts.

• are very slow–adapting receptors.

B. Cutaneous mechanoreceptors

• are endings that respond to touch and pressure.

1. Merkel tactile disks

• are nonencapsulated endings found in the basal layer of the epidermis in hairy and glabrous skin.

• mediate light (crude) touch (e.g., stroking the skin with a wisp of cotton).

• are associated with group II fibers.

• project centrally via the spinothalamic tracts and the dorsal column–medial lemniscus pathway.

• are slow-adapting receptors.

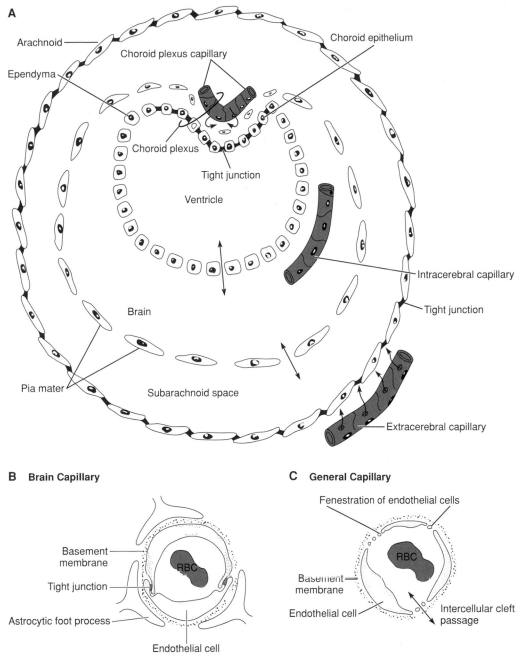

A

Arachnoid

Choroid plexus capillary

Choroid epithelium

Ependyma

Choroid plexus

Tight junction

Ventricle

Intracerebral capillary

Tight junction

Brain

Pia mater

Subarachnoid space

Extracerebral capillary

B **Brain Capillary**

Basement membrane

Tight junction

RBC

Astrocytic foot process

Endothelial cell

C **General Capillary**

Fenestration of endothelial cells

RBC

Basement membrane

Endothelial cell

Intercellular cleft passage

Figure 5-5. The blood–brain barrier and the blood-CSF barrier. Compare the difference between the intracerebral capillaries (**B**), the extracerebral capillaries (**C**), and the capillaries of the choroid plexus (**A**). Barrier function is mediated by tight junctions between the endothelial cells and between choroid plexus epithelial cells. Arachnoid cells have barrier function. Tumors and cerebrovascular accidents disrupt the endothelial wall and cause cerebral edema (vasculotoxic edema). (Adapted from Nolte J: *Human Brain,* 2nd ed. Washington, DC, Mosby, 1988.)

2. Meissner corpuscles (Figure 5-6)
- are encapsulated endings found in the dermal papillae of glabrous skin.
- mediate fine discriminative tactile sensation via the dorsal column–medial lemniscus pathway.
- are associated with group II fibers.
- are fast-adapting receptors.

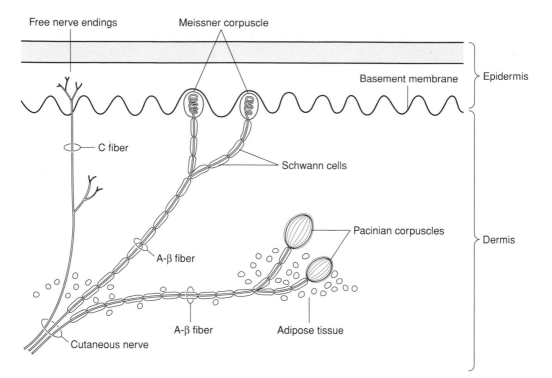

Figure 5-6.   Four important cutaneous receptors: free nerve endings, which mediate pain and temperature sensation; Meissner corpuscles of the dermal papillae, which mediate tactile two-point discrimination; pacinian corpuscles of the dermis, which mediate touch, pressure, and vibration sensation; and Merkel disks (not shown), which mediate light touch. (Modified from Fix JD: *High-Yield Neuroanatomy,* 3rd ed. Philadelphia, Lippincott Williams & Wilkins, 2005, p 53.)

3. **Pacinian corpuscles**
   - are found in the dermis, mesenteries, and periosteum.
   - respond to pressure and vibration sensation via the dorsal column–medial lemniscus pathway.
   - are associated with group II fibers.
   - are very fast–adapting receptors.

C. **Muscle and tendon receptors**
   - are encapsulated mechanoreceptors and proprioceptors.
   1. **Muscle receptors**
      - consist of capsules containing intrafusal fibers (i.e., nuclear bag and nuclear chain fibers).
      - are arranged parallel with the extrafusal fibers of the muscle.
      - mediate, via group Ia afferents, the muscle stretch reflex (MSR) and the myotatic reflex (e.g., patellar reflex).
      - sense the relative length of the muscle (static function) and the rate of change of length (dynamic function).
      - The activity of the gamma motor neurons regulates the sensitivity of the muscle spindle to stretch.
      - contain the following structures:
        a. **Nuclear bag fibers**
           - receive group IA primary afferent fibers (annulospiral endings) and static and dynamic gamma efferent fibers.
           - respond primarily to the rate of change of muscle length.

    b. Nuclear chain fibers
- receive group Ia primary and group II secondary afferent fibers (flower spray endings) and static gamma efferent fibers.
- respond primarily to muscle length.

2. Gamma motor neurons
- consist of static and dynamic motor neurons.
- are found in the ventral horn with the larger alpha motor neurons.
- receive input from descending motor pathways (e.g., corticospinal and reticulospinal tracts).
- modify the sensitivity of muscle spindles.
- are coactivated along with alpha motor neurons.

3. Golgi tendon organs (GTOs)
- are found at the junction of the muscle and its tendon and are connected with the muscle fibers in series.
- respond to muscle tension during muscle stretch and contraction and are also sensitive to the velocity of tension development.
- are innervated by group Ib fibers.

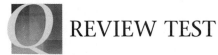

REVIEW TEST

1. Peripheral nerve fibers regenerate at the rate of

(A) 0.1 mm/day
(B) 3 mm/day
(C) 100 mm/day
(D) 200 mm/day
(E) 400 mm/day

2. Fast pain has a conduction velocity of

(A) 1 m/sec
(B) 5 m/sec
(C) 15 m/sec
(D) 30 m/sec
(E) 100 m/sec

3. A 10-year-old boy has severed his radial nerve. Which of the following cells plays a major role in axonal regrowth?

(A) Fibrous astrocytes
(B) Fibroblasts
(C) Oligodendrocytes
(D) Protoplasmic astrocytes
(E) Schwann cells

4. The MSR is initiated by which of the following receptors?

(A) End bulbs of Krause
(B) Merkel disks
(C) Muscle spindles
(D) Ruffini end bulbs
(E) Vater-Pacini corpuscles

5. Wallerian degeneration involves

(A) the proximal end of the axon
(B) only the CNS
(C) chromatolysis
(D) swelling of the cell body
(E) successive fragmentation of the axon

6. A 46-year-old female nurse complains of right-sided hearing loss and vertigo (dizziness). A small tumor was demonstrated within the internal auditory canal. Which structure listed below accounts for the hearing loss and vertigo?

(A) arachnoid cyst
(B) ependymoma
(C) epidermoid cyst
(D) meningioma
(E) Schwannoma

7. A 9-year-old boy has a stumbling gait, dizziness, diplopia, headache, vomiting, and coarse nystagmus toward the side of the lesion. He scans his speech. Tests for dysdiadochokinesia, papilledema, elevated CSF protein, and intention tremor are positive. Match this symptom complex with the best-fitting choice.

(A) meningioma
(B) oligodendroglia
(C) medulloblastoma
(D) craniopharyngioma
(E) von Hippel-Lindau disease

Questions 8 to 12

The response options for items 8 to 12 are the same. Select one answer for each item in the set.

(A) Astrocytes
(B) Oligodendrocytes
(C) Microglial cells
(D) Schwann cells
(E) Tanycytes

Match each of the following descriptions with the corresponding type of nerve cell.

8. Are a variety of ependymal cell found in the wall of the third ventricle

9. Arise from monocytes

10. Are neural crest derivatives

11. Contain glial filaments and glycogen granules

12. Are perineuronal satellite cells in the CNS

ANSWERS AND EXPLANATIONS

1–B. Peripheral nerve fibers regenerate at 3 mm/day.

2–C. Fast pain has a nerve fiber (A delta) conduction velocity of 12 to 30 m/sec. Slow pain has a nerve fiber (C) conduction velocity of 0.5 to 2 m/sec.

3–E. Schwann cells play a major role in axon regeneration (axon regrowth) in the PNS.

4–C. The muscle stretch reflex is initiated by muscle spindles.

5–E. Wallerian, or anterograde, degeneration occurs toward the distal end of the axon in both the CNS and PNS and is characterized by successive fragmentation and disappearance of axons and myelin sheaths and by secondary proliferation of Schwann cells. Retrograde degeneration occurs toward the proximal end of the axon and in the cell body. It takes place in both the CNS and PNS and is characterized by chromatolysis, cell body swelling, and flattening and displacement of the nucleus to the periphery.

6–E. A schwannoma is a benign tumor derived from Schwann cells of the vestibular division of CN VIII (acoustic neuroma of CN VIII). Schwannomas occur twice as frequently in females as in males. Symptoms arise from pressure on the vestibular division, resulting in vertigo, and pressure on the cochlear division, resulting in nerve deafness (sensorineural). Acoustic neurinomas represent 8% of intracranial neoplasms. When bilateral they are diagnostic of type 2 neurofibromatosis. The internal auditory canal contains the facial and vestibulocochlear nerves and the labyrinthine artery, a branch of the anterior inferior cerebellar artery. An arachnoid cyst is a congenital disorder; it is a CSF sac that forms in the cranium or spinal cord. An ependymoma is a slow-growing, benign circumscribed neoplasm typically found within the ventricles. An epidermoid cyst is a benign cyst derived from ectodermal tissue. A meningioma is a slow-growing intracranial tumor of mesenchymal origin.

7–C. The medulloblastomas are malignant neoplasms comprising one-third of the tumors in the posterior fossa of children. They are radiosensitive. Metastatic spread within the neuraxis is frequent. Meningiomas are benign tumors originating from arachnoid cells; they contain psammoma bodies that are calcified and visible on computed tomography. Oligodendroglia are the myelin-producing cells of the CNS. Craniopharyngiomas, congenital epidermoid tumors, are the most common supratentorial tumors found in children. Von Hippel-Lindau disease is a rare genetic disorder that results in tumor growth in blood-rich areas of the body.

8–E. Tanycytes are a variety of ependymal cell found in the wall of the third ventricle. The processes of these cells extend from the lumen of the third ventricle to the capillaries of the hypophyseal portal system and also to the neurosecretory neurons of the arcuate nucleus.

9–C. Microglial cells, the scavenger cells of the CNS, arise from monocytes and enter the CNS via abnormal blood vessels.

10–D. Schwann cells are derived from the neural crest; they myelinate the axons of the PNS.

11–A. Astrocytes are characterized by the presence of glial filaments and glycogen; glial filaments contain GFAP, a marker for astrocytes.

12–B. Oligodendrocytes are perineuronal satellite cells; they myelinate the axons of the central nervous system (CNS).

CHAPTER

6

Spinal Cord

I. Introduction: Spinal Cord

- is derived from the caudal part of the neural tube.
- maintains segmental organization throughout development.
- is surrounded by three membranes, the **meninges**.
- weighs about 30 g, comprising 2% of the weight of the adult brain.

II. External Morphology

A. Location: the spinal cord (Figure 6-1)
- extends, in adults, from the foramen magnum to the lower border of the first lumbar vertebra; in newborns, it extends to the third lumbar vertebra.
- is continuous with the **medulla oblongata** at the spinomedullary junction, a plane defined by three structures: the foramen magnum, the pyramidal decussation, and the emergence of the first cervical nerve ventral rootlets.
- lies within the **subarachnoid space**, which extends caudally to the level of the second sacral vertebra (see Figure 2-2).

B. Attachments
- suspend and anchor the spinal cord within the dural sac.
- arise from the vascular **pia mater**, which closely invests the spinal cord.
  1. **Denticulate ligaments**
     - are two flattened bands of pial tissue that attach to the spinal dura with about 21 attachments.
  2. **Filum terminale**
     - is a pial filament extending from the conus medullaris to the end of the dural sac, with which it fuses.
  3. **Spinal nerve roots**
     - provide the strongest anchorage and fixation of the spinal cord to the vertebral canal.

C. Shape: the spinal cord (see Figure 6-1)
- is an elongated nearly cylindrical structure, flattened dorsoventrally, and is approximately 1 cm in diameter.
- has **cervical** (C5–T1) and **lumbar** (L1–S2) **enlargements** for the nerve supply of the upper and lower extremities (the brachial and lumbosacral plexuses).
- terminates caudally as the **conus medullaris**.
- averages, in length, 45 cm in males and 42 cm in females.

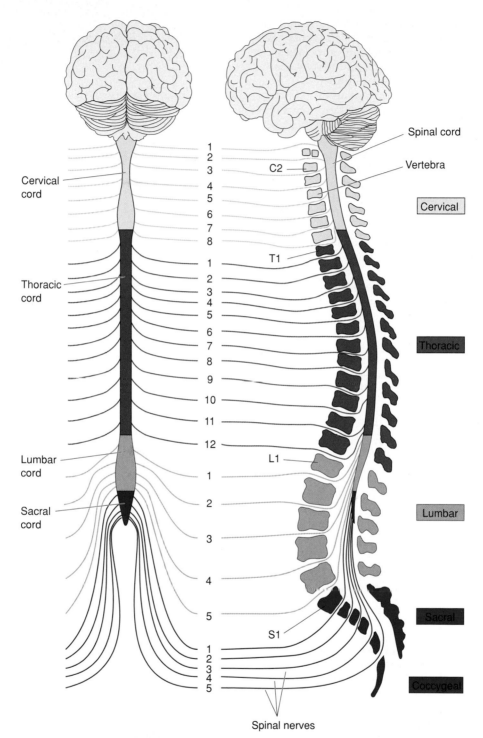

Figure 6-1. Diagram of the position of the spinal cord with reference to the vertebral bodies and spinous processes. The conus medullaris lies in the L1–L2 interspace. The dural cul-de-sac ends at S2. (Adapted with permission from Bear MF, Connors BW, Paradiso MA. *Neuroscience: Exploring the Brain,* 2nd ed. Philadelphia: Lippincott Williams & Wilkins, 2001, Fig. 12-10.)

D. Spinal nerves (Figure 6-2; see Figure 5-1)
- consist of 31 pairs of nerves that emerge from the spinal cord: **8 cervical**, **12 thoracic**, **5 lumbar**, **5 sacral**, and **1 coccygeal**.
- contain both motor and sensory fibers.
  1. **Special considerations**
     a. The first cervical nerve and the coccygeal nerve usually have no dorsal (sensory) roots and no corresponding dermatomes.
     b. The first cervical nerve passes between the atlas and the skull.
     c. The second cervical nerve passes between the atlas and the axis.
     d. With the exception of C1, spinal nerves exit the vertebral canal via intervertebral or sacral foramina.
  2. **Functional components of spinal nerve fibers** (Figure 6-3)
     a. **General somatic afferent (GSA) fibers**
        - convey sensory input from skin, muscle, bone, and joints to the central nervous system (CNS).
     b. **General visceral afferent (GVA) fibers**
        - convey sensory input from visceral organs to the CNS.
     c. **General somatic efferent (GSE) fibers**
        - convey motor output from ventral horn motor neurons to skeletal muscle.
     d. **General visceral efferent (GVE) fibers**
        - convey motor output from intermediolateral cell column neurons, via paravertebral or prevertebral ganglia, to glands, smooth muscle, and visceral organs (sympathetic divisions of the autonomic nervous system).
        - convey motor output from the sacral parasympathetic nucleus to the pelvic viscera via intramural ganglia.

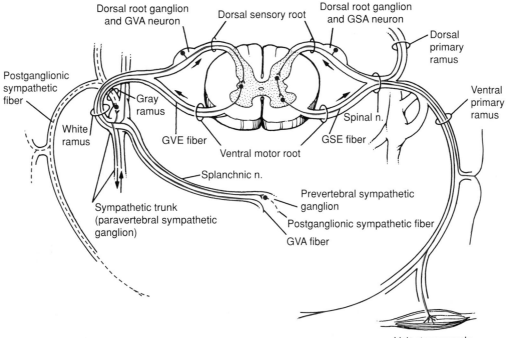

Figure 6-2. The typical thoracic spinal nerve and its branches and reflex connections. White communicating rami are found only at thoracolumbar levels T1 to L3. Gray communicating rami are found at all spinal cord levels. GVA = general visceral afferent; GSA = general somatic afferent; GSE = general somatic efferent; GVE = general visceral efferent.

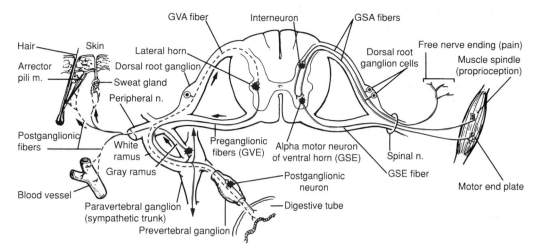

Figure 6-3. Diagram of the four functional components of the thoracic spinal nerve: general visceral afferent (GVA), general somatic afferent (GSA), general somatic efferent (GSE), and general visceral efferent (GVE). Proprioceptive, cutaneous, and visceral reflex arcs are shown. The muscle stretch (myotatic) reflex (MSR) includes the muscle spindle, GSA dorsal root ganglion cell, GSE ventral horn motor neuron, and skeletal muscle.

3. Components and branches of spinal nerves
- The spinal nerve is formed by the union of dorsal and ventral roots within the intervertebral foramen, resulting in a mixed nerve.
  a. Dorsal root
  - enters the dorsal lateral sulcus as dorsal rootlets, conveying sensory input from the body via the dorsal root ganglion.
  - contains, distally, the dorsal root ganglion.
  - joins the ventral root distal to the dorsal root ganglion and within the intervertebral foramen to form the spinal nerve.
  b. Dorsal root ganglion
  - is located within the dorsal root and within the **intervertebral foramen**.
  - contains **pseudounipolar neurons** of neural crest origin, which transmit sensory input from the periphery (GSA and GVA) to the spinal cord via the dorsal roots.
  c. Ventral root
  - emerges as ventral rootlets from the ventral lateral sulcus, conveying motor output from visceral and somatic motor neurons.
  - joins the dorsal roots distal to the dorsal root ganglion and within the intervertebral foramen to form the spinal nerve.
  d. Cauda equina
  - consists of lumbosacral (dorsal and ventral) nerve roots (L2–Co) that descend from the spinal cord through the subarachnoid space to exit through their respective intervertebral or sacral foramina.
  e. Spinal nerve rami
    (1) Dorsal primary ramus
    - innervates the skin and muscles of the back.
    (2) Ventral primary ramus
    - innervates the ventral lateral muscles and skin of the trunk, extremities, and visceral organs.
    (3) Meningeal ramus
    - innervates the meninges and vertebral column.
    (4) Gray communicating rami
    - contain **unmyelinated** postganglionic sympathetic fibers.
    - are associated with *all* spinal nerves.

(5) White communicating rami
- contain **myelinated** preganglionic sympathetic fibers and myelinated GVA fibers (splanchnic nerves).
- are found only in thoracolumbar segments of the spinal cord (T1–L3).

E. Spinal nerve innervation (Figure 6-4)
- one spinal nerve innervates the derivatives from one **somite**, which includes:
  1. **Dermatome** (see Figure 6-4)
     - consists of a **cutaneous area** innervated by the fibers of one spinal nerve.
  2. **Myotome**
     - consists of **muscles** innervated by the fibers of one spinal nerve.
  3. **Sclerotome**
     - consists of **bones and ligaments** innervated by the fibers of one spinal nerve.

F. Surface structures and sulci (Figure 6-5)
- underlie the pia mater and include:
  1. **Ventral median fissure**
     - is a deep ventral midline groove underlying the ventral spinal artery.

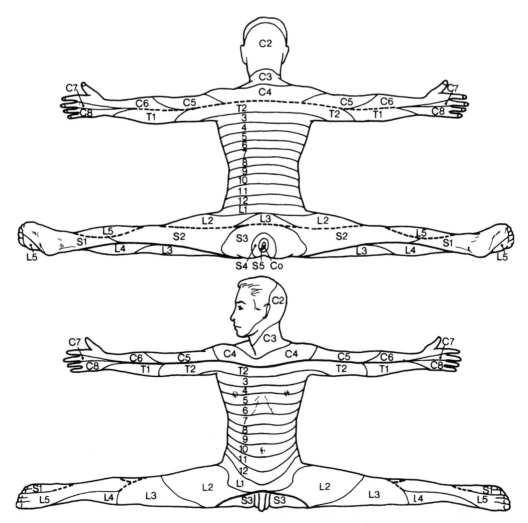

Figure 6-4. Cutaneous distribution of spinal nerves, the dermatomes. (Reprinted with permission from Haymaker W, Woodhall B: *Peripheral Nerve Injuries,* 2nd ed. Philadelphia, WB Saunders, 1952, p 32.)

2. **Ventral lateral sulcus**
   - is a shallow groove from which the ventral rootlets emerge.
3. **Dorsal lateral sulcus**
   - is a shallow groove into which the dorsal rootlets enter.
4. **Dorsal intermediate sulcus**
   - is a shallow groove that is continuous with the dorsal intermediate septum.
   - is found between the dorsal lateral and dorsal median sulci but only rostral to T6.
   - separates the fasciculus gracilis from the fasciculus cuneatus.
5. **Dorsal median sulcus**
   - is a shallow dorsal midline groove that is continuous with the dorsal median septum.

III. Internal Morphology (see Figure 6-5)

- In transverse sections, the spinal cord consists of central gray matter and peripheral white matter.

A. **Gray matter**
   - is in the center of the spinal cord.
   - is butterfly- or **H**-shaped in a configuration that varies according to spinal cord level.
   - contains a central canal.
   - is divided into cytoarchitectural areas called **Rexed laminae**, expressed with Roman numerals (see Figure 6-5).
   - is divided into three horns or cell columns on each side:
     1. **Dorsal horn (column)**
        - receives and processes sensory input.
        - is found at all levels.

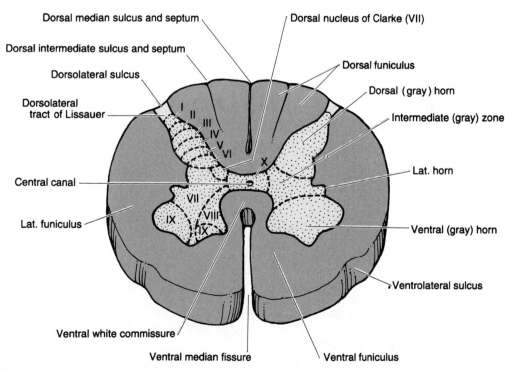

Figure 6-5. Topography of the spinal cord in transverse section: horns (columns), sulci, funiculi, and Rexed laminae. The lateral horn is found only at thoracolumbar cord levels (T1–L3). The dorsal intermediate sulcus and septum are found only above T6.

- includes the following nuclei:
    a. **Dorsomarginal nucleus (Rexed lamina I)**
        - is found at all cord levels.
        - is associated with light touch, pain, and temperature sensation.
        - is one site of origin of the ventral and lateral spinothalamic tracts.
    b. **Substantia gelatinosa (Rexed lamina II)**
        - is found at all cord levels.
        - is homologous to the spinal trigeminal nucleus.
        - is associated with light touch, pain, and temperature sensation.
        - integrates input for the ventral and lateral spinothalamic tracts.
    c. **Nucleus proprius (Rexed laminae III and IV)**
        - is found at all cord levels.
        - is associated with light touch, pain, and temperature sensation.
        - gives rise (from Rexed lamina IV) to the ventral and lateral spinothalamic tracts.
    d. **Nucleus dorsalis of Clarke (Rexed lamina VII)**
        - is found at the base of the dorsal horn.
        - extends from (C8) T1 to L3.
        - is homologous to the **accessory cuneate nucleus** of the medulla.
        - subserves unconscious proprioception from muscle spindles and Golgi tendon organs (GTOs).
        - is the origin of the dorsal spinocerebellar tract.

2. **Lateral horn (column) (Rexed lamina VII)**
    - receives viscerosensory input.
    - is found between the dorsal and ventral horns.
    - extends from (C8) T1 to L3.
    - contains the **intermediolateral nucleus** (column), a visceromotor nucleus that extends from T1 to L3.
    - contains preganglionic sympathetic neurons (GVE).
    - contains, at T1–T2, the ciliospinal **center of Budge** (sympathetic innervation of the eye).

3. **Ventral horn (column) (Rexed laminae VII, VIII, and IX)**
    - contains predominantly motor nuclei.
    - is found at all levels.
    - includes the following nuclei:
        a. **Spinal border cells (Cooper-Sherrington border cells)**
            - extend from L2 to S3.
            - subserve unconscious proprioception from GTOs and muscle spindles.
            - are the origin of the ventral spinocerebellar tract.
        b. **Sacral parasympathetic nucleus (Rexed lamina VII)**
            - extends from S2 to S4.
            - gives rise to preganglionic parasympathetic fibers that innervate the pelvic viscera via the pelvic nerve.
        c. **Somatic motor nuclei (Rexed lamina IX)**
            - are found at all levels.
            - are subdivided into medial and lateral groups that innervate axial and appendicular muscles, respectively.
        d. **Spinal accessory nucleus (Rexed lamina IX)**
            - extends from C1 to C6.
            - gives rise to the spinal root of the **spinal accessory nerve** (cranial nerve [CN] XI).
            - innervates the sternocleidomastoid and trapezius muscles.
        e. **Phrenic nucleus (Rexed lamina IX)**
            - extends from C3 to C6.
            - innervates the diaphragm.

B. **White matter** (see Figure 6-5)
    - consists of bundles of myelinated fibers that surround the central gray matter.
    - consists of ascending and descending fiber pathways called tracts.

- is divided bilaterally by sulci into three major divisions.
  1. **Dorsal funiculus (dorsal column)**
     - is located between the dorsal median sulcus and the dorsal lateral sulcus.
     - is subdivided above T6 into two fasciculi:
       a. **Fasciculus gracilis**
          - is located between the dorsal median sulcus and the dorsal intermediate sulcus and septum.
          - is found at all cord levels.
       b. **Fasciculus cuneatus**
          - is located between the dorsal intermediate sulcus and septum and the dorsal lateral sulcus.
          - is found only at the upper thoracic and cervical cord levels (C1–T6).
  2. **Lateral funiculus**
     - is located between the dorsal lateral and ventral lateral sulci.
  3. **Ventral funiculus**
     - is located between the ventral median fissure and the ventral lateral sulcus.
     - contains the **ventral white commissure**, which:
       a. is located between the central canal and the ventral medial fissure.
       b. contains decussating spinothalamic tracts.

C. **Determination of spinal cord levels**
   - is based on regional variation in the shape of gray matter and on the presence of dorsal intermediate sulci and septa.
   1. **Cervical cord**
      - dorsal intermediate sulci and septa are present.
      - ventral horns are massive from C3 to C8.
   2. **Thoracic cord**
      - dorsal intermediate sulci and septa are present from T1 to T6.
      - The nucleus dorsalis of Clarke is present at all thoracic levels but is most prominent at T11 and T12.
      - Lateral horns are present at all thoracic levels.
      - Dorsal and ventral horns are typically slender and **H**-shaped.
   3. **Lumbar cord**
      - The nucleus dorsalis of Clarke is very prominent at L1 and L2.
      - contains massive ventral and dorsal horns from L2 to L5; the substantia gelatinosa is greatly enlarged.
      - The lumbar section is difficult to distinguish from the upper sacral segments.
      - The lateral horn is prominent only at L1.
   4. **Sacral cord**
      - contains massive ventral and dorsal horns; the substantia gelatinosa is greatly enlarged.
      - is greatly reduced in diameter from S3 to S5.
   5. **Coccygeal segment**
      - contains dorsal horns that are more voluminous than the ventral horns.
      - has a greatly reduced diameter.

IV. Myotatic Reflex (see Figure 6-3)

- is a monosynaptic and ipsilateral muscle stretch reflex (MSR).
- is incorrectly called a deep tendon reflex.
- has an afferent and an efferent limb, like all reflexes.
- Interruption of either limb results in areflexia.

A. **Afferent limb**
   - includes a muscle spindle (receptor) and a dorsal root ganglion neuron and its Ia fiber.

B. Efferent limb
  • includes a ventral horn motor neuron that innervates striated muscle (effector).

C. The five most commonly tested MSRs
  1. **Ankle jerk (Achilles reflex):** cord segment S1; gastrocnemius muscle
  2. **Knee jerk:** cord segments L2 to L4; quadriceps muscle
  3. **Biceps jerk:** cord segments C5 and C6; biceps muscle
  4. **Forearm jerk:** cord segments C5 and C6: brachioradialis muscle
  5. **Triceps jerk:** cord segments C7 and C8; triceps muscle

REVIEW TEST

1. Which of the following reflexes is monosynaptic?

(A) Achilles reflex
(B) Babinski reflex
(C) Corneal reflex
(D) Extensor plantar reflex
(E) Pupillary light reflex

2. The spinal cord of a newborn baby terminates at

(A) VL1
(B) VL3
(C) VS1
(D) VS3
(E) VS5

3. Which spinal nerve rami contain unmyelinated postganglionic sympathetic nerve fibers?

(A) White communicating
(B) Dorsal primary
(C) Gray communicating
(D) Ventral primary
(E) Meningeal

4. The efferent limb of a myotatic reflex includes a

(A) ventral horn motor neuron
(B) muscle spindle
(C) dorsal root ganglion neuron
(D) lateral horn visceromotor nucleus
(E) preganglionic sympathetic neuron

Questions 5 to 9

The response options for the items 5 to 9 are the same. Select one answer for each item in the set.

(A) Cervical cord
(B) Upper thoracic cord
(C) Lumbar cord
(D) Lower thoracic cord
(E) Coccygeal cord
(F) Sacral cord

Match each characteristic below with the spinal cord level it best describes.

5. Contains preganglionic parasympathetic neurons

6. Contains the brachial plexus

7. Has a ciliospinal center of Budge

8. Contains the spinal accessory nucleus (CN XI)

9. Contains the phrenic nucleus

ANSWERS AND EXPLANATIONS

1–A. The Achilles reflex, or ankle jerk reflex, is a myotatic monosynaptic reflex that is mediated by cord segment S1.

2–B. In the newborn, the spinal cord ends at the level of the third lumbar vertebra (VL3). In the adult, the spinal cord ends at the lower border of the first lumbar vertebra (VL1), and the dural cul-de-sac ends at the level of the second sacral vertebra (VS2). The pia mater is the innermost meningeal layer of the spinal cord; spinal cord, pia mater, arachnoid, dura mater, ligamenta flava, periosteum.

3–D. Gray communicating rami contain unmyelinated preganglionic sympathetic fibers, whereas white communicating rami contain myelinated preganglionic sympathetic fibers and myelinated GVA fibers. The meningeal ramus innervates the meninges and vertebral column; the dorsal primary ramus innervates the skin and muscles of the back; and the ventral primary ramus innervates the ventral lateral muscles and skin of the trunk, extremities, and visceral organs.

4–A. The myotatic reflex is a monosynaptic and ipsilateral MSR (incorrectly called a deep tendon reflex). The efferent limb consists of the axon of a ventral horn alpha motor neuron that innervates striated muscle fibers (effector); the afferent limb consists of a muscle spindle (receptor) and an Ia fiber (axon) of a dorsal root ganglion neuron. The quadriceps (patellar) and triceps surae (ankle) MSRs are myotatic reflexes.

5–F. The sacral cord contains the sacral parasympathetic nucleus (S2–S4); this gives rise to preganglionic fibers that synapse in the intramural ganglia of the pelvic viscera.

6–A. The cervical cord contains massive ventral horns, which give rise to the brachial plexus (C5–C8).

7–B. The ciliospinal center of Budge is found in the lateral horn at T1. This sympathetic nucleus innervates the radial muscle of the iris (dilator pupillae) and the nonstriated superior and inferior tarsal (Müller) muscles.

8–A. The spinal accessory nucleus extends from C1 to C6 and gives rise to the spinal root of the spinal accessory nerve; it innervates the sternocleidomastoid and trapezius muscles.

9–A. The phrenic nucleus extends from C3 to C6 and innervates the diaphragm.

Tracts of the Spinal Cord

I. Introduction: Tracts of the Spinal Cord

- consist of fiber bundles that have a common origin and a common termination.
- are somatotopically organized.
- are divided into **ascending and descending pathways**.

II. Ascending Spinal Tracts

- represent functional pathways that convey sensory information from soma or viscera to higher levels of the neuraxis.
- usually consist of a chain of three neurons: first-, second-, and third-order neurons. The first-order neuron is always in the dorsal root ganglion.
- may decussate before reaching their final destination.
- give rise to collateral branches that serve in local spinal reflex arcs.
- include six major tracts:

A. Dorsal column–medial lemniscus pathway (Figure 7-1)
- mediates tactile discrimination, vibration, form recognition, and joint and muscle sensation.
- mediates conscious proprioception.
- receives input from Pacini and Meissner corpuscles, joint receptors, muscle spindles, and Golgi tendon organs (GTOs).
    1. First-order neurons
    - are located in dorsal root ganglia at all levels.
    - give rise to the **fasciculus gracilis** from the lower extremity.
    - give rise to the **fasciculus cuneatus** from the upper extremity.
    - give rise to axons that ascend in the dorsal columns and terminate in the gracile and cuneate nuclei of the medulla.
    2. Second-order neurons
    - are located in the gracile and cuneate nuclei of the caudal medulla.
    - give rise to axons, **internal arcuate fibers** that decussate and form a compact fiber bundle, the **medial lemniscus**. The medial lemniscus ascends through the contralateral brainstem to terminate in the ventral posterolateral (**VPL**) nucleus of the thalamus.
    3. Third-order neurons
    - are located in the VPL nucleus of the thalamus.
    - project via the posterior limb of the internal capsule to the postcentral gyrus, the **somatosensory cortex** (areas 3, 1, and 2).

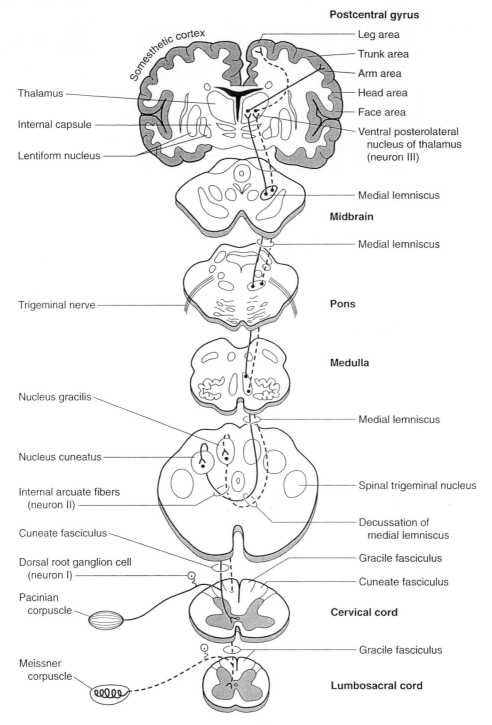

Figure 7-1. The dorsal column–medial lemniscus pathway. Impulses conducted by this pathway mediate discriminatory tactile sense (e.g., touch, vibration, pressure) and kinesthetic sense (e.g., position, movement). The dorsal column system mediates conscious proprioception. (Adapted with permission from Carpenter MB, Sutin J: *Human Neuroanatomy,* 8th ed. Baltimore, Williams & Wilkins, 1983, p 266.)

B. **Ventral spinothalamic tract**
   - with lateral spinothalamic tract comprises anterolateral system.
   - is concerned with **light touch**, the sensation produced by stroking glabrous skin with a wisp of cotton.
   - receives input from free nerve endings and from Merkel tactile disks.
      1. **First-order neurons**
         - are found in dorsal root ganglia at all levels.
         - project axons into the medial root entry zone to second-order neurons in the dorsal horn.
      2. **Second-order neurons**
         - are located in the **dorsal horn**.
         - give rise to axons that decussate in the ventral white commissure and ascend in the contralateral ventral funiculus.
         - terminate in the VPL nucleus of the thalamus.
      3. **Third-order neurons**
         - are found in the **VPL nucleus** of the thalamus.
         - project via the posterior limb of the internal capsule and corona radiata to the post-central gyrus (areas 3, 1, and 2).

C. **Lateral spinothalamic tract** (Figure 7-2)
   - mediates itch, pain, and temperature sensation.
   - receives input from free nerve endings and thermal receptors.
   - receives input from A-δ and C fibers (i.e., fast- and slow-conducting pain fibers, respectively).
   - is somatotopically organized with sacral fibers dorsolaterally and cervical fibers ventromedially.
      1. **First-order neurons**
         - are found in dorsal root ganglia at all levels.
         - project axons via the **dorsolateral tract of Lissauer** to second-order neurons in the dorsal horn.
         - synapse with second-order neurons in the dorsal horn.
      2. **Second-order neurons**
         - are found in the dorsal horn.
         - give rise to axons that decussate in the **ventral white commissure** and ascend in the ventral half of the lateral funiculus.
         - project collaterals to the reticular formation.
         - terminate contralaterally in the VPL nucleus and bilaterally in the intralaminar nuclei of the thalamus.
      3. **Third-order neurons**
         - are found in the VPL nucleus and in the intralaminar nuclei.
            a. **VPL neurons**
               - project via the posterior limb of the internal capsule to the somatesthetic cortex of the postcentral gyrus (areas 3, 1, and 2).
            b. **Intralaminar neurons**
               - project to the caudatoputamen and to the frontal and parietal cortex.

D. **Dorsal spinocerebellar tract** (Figure 7-3)
   - transmits unconscious proprioceptive information to the cerebellum.
   - receives input from muscle spindles, GTOs, and pressure receptors.
   - is involved in fine coordination of posture and the movement of individual muscles of the lower extremity.
   - is an uncrossed tract.
      1. **First-order neurons**
         - are found in dorsal root ganglia from C8 to S3.
         - provide the afferent limb for muscle stretch reflexes (MSRs) (e.g., the patellar reflex).
         - project via the medial root entry zone to synapse in the **nucleus dorsalis of Clarke**.

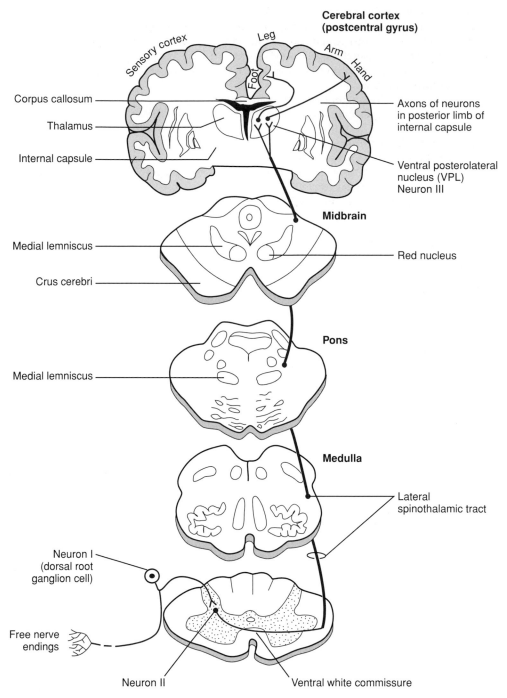

Figure 7-2. The lateral spinothalamic tract. Impulses conducted by this tract mediate pain and thermal sense. Numerous collaterals are distributed to the brainstem reticular formation. (Adapted with permission from Carpenter MB, Sutin J: *Human Neuroanatomy,* 8th ed. Baltimore, Williams & Wilkins, 1983, p 274.)

2. **Second-order neurons**
   - are found in the nucleus dorsalis of Clarke (C8–L3).
   - give rise to axons that ascend in the lateral funiculus and reach the cerebellum via the inferior cerebellar peduncle.
   - contain axons that terminate ipsilaterally as mossy fibers in the cortex of the rostral and caudal cerebellar vermis.

E. **Ventral spinocerebellar tract** (see Figure 7-3)
- transmits unconscious proprioceptive information to the cerebellum.
- is concerned with coordinated movement and posture of the entire lower extremity.
- receives input from muscle spindles, GTOs, and pressure receptors.
- is a crossed tract.
  1. **First-order neurons**
     - are found in the dorsal root ganglia from L1 to S2.
     - provide the afferent limb for MSRs (e.g., the patellar reflex).
     - synapse on **spinal border cells.**
  2. **Second-order neurons**
     - are spinal border cells found in the ventral horns (L1–S2).
     - give rise to axons that decussate in the ventral white commissure and ascend lateral to the lateral spinothalamic tract in the lateral funiculus.
     - give rise to axons that enter the cerebellum via the **superior cerebellar peduncle** and terminate contralaterally as mossy fibers in the cortex of the rostral cerebellar vermis.

F. **Cuneocerebellar tract** (see Figure 7-3)
- is the upper-extremity equivalent of the dorsal spinocerebellar tract.
  1. **First-order neurons**
     - are found in the dorsal root ganglia from C2 to T7.
     - project their axons via the fasciculus cuneatus to the caudal medulla, where they synapse in the **accessory cuneate nucleus**, a homolog of the nucleus dorsalis of Clarke.
  2. **Second-order neurons**
     - are located in the accessory cuneate nucleus of the medulla.
     - give rise to axons that project to the cerebellum via the **inferior cerebellar peduncle**. These axons terminate ipsilaterally in the arm region of the anterior lobe of the cerebellum.

III. Descending Spinal Tracts (Figures 7-4 and 7-5)

- are concerned with somatic and visceral motor activities.
- have their cells of origin in the cerebral cortex or in the brainstem.

A. **Lateral corticospinal (pyramidal) tract** (see Figure 7-4)
- is not fully myelinated until the end of the second year.
  1. **Function: the lateral corticospinal tract**
     - is concerned with **volitional skilled motor activity**, primarily of the digits of the upper limb.
     - modulates the transmission of sensory input via the ascending sensory pathways.
     - receives input from the **paracentral lobule**, a medial continuation of the motor and sensory cortices, and subserves the muscles of the contralateral leg and foot.
  2. **Origin and termination: the lateral corticospinal tract**
     - arises from lamina V of the cerebral cortex from three cortical areas, in equal proportions: the **premotor cortex** (area 6); the **precentral motor cortex** (area 4); and the **postcentral sensory cortex** (areas 3, 1, and 2).
     - terminates via interneurons on ventral horn motor neurons and sensory neurons of the dorsal horn.
  3. **Fibers of the lateral corticospinal tract**
     - number approximately 1 million.
     - are usually (90%) between 1 and 4 μm in diameter.
     - are usually (67%) myelinated.

(text continues on page 114)

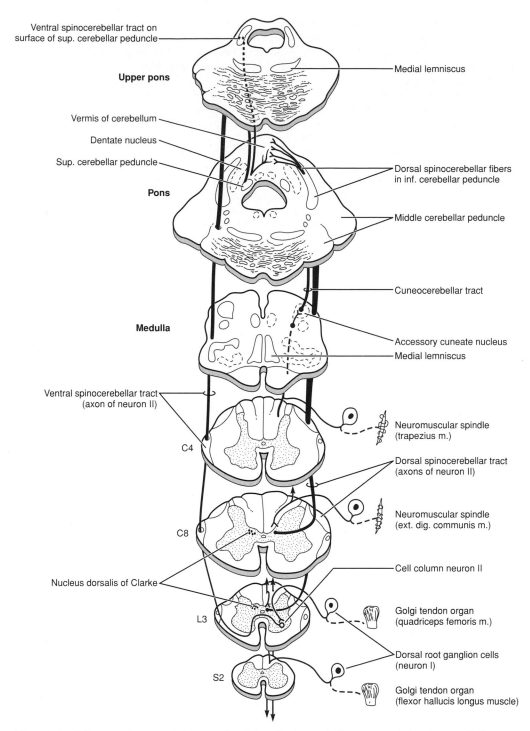

Figure 7-3. Schematic diagram of the ventral and dorsal spinocerebellar tracts and the cuneocerebellar tract. Impulses conducted by these tracts arise from the muscle spindles and the Golgi tendon organs and are conveyed to the spinocerebellum. These tracts mediate unconscious proprioception. Their first-order neurons mediate the myotatic reflexes. (Adapted with permission from Carpenter MB, Sutin J: *Human Neuroanatomy*, 8th ed. Baltimore, Williams & Wilkins, 1983, p 277.)

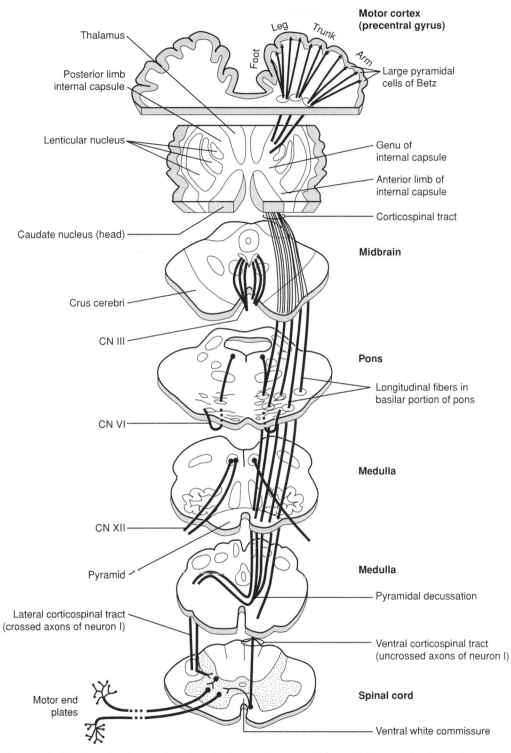

Figure 7-4. The lateral and ventral corticospinal tracts (the pyramidal tracts). These major descending motor pathways mediate volitional motor activity. The cells of origin are located in the premotor, the motor, and the sensory cortices. (Adapted with permission from Carpenter MB, Sutin J: *Human Neuroanatomy*, 8th ed. Baltimore, Williams & Wilkins, 1983, p 285.)

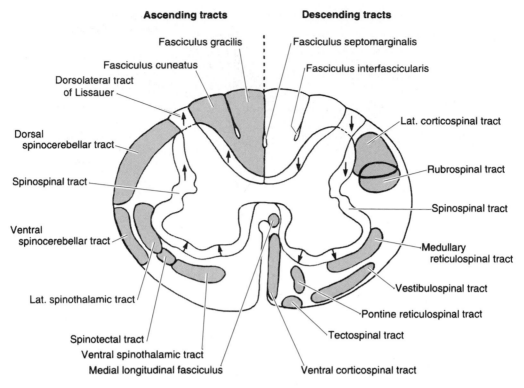

Ascending tracts

Fasciculus gracilis

Fasciculus cuneatus

Dorsolateral tract of Lissauer

Dorsal spinocerebellar tract

Spinospinal tract

Ventral spinocerebellar tract

Lat. spinothalamic tract

Spinotectal tract
Ventral spinothalamic tract
Medial longitudinal fasciculus

Descending tracts

Fasciculus septomarginalis

Fasciculus interfascicularis

Lat. corticospinal tract

Rubrospinal tract

Spinospinal tract

Medullary reticulospinal tract

Vestibulospinal tract

Pontine reticulospinal tract

Tectospinal tract

Ventral corticospinal tract

Figure 7-5. Schematic diagram of the major ascending and descending pathways of the spinal cord. The spinospinal system surrounds the spinal gray matter. Ascending tracts are shown on the *left*; descending tracts are shown on the *right*. (Adapted with permission from Carpenter MB: *Core Text of Neuroanatomy*, 3rd. ed. Baltimore, Williams & Wilkins, 1985, p 97.)

- represent 4% of the fibers of the tract, with diameters greater than 20 μm. These are the axons of the **giant cells of Betz.**
- Betz cells are found in the precentral gyrus and in the anterior paracentral lobule.
4. **Course: the lateral corticospinal tract**
    - passes through the posterior limb of the internal capsule.
    - passes through the middle three-fifths of the **crus cerebri** (basis pedunculi) of the midbrain.
    - passes through the base of the pons.
    - constitutes the pyramid of the medulla.
    - undergoes a 90% decussation in the caudal medulla.
    - lies in the dorsal quadrant of the lateral funiculus of the spinal cord.
5. **Transection**
    - results in **spastic hemiparesis** with the Babinski sign.

B. **Ventral corticospinal tract** (see Figure 7-4)
    - is a small uncrossed tract that decussates at spinal cord levels in the ventral white commissure.
    - is concerned with the control of axial muscles.

C. **Rubrospinal tract** (see Figure 7-5)
    - arises in the contralateral red nucleus of the midbrain.
    - plays a role in the control of flexor tone.
    - is ventral to the lateral corticospinal tract.

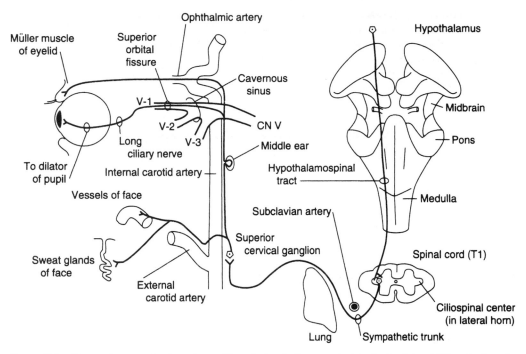

Figure 7-6. The oculosympathetic pathway. Hypothalamic fibers project to the ipsilateral ciliospinal center of the intermediolateral cell column at T1. The ciliospinal center projects preganglionic sympathetic fibers to the superior cervical ganglion. The superior cervical ganglion projects perivascular postganglionic sympathetic fibers through the tympanic cavity, cavernous sinus, and superior orbital fissure to the dilator muscle of the iris. Interruption of this pathway at any level results in Horner syndrome. *CN* = cranial nerve. (Reprinted with permission from Fix, JD: *High-Yield Neuroanatomy,* 3rd ed. Philadelphia, Lippincott Williams & Wilkins, 2005, p 67.)

D. **Vestibulospinal tract** (see Figure 7-5)
   - arises from the giant cells of Deiters in the ipsilateral lateral vestibular nucleus.
   - plays a role in the control of extensor tone.
   - is located in the ventral funiculus.

E. **Descending autonomic tracts** (Figure 7-6)
   - project to sympathetic (T1–L3) and parasympathetic (S2–S4) centers in the spinal cord.
   - innervate the ciliospinal center (T1–T2), a pupillary center; interruption of this hypothalamospinal tract (found in the dorsal quadrant of the lateral funiculus) results in **Horner syndrome.**

IV. Clinical Correlations

A. **Upper motor neurons (UMNs)**
   - are cortical neurons that give rise to corticobulbar or corticospinal tracts.
   - are found in brainstem nuclei that influence lower motor neurons (LMNs) (e.g., lateral vestibular nucleus, red nucleus).
   - terminate directly on or via interneurons on LMNs.

B. **UMN lesions**
   - are caused by damage to the neurons (or their axons) that innervate LMNs.

1. **Acute-stage lesions**
   - result in transient spinal shock, including:
     a. **Flaccid paralysis**
     b. **Areflexia**
     c. **Hypotonia**
2. **Chronic-stage lesions**
   - result in:
     a. **Spastic paresis**
     b. **Hypertonia**
        - occurs with increased tone in antigravity muscles (i.e., flexors of arms and extensors of legs).
     c. **Reduction or loss of superficial abdominal and cremasteric reflexes**
     d. **Extensor toe response (Babinski sign)**
     e. **Clonus**
        - is a repetitive, sustained MSR (e.g., ankle clonus).

C. **LMNs**
   - are neurons that directly innervate skeletal muscles.
   - are found in the ventral horns of the spinal cord.
   - are found in the motor nuclei of CN III, CN IV to CN VII, and CN IX to CN XII.

D. **LMN lesions**
   - result from damage to motor neurons or their peripheral axons.
   - result in:
   1. **Flaccid paralysis**
   2. **Areflexia**
   3. **Muscle atrophy**
   4. **Fasciculations and fibrillations**

1. The ability to recognize an unseen familiar object placed in the hand depends on the integrity of which pathway?

(A) Spinospinal tract
(B) Dorsal column
(C) Dorsal spinocerebellar tract
(D) Spino-olivary tract
(E) Spinothalamic tract

2. The spinal tract involved with the control of trunk muscles is the

(A) cuneocerebellar
(B) vestibulospinal
(C) ventral corticospinal
(D) lateral corticospinal
(E) ventral spinocerebellar

3. The sensation produced by a wisp of cotton on one's fingertip is mediated by the

(A) cuneocerebellar tract
(B) dorsal column–medial lemniscus pathway
(C) ventral spinocerebellar tract
(D) ventral corticospinal tract
(E) ventral spinothalamic tract

4. First-order neurons of the ventral spinocerebellar tract

(A) are found in dorsal root ganglia at all levels
(B) provide the afferent limb for muscle stretch reflexes
(C) project axons into the medial root entry zone
(D) give rise to the fasciculus cuneatus
(E) project axons via the tract of Lissauer

5. Acute-stage upper motor neuron lesions result in

(A) hypertonia
(B) spastic paresis
(C) flaccid paralysis
(D) extensor toe response
(E) clonus

Questions 6 to 10

The response options for items 6 to 10 are the same. Select one answer for each item in the set.

(A) Cuneocerebellar tract
(B) Cuneate fasciculus
(C) Dorsal spinocerebellar tract
(D) Lateral corticospinal tract
(E) Lateral spinothalamic tract
(F) Lissauer tract
(G) Vestibulospinal tract

Match each statement below with the appropriate spinal cord tract.

6. Contains axons from the giant cells of Deiters

7. Is the upper extremity equivalent of a tract that arises from the cells of Clarke column

8. Conveys nociceptive input from the contralateral side of the body

9. Contains axons from the giant cells of Betz

10. Contains ipsilateral pain fibers that have their second-order neurons in the dorsal horn

Questions 11 to 18

Match the description of a spinal cord tract in items 11 to 18 with the appropriate lettered structure shown in the figure.

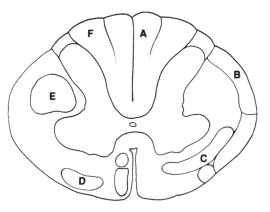

11. Projects to the cerebellum via the inferior cerebellar peduncle

12. Mediates pain and temperature sensation

13. Cells of origin are found in the precentral gyrus

14. Mediates two-point tactile discrimination from the hand

15. Myelination is not fully achieved until the end of the second year

16. Transection results in spasticity

17. Plays a role in regulating extensor tone

18. Transmits vibration sensation from the ankle

ANSWERS AND EXPLANATIONS

1–B. The ability to recognize the form and texture of an unseen familiar object is called stereognosis. This is an important function of the dorsal column–medial lemniscus system.

2–C. The ventral corticospinal tract is concerned with the control of axial muscles, including the muscles of the trunk and head.

3–E. The ventral spinothalamic tract is concerned with light touch, the sensation produced by stroking glabrous skin with a wisp of cotton.

4–B. First-order neurons of the ventral spinocerebellar tract provide the afferent limb for muscle stretch reflexes. They are found in the dorsal root ganglia from L1 to S2 and synapse on spinal border cell. First-order neurons of the ventral spinothalamic and dorsal spinocerebellar tracts project axons into the medial root entry zone; first-order neurons of the dorsal column–medial lemniscus pathway give rise to the fasciculus gracilis and cuneatus; and first-order neurons of the lateral spinothalamic tract project axons via the dorsolateral tract of Lissauer.

5–C. Acute-stage upper motor neuron lesions result in transient spinal shock, which includes flaccid paralysis, areflexia, and hypotonia. Chronic-stage lesions result in spastic paresis, hypertonia, reduction or loss of superficial abdominal and cremasteric reflexes and extensor toe response, and clonus.

6–G. The vestibulospinal tract arises from the giant cells of Deiters found in the ipsilateral lateral vestibular nucleus of the pons. The vestibulospinal tract facilitates extensor muscle tone.

7–A. The cuneocerebellar tract is the upper extremity equivalent of the dorsal spinocerebellar tract, which arises from the cells of the Clarke column. The cuneocerebellar tract arises from cells of the accessory cuneate nucleus, a homolog of the nucleus of Clarke.

8–E. The lateral spinothalamic tract conveys nociceptive input from the contralateral side of the body.

9–D. The lateral corticospinal tract contains axons from the giant cells of Betz. The giant pyramidal cells of Betz are found in the precentral gyrus and in the anterior paracentral lobule.

10–F. The dorsolateral tract of Lissauer contains ipsilateral pain fibers that have their second-order neurons in the dorsal horn.

11–B. The dorsal spinocerebellar tract projects unconscious proprioceptive information (muscle spindles and GTOs) to the cerebellum via the inferior cerebellar peduncle.

12–C. The lateral spinothalamic tract lies between the ventral spinocerebellar tract and the ventral horn. It mediates pain and temperature sensation.

13–E. The lateral corticospinal tract has its cells of origin in the premotor, motor, and sensory cortices. The precentral gyrus and the anterior paracentral lobule are motor cortices and contain the motor homunculus. The lateral corticospinal gives rise to one-third of the fibers of the corticospinal (pyramidal) tract.

14–F. The fasciculus cuneatus mediates two-point tactile discrimination from the hand.

15–E. The corticospinal (pyramidal) tracts are not fully myelinated until the end of the second year. For this reason, the Babinski sign may be elicited in young children.

16–E. Transection of the lateral corticospinal tract results in spastic paresis (exaggerated MSRs and clonus).

17–D. The vestibulospinal (lateral) tract, found ventral to the ventral horn, plays a role in regulating extensor tone.

18–A. The fasciculus gracilis transmits vibratory sensation (pallesthesia) from the lower extremities.

Some authors refer to the spinothalamic tracts as the anterolateral system.

Lesions of the Spinal Cord

I. Overview: Lesions of the Spinal Cord (Figure 8-1)

- may be classified according to the area of origin or the area affected.

A. Lower motor neuron (LMN) lesions

B. Upper motor neuron (UMN) lesions

C. Sensory pathway lesions

D. Peripheral nervous system (PNS) lesions

E. Combined upper and lower motor neuron lesions

F. Combined motor and sensory lesions

G. Herniations of the intervertebral disk

II. Lower Motor Neuron Lesions (Figure 8-2A)

- result from damage to motor neurons of the ventral horns or motor neurons of the cranial nerve nuclei.
- result from interruption of the final common pathway connecting the neuron via its axon with the muscle fibers it innervates (the motor unit).

A. Neurologic deficits resulting from LMN lesions
  1. **Flaccid paralysis**
  2. **Muscle atrophy (amyotrophy)**
  3. **Hypotonia**
  4. **Areflexia**
     - consists of loss of muscle stretch reflexes (MSRs) (knee and ankle jerks) and loss of superficial reflexes (abdominal and cremasteric reflexes).
  5. **Fasciculations (visible muscle twitches)**
  6. **Fibrillations** (seen only on electromyogram)

B. Diseases of LMNs (see Figure 8-2A)
  1. **Poliomyelitis**
     - is an acute inflammatory viral infection affecting the LMNs; it is caused by an enterovirus.
     - results in a flaccid paralysis.

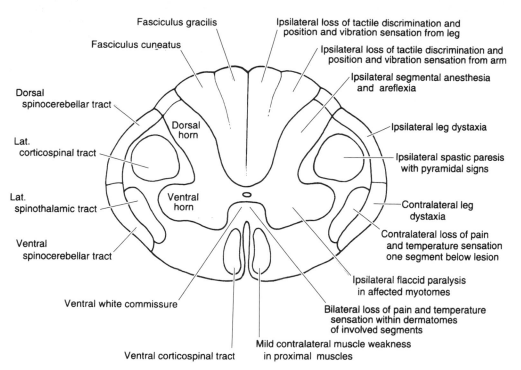

Figure 8-1. Transverse section of the cervical spinal cord. Clinically important pathways are shown on the left side; clinical deficits resulting from the interruption of these pathways are shown on the right side. Destructive lesions of the dorsal horns result in anesthesia and areflexia, and destructive lesions of the ventral horns result in LMN lesions and areflexia. Destruction of the ventral white commissure interrupts the central transmission of pain and temperature impulses bilaterally via the lateral spinothalamic tracts.

  2. **Progressive infantile muscular atrophy (Werdnig-Hoffmann disease)**
     • is a heredofamilial degenerative disease of infants that affects LMNs.
  3. **Kugelberg-Welander disease** (juvenile hereditary LMN disease)
     • appears at 3 to 20 years of age.
     • affects the large girdle muscles first and then the distal muscles.

III. Upper Motor Neuron Lesions

• result from damage to cortical neurons that give rise to corticospinal and corticobulbar tracts.
• are lesions of the corticospinal and corticobulbar tracts, called **pyramidal tract lesions**.
• may occur at all levels of the neuraxis from the cerebral cortex to the spinal cord.
• When rostral to the pyramidal decussation of the caudal medulla, they result in deficits below the lesion, on the contralateral side.
• When caudal to the pyramidal decussation, they result in deficits below the lesion, on the ipsilateral side.

A. **Lateral corticospinal tract lesion**
     • results in the following ipsilateral motor deficits found below the lesion:
     1. **Spastic hemiparesis with muscle weakness**
     2. **Hyperreflexia (exaggerated muscle stretch reflexes)**
     3. **Clasp-knife spasticity**
        • When a joint is moved briskly, resistance occurs initially and then fades (like the opening of a pocketknife blade).

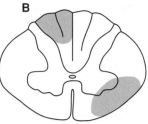
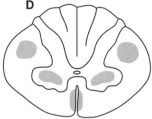
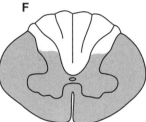
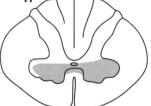
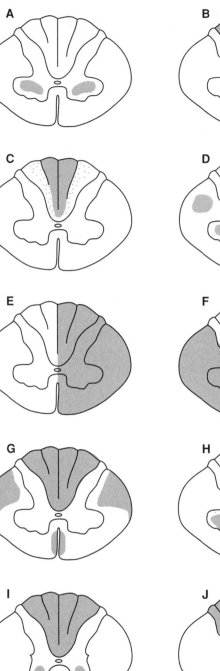
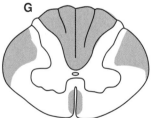
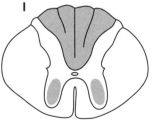
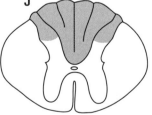

Figure 8-2. Lesions of the spinal cord: **(A)** poliomyelitis and progressive infantile muscular atrophy (Werdnig-Hoffmann disease); **(B)** multiple sclerosis; **(C)** dorsal column disease (tabes dorsalis); **(D)** amyotrophic lateral sclerosis; **(E)** hemisection of the spinal cord (Brown-Séquard syndrome); **(F)** complete ventral spinal artery occlusion of the spinal cord; **(G)** subacute combined degeneration (vitamin B_{12} neuropathy); **(H)** syringomyelia; **(I)** Charcot-Marie-Tooth disease (hereditary motor–sensory neuropathy type 1); **(J)** complete dorsal spinal artery occlusion. (Modified from Fix JD: *High-Yield Neuroanatomy,* 3rd ed. Philadelphia, Lippincott Williams & Wilkins, 2005, p 70.)

4. **Loss of superficial (abdominal and cremasteric) reflexes**
5. **Clonus**
   - consists of rhythmic contractions of muscles in response to sudden, passive movements (wrist, patellar, or ankle clonus).
6. **Babinski sign**
   - consists of plantar reflex response that is extensor (dorsiflexion of big toe).

B. **Ventral corticospinal tract lesion**
   - results in **mild contralateral motor deficit**. Ventral corticospinal tract fibers decussate at spinal levels in the ventral white commissure.

C. **Hereditary spastic paraplegia or diplegia**
   - is caused by bilateral degeneration of the corticospinal tracts.
   - results in gradual development of spastic weakness of the legs with increased difficulty in walking.

IV.   Sensory Pathway Lesions

A. **Dorsal column syndrome** (see Figure 8-2C)
   - includes the fasciculi gracilis (T6–S5) and cuneatus (C2–T6) and the dorsal roots.
   - is seen in subacute combined degeneration (vitamin B_{12} neuropathy).
   - is seen in neurosyphilis as **tabes dorsalis** and in nonsyphilitic sensory neuropathies.
   - results in the following **ipsilateral sensory deficits** found below the lesion:
     1. **Loss of tactile discrimination**
     2. **Loss of position (joint) and vibratory sensation**
     3. **Stereoanesthesia** (astereognosis)
     4. **Sensory (dorsal column) dystaxia**
     5. **Paresthesias and pain** (dorsal root irritation)
     6. **Hyporeflexia or areflexia** (dorsal root deafferentation)
     7. **Urinary incontinence, constipation, and impotence** (dorsal root deafferentation)
     8. **Romberg sign** (sensory dystaxia) (standing patient is more unsteady with eyes closed)

B. **Lateral spinothalamic tract lesion**
   - results in contralateral loss of pain and temperature sensation one segment below the level of the lesion.

C. **Ventral spinothalamic tract lesion**
   - results in contralateral loss of light (crude) touch sensation three or four segments below the level of the lesion.
   - does not appreciably reduce touch sensation if the dorsal columns are intact.

D. **Dorsal spinocerebellar tract lesion**
   - results in ipsilateral leg dystaxia; patient has difficulty performing the heel-to-shin test.

E. **Ventral spinocerebellar tract lesion**
   - results in contralateral leg dystaxia; patient has difficulty performing the heel-to-shin test.

V.   Peripheral Nervous System Lesions

- may be sensory, motor, or combined.
- affect spinal roots, dorsal root ganglia, and peripheral nerves.

A. **Herpes zoster (shingles)**
   - is a common **viral infection** of the nervous system.
   - consists of an acute inflammatory reaction in the dorsal root or cranial nerve ganglia.
   - is usually limited to the territory of one dermatome; the most common sites are **T5 to T10.**
   - causes irritation of dorsal root ganglion cells, resulting in pain, itching, and burning sensations in the involved dermatomes.
   - produces the characteristic vesicular eruption in the affected dermatome.

B. Acute idiopathic polyneuritis (Guillain-Barré syndrome)
- is also called **postinfectious polyneuritis**.
- usually follows an infectious illness.
- results from a cell-mediated immunologic reaction directed at peripheral nerves.
- affects primarily motor fibers and causes segmental demyelination and wallerian degeneration.
- produces **LMN symptoms** (muscle weakness, flaccid paralysis, and areflexia).
- results in symmetric paralysis that begins in the lower extremities and ascends to involve the trunk and upper extremities; the facial nerve frequently is involved bilaterally.
- elevates cerebrospinal fluid (CSF) protein; however, the CSF cell count remains normal (**albuminocytologic dissociation**).

VI.   Combined Upper and Lower Motor Neuron Lesions

A. Characteristics
- are muscle weakness and wasting without sensory deficits.

B. Prototypic disease—amyotrophic lateral sclerosis (AML) (see Figure 8-2D)
- is also called **Lou Gehrig disease**, motor neuron disease, or motor system disease.
- usually occurs in persons 50 to 70 years of age.
- affects twice as many men as women.
- involves both LMNs and UMNs; either component may dominate the clinical picture.
- progressive (spinal) muscular atrophy or progressive bulbar palsy refers to an LMN component.
- pseudobulbar palsy or primary lateral sclerosis refers to a UMN component.

VII.   Combined Motor and Sensory Lesions

A. Spinal cord hemisection (Brown-Séquard syndrome) (Figure 8-3; see Figures 8-1 and 8-2E)
  1. **Dorsal column transection**
     - results in ipsilateral loss of tactile discrimination, form perception, and position and vibration sensation below the lesion.
  2. **Lateral spinothalamic tract transection**
     - results in contralateral loss of pain and temperature sensation, starting one segment below the lesion.
  3. **Ventral spinothalamic tract transection**
     - results in contralateral loss of crude touch sensation starting three or four segments below the lesion.
  4. **Dorsal spinocerebellar tract transection**
     - results in ipsilateral leg dystaxia.
  5. **Ventral spinocerebellar tract transection**
     - results in contralateral leg dystaxia.
  6. **Hypothalamospinal tract transection rostral to T2**
     - results in Horner syndrome.
  7. **Lateral corticospinal tract transection**
     - results in ipsilateral spastic paresis below the UMN lesion with the Babinski sign.
  8. **Ventral corticospinal tract transection**
     - results in minor contralateral muscle weakness below the lesion.
  9. **Ventral horn destruction**
     - results in ipsilateral flaccid paralysis of somatic muscles (LMN lesion).
  10. **Dorsal horn destruction**
     - results in ipsilateral dermatomic anesthesia and areflexia.

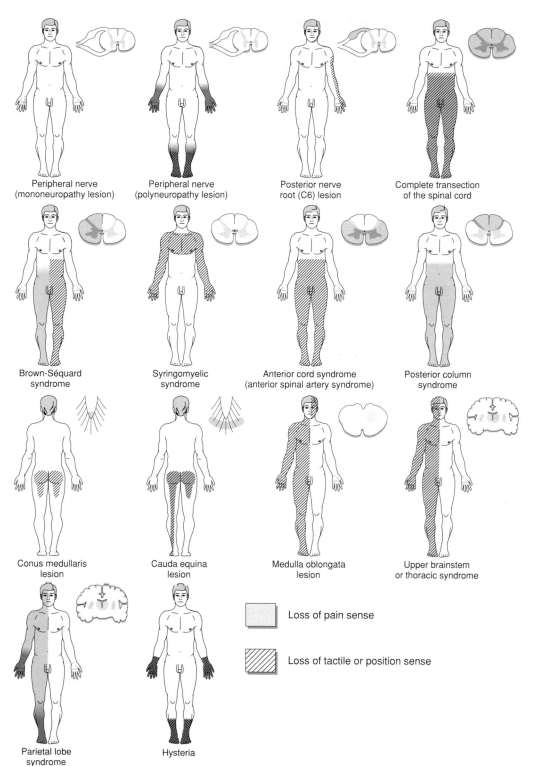

Figure 8-3. Localization of sensory disorders.

B. **Complete transection of the spinal cord**
- results in the following conditions:
  1. **Exitus lethalis** between C1 and C3
  2. **Quadriplegia** between C4 and C5
  3. **Paraplegia** below T1
  4. **Spastic paralysis** of all voluntary movements below the lesion
  5. **Complete anesthesia** below the lesion
  6. **Urinary and fecal incontinence**, although reflex emptying may occur
  7. **Anhidrosis and loss of vasomotor tone**
  8. **Paralysis of volitional and automatic breathing** if the transection is above C5 (the phrenic nucleus is found at C3–C5)

C. **Ventral (anterior) spinal artery occlusion** (see Figure 8-2F)
- causes infarction of the ventral two-thirds of the spinal cord.
- usually spares the dorsal columns and dorsal horns.
- results in paralysis of voluntary and automatic respiration in cervical segments; it also results in bilateral Horner syndrome.
- results in loss of voluntary bladder and bowel control, with preservation of reflex emptying.
- results in anhidrosis and loss of vasomotor tone.
  1. **Ventral horn destruction**
     - results in complete flaccid paralysis and areflexia at the level of the lesion.
  2. **Corticospinal tract transection**
     - results in a spastic paresis below the lesion.
  3. **Spinothalamic tract transection**
     - results in loss of pain and temperature sensations, starting one segment below the lesion.
  4. **Dorsal spinocerebellar tract and ventral spinocerebellar tract transection**
     - results in cerebellar incoordination, which is masked by LMN and UMN paralysis.

D. **Conus medullaris and epiconus syndromes**
- include neurologic deficits and signs that are most always bilateral.
  1. **Conus medullaris syndrome**
     - involves segments S3 to Co.
     - is usually caused by small intramedullary tumor metastases or hemorrhagic infarcts.
     - results in destruction of the sacral parasympathetic nucleus, which causes paralytic bladder, fecal incontinence, and impotence.
     - causes perianogenital sensory loss in dermatomes S3 to Co (saddle anesthesia).
     - shows an absence of motor deficits in the lower limbs.
  2. **Epiconus syndrome**
     - involves segments L4 to S2.
     - results in reflex functioning of the bladder and rectum but loss of voluntary control.
     - is characterized by considerable **motor disability** (external rotation and extension of the thigh are most affected).
     - affects the ventral horns and long tracts.
     - is associated with absent Achilles tendon reflex.

E. **Cauda equina syndrome**
- classically involves spinal roots L3 to Co.
- produces neurologic deficits similar to those seen in conus or epiconus lesions.
- results in signs that frequently predominate on one side.
- may result from intervertebral disk herniation.
- commonly results in severe spontaneous radicular pain.

F. **Filum terminale (tethered cord) syndrome**
- results from a thickened, shortened filum terminale that adheres to the sacrum and causes traction on the conus medullaris.
- results in sphincter dysfunction, gait disorders, and deformities of the feet.

G. **Subacute combined degeneration (vitamin B$_{12}$ neuropathy)** (see Figure 8-2G)
- is a spinal cord disease associated with pernicious anemia.
- consists of demyelination of dorsal columns, resulting in loss of vibration and position sensation.
- consists of demyelination of spinocerebellar tracts, resulting in arm and leg dystaxia.
- consists of demyelination of corticospinal tracts resulting in spastic paresis (UMN signs).

H. **Friedreich hereditary ataxia** (see Figure 8-2G)
- is the most common hereditary ataxia with autosomal recessive inheritance.
- results in spinal cord pathology and spinal cord symptoms that are similar to subacute combined degeneration with dorsal column, spinocerebellar, and corticospinal tract involvement.
- cerebellar involvement (Purkinje cells and dentate nucleus) is frequent with progressive ataxia.
- commonly leads to cardiomyopathy, pes cavus, and kyphoscoliosis.

I. **Syringomyelia** (see Figures 8-2H and 8-3)
- is a central cavitation of the cervical spinal cord of unknown etiology.
- results in destruction of the ventral white commissure and interruption of decussating spinothalamic fibers, causing bilateral loss of pain and temperature sensation.
- can result in extension of the syrinx into the ventral horn, causing an LMN lesion with muscle wasting and hyporeflexia. Atrophy of lumbricals and interosseous muscles of the hand is a common finding.
- can result in extension of the syrinx into the lateral funiculus, affecting the lateral corticospinal tract and resulting in spastic paresis (a UMN lesion).
- can result in caudal extension of the syrinx into the lateral horn at T1 or lateral extension into the lateral funiculus (interruption of descending autonomic pathways), resulting in Horner syndrome.

J. **Multiple sclerosis** (see Figure 8-2B)
- is the most common form of demyelinating disease.
- has asymmetric lesions and may affect all tracts of the spinal cord white matter. Spinal cord lesions occur most frequently in the cervical segments.

K. **Charcot-Marie-Tooth disease** (hereditary motor–sensory neuropathy type I) (see Figure 8-2I)
- is also called peroneal muscular atrophy.
- is the most common inherited neuropathy.
- affects the posterior columns, resulting in a loss of conscious proprioception.
- affects the anterior horn motor neurons, resulting in muscle weakness (atrophy).

VIII. Intervertebral Disk Herniation

A. **Overview: intervertebral disk herniation**
- consists of prolapse or herniation of the **nucleus pulposus** through the defective **annulus fibrosus** into the vertebral canal. The nucleus pulposus impinges on spinal roots, resulting in root pain (radiculopathy) or muscle weakness.
- may compress the spinal cord with a large central protrusion (above VL1).
- is recognized as the major cause of severe and chronic low back and leg pain.
- appears in 90% of cases at the L4–L5 or L5–S1 interspaces; usually a single nerve root is compressed, but several may be involved at the L5–S1 interspace (cauda equina).
- appears in 10% of cases in the cervical region, usually at the C5–C6 or C6–C7 interspaces.
- is characterized by **spinal root symptoms**, which include paresthesias, pain, sensory loss, hyporeflexia, and muscle weakness.

B. Cervical spondylosis with myelopathy

- is the most commonly observed myelopathy.
- consists of spinal cord or spinal cord root compression by calcified disk material extruded into the spinal vertebral canal.
- presents as painful stiff neck, arm pain and weakness, and spastic leg weakness with dystaxia; sensory disorders are frequent.

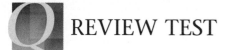
Questions 1 to 3

Questions 1 to 3 relate to the figure.

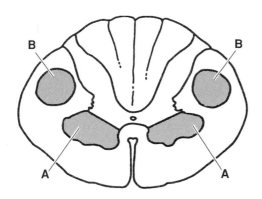

Neuropathologic examination of the spinal cord reveals two lesions labeled A and B. Lesion A is restricted to five segments.

1. The result of lesion A is best described as

(A) bilateral arm dystaxia with dysdiadochokinesia
(B) spastic paresis of the legs
(C) flaccid paralysis of the upper extremities
(D) loss of pain and temperature sensation below the lesion
(E) urinary and fecal incontinence

2. The result of lesion B is best described as

(A) dyssynergia of movements affecting both arms and legs
(B) flaccid paralysis of the upper extremities
(C) impaired two-point tactile discrimination in both arms
(D) spastic paresis affecting primarily the muscles distal to the knee joint
(E) bilateral apallesthesia

3. Lesions A and B result from

(A) an intramedullary tumor
(B) an extramedullary tumor
(C) thrombosis of a spinal artery
(D) multiple sclerosis
(E) amyotrophic lateral sclerosis

4. Neurologic examination reveals an extensor plantar reflex on the left side, hyperreflexia on the left side, a loss of pain and temperature sensation on the right side, and ptosis and miosis on the left side. A lesion that causes this constellation of deficits would most likely be found in the

(A) paracentral lobule, left side
(B) crus cerebri, right side
(C) dorsolateral medulla, left side
(D) cervical spinal cord
(E) lumbar spinal cord

5. A 50-year-old woman complains of clumsiness in her hands while working in the kitchen: she recently burned her hands on the stove without experiencing any pain. Neurologic examination reveals bilateral weakness of the shoulder girdles, arms, and hands, as well as a loss of pain and temperature sensation covering the shoulder and upper extremity in a cape-like distribution. Severe atrophy is present in the intrinsic muscles of the hands. The most likely diagnosis is

(A) amyotrophic lateral sclerosis
(B) subacute combined degeneration
(C) Werdnig-Hoffmann disease
(D) syringomyelia
(E) tabes dorsalis

6. A 50-year-old man has a 2-year history of progressive muscle weakness in all extremities, with severe muscle atrophy and reduced MSRs in both legs. In his arms, the muscle atrophy is less pronounced and the MSRs are exaggerated. Which of the following types of neuronal degeneration would postmortem examination most likely show?

(A) Loss of Purkinje cells
(B) Loss of neurons from the globus pallidus
(C) Loss of neurons from the paracentral lobule and from the anterior horns of the spinal cord
(D) Demyelination of axons in the posterior and lateral columns
(E) Demyelination of axons in the posterior limb of the internal capsule

7. Transection of the spinothalamic tract results in

(A) Loss of pain and temperature sensation
(B) Complete flaccid paralysis
(C) Spastic paresis
(D) Cerebellar incoordination
(E) Areflexia

8. Which of the following is a characteristic of Lou Gehrig disease?

(A) Loss of tactile discrimination
(B) Loss of vibratory sensation
(C) Dorsal root irritation
(D) Progressive bulbar palsy
(E) Stereoanesthesia

9. Clasp-knife spasticity results from a lesion in the

(A) Ventral corticospinal tract
(B) Ventral spinothalamic tract
(C) Lateral corticospinal tract
(D) Dorsal spinocerebellar tract
(E) Lateral spinothalamic tract

10. Which of the following syndromes is associated with an absent Achilles tendon reflex?

(A) Filum terminale
(B) Cauda equina
(C) Conus medullaris
(D) Epicomus
(E) Syringomyelia

11. An example of a peripheral nervous system lesion is

(A) Guillain-Barré syndrome
(B) Charcot-Marie-Tooth disease
(C) Friedreich ataxia
(D) Lou Gehrig disease
(E) Brown-Séquard syndrome

12. A patient has the ability to stand with open eyes but falls with closed eyes. A lesion of which pathway is likely responsible for this symptom?

(A) Ventral spinothalamic tract
(B) Dorsal spinocerebellar tract
(C) Lateral spinothalamic tract
(D) Ventral spinocerebellar tract
(E) Dorsal column syndrome

Questions 13 to 18

The response options for items 13 to 18 are the same. Select one answer for each item in the set.

(A) Amyotrophic lateral sclerosis
(B) Cauda equina syndrome
(C) Cervical spondylosis
(D) Friedreich ataxia
(E) Guillain-Barré syndrome
(F) Multiple sclerosis
(G) Subacute combined degeneration
(H) Tabes dorsalis
(I) Werdnig-Hoffmann disease

Match each statement below with the syndrome that corresponds best to it.

13. A pure lower motor neuron disease

14. Elevated CSF protein with a normal CSF cell count

15. Characterized by asymmetric lesions found in the white matter of cervical segments

16. May result from intervertebral disk herniation

17. Symptoms include a painful stiff neck, arm pain and weakness, spastic leg weakness with dystaxia; sensory disorders are frequent

18. Associated with a loss of Purkinje cells

Questions 19 to 26

Match the statement in items 19 to 26 with the lesion shown in the figure that corresponds best to it.

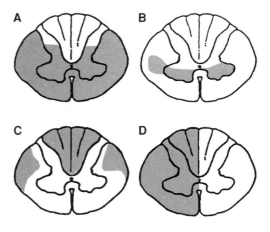

19. Neurologic manifestation of vitamin B_{12} deficiency

20. Lesion due to vascular occlusion

21. Loss of vibration sensation on the right side; loss of pain and temperature sensation on the left side

22. Bilateral loss of pain and temperature sensation in the legs

23. Bilateral loss of pain and temperature sensation in the hands; muscle atrophy in both hands; spastic paresis on the right side only

24. Urinary incontinence and quadriplegia

25. No muscle atrophy or fasciculations

26. Demyelinating disease

ANSWERS AND EXPLANATIONS

1–C. Lesion A involves degeneration of the ventral horns bilaterally at midcervical levels, resulting in flaccid paralysis in the upper extremities.

2–D. Lesion B involves degeneration of the lateral corticospinal tracts bilaterally, resulting in spastic paresis of the lower extremities and primarily affecting the muscles distal to the knee. Spastic paresis of the upper extremities is masked by flaccid paralysis resulting from lesion A. Apallesthesia is the inability to perceive a vibrating tuning fork.

3–E. Lesions A and B are the result of amyotrophic lateral sclerosis, a pure motor disease.

4–D. A lesion of the cervical spinal cord could result in ipsilateral Horner syndrome, ipsilateral spastic paresis, and contralateral loss of pain and temperature sensation. Horner syndrome is always manifested on the ipsilateral side. This lesion produces a classic Brown-Séquard syndrome.

5–D. Syringomyelia is a cavitation of the spinal cord most commonly seen in the cervicothoracic segments. This condition results in bilateral loss of pain and temperature sensation in a cape-like distribution as well as wasting of the intrinsic muscles of the hands. Amyotrophic lateral sclerosis is a pure motor syndrome; subacute combined degeneration includes both sensory and motor deficits; Werdnig-Hoffmann disease is a pure motor disease; and tabes dorsalis is a pure sensory syndrome (neurosyphilis).

6–C. Amyotrophic lateral sclerosis affects both the upper and lower motor neurons. It is also referred to as motor systems disease. A loss of Purkinje cells as seen in cerebellar cortical atrophy (cerebello-olivary atrophy) results in cerebellar signs. Cell loss in the globus pallidus and putamen is seen in Wilson disease (hepatolenticular degeneration). Demyelination of axons in the posterior and lateral columns is seen in subacute combined degeneration. Demyelination of axons in the posterior limb of the internal capsule results in contralateral spastic hemiparesis.

7–A. Transection of the spinothalamic tract results in loss of pain and temperature sensations, starting one segment below the lesion. Ventral horn destruction results in complete flaccid paralysis and areflexia at the level of the lesion. Corticospinal tract transection results in spastic paresis below the lesion. Dorsal spinocerebellar tract and ventral spinocerebellar tract transection results in cerebellar incoordination.

8–D. Progressive bulbar palsy is a lower motor neuron component of amyotrophic lateral sclerosis, or Lou Gehrig disease. Disease characteristics are muscle weakness and wasting without sensory deficits. Loss of tactile discrimination, loss of vibratory sensation, stereoanesthesia, and dorsal root irritation are all sensory deficits found in dorsal column syndrome.

9–C. Clasp-knife spasticity is an ipsilateral motor deficit found below a lesion of the lateral corticospinal tract. It is characterized by initial but fading resistance of a briskly moved joint.

10–D. Epicomus syndrome involves segments L4 to S2 and results in loss of voluntary control of the bladder and rectum, motor disability, and an absent Achilles tendon reflex.

11-A. Acute idiopathic polyneuritis, or Guillain-Barré syndrome, is a peripheral nervous system lesion. It typically follows an infectious illness and results from a cell-mediated immunologic reaction.

12-E. Dorsal column syndrome results in a sensory deficit known as sensory dystaxia, or Romberg sign. Patients are Romberg positive when they are able to stand with the eyes open but fall with the eyes closed.

13–I. Werdnig-Hoffmann disease is a heredofamilial degenerative disease of infants that affects only LMNs.

14–E. Guillain-Barré syndrome is characterized by elevated CSF protein with normal CSF cell count (albuminocytologic dissociation).

15–F. Multiple sclerosis is characterized by asymmetric lesions frequently found in the white matter of cervical segments.

16–B. The cauda equina syndrome frequently results from intervertebral disk herniation; severe spontaneous radicular pain is common.

17–C. Cervical spondylosis is the most commonly observed myelopathy. Its symptoms include a painful stiff neck, arm pain and weakness, and spastic leg weakness with dystaxia; sensory disorders are frequent.

18–D. Friedreich ataxia is the most common hereditary ataxia with autosomal recessive inheritance. Dorsal columns, spinocerebellar tracts, and the corticospinal tracts show demyelination. Friedreich ataxia results in a loss of Purkinje cells in the cerebellar cortex and a loss of neurons in the dentate nucleus.

19–C. A neurologic manifestation of vitamin B_{12} deficiency is subacute combined degeneration. There is no involvement of LMNs.

20–A. Lesion A shows the territory of infarction resulting from occlusion of the ventral (anterior) spinal artery.

21–D. A spinal cord hemisection (Brown-Séquard syndrome) on the right side results in a loss of vibration sensation on the right side and a loss of pain and temperature sensation on the left side (dissociated sensory loss).

22–A. Total occlusion of the ventral spinal artery, involving five cervical segments, results in infarction of the ventral two-thirds of the spinal cord and interrupts both lateral spinothalamic tracts. The patient would have a loss of pain and temperature sensation caudal to the lesion.

23–B. Lesion B shows a cervical syringomyelic lesion involving the ventral white commissure, both ventral horns, and the right corticospinal tract. The patient would have a bilateral loss of pain and temperature sensation in the hands, muscle wasting in both hands, and a spastic paresis on the right side.

24–A. In lesion A, both lateral and ventral funiculi have been infarcted by arterial occlusion. Bilateral destruction of the lateral corticospinal tracts at upper cervical levels results in quadriplegia (spastic paresis in upper and lower extremities). Bilateral destruction of the ventrolateral quadrants results in urinary and fecal incontinence.

25–C. In lesion C, subacute combined degeneration, there is no involvement of LMNs, hence no flaccid paralysis, muscle atrophy, or fasciculations.

26–C. In lesion C, subacute combined degeneration, there is symmetric degeneration of the white matter, both in the dorsal columns (fasciculi gracilis) and in the lateral funiculi (corticospinal tracts). In this degenerative disease, both the myelin sheaths and the axis cylinders are involved. Subacute combined degeneration is classified under nutritional diseases (in this case a vitamin B_{12} neuropathy). In true demyelinative diseases (e.g., multiple sclerosis), the myelin sheaths are involved but the axis cylinders and nerve cells are relatively spared.

CHAPTER

9

Brainstem

I. Introduction: The Brainstem (Figure 9-1)

- includes the **medulla**, **pons**, and **mesencephalon** (midbrain).
- extends from the pyramidal decussation to the posterior commissure.
- gives rise to cranial nerve (CN) III to CN XII.
- receives its blood supply from the vertebrobasilar system.

II. Medullar Oblongata (Myelencephalon)

A. **Overview: the medulla**
- contains autonomic centers that regulate respiration, circulation, and gastrointestinal motility.
- extends from the pyramidal decussation to the inferior pontine sulcus.
- gives rise to CN IX to CN XII. The nuclei of CN V and CN VIII extend caudally into the medulla.
- is connected to the cerebellum by the inferior cerebellar peduncle.

B. **Internal structures of the medulla** (Figures 9-2 through 9-5)
1. **Ascending sensory pathways and relay nuclei**
   a. **Fasciculus gracilis and fasciculus cuneatus**
      - convey dorsal column modalities.
      - terminate in the nucleus gracilis and nucleus cuneatus.
   b. **Nucleus gracilis and nucleus cuneatus**
      - contain second-order neurons of the dorsal column–medial lemniscus pathway.
      - give rise to internal arcuate fibers.
      - project via the medial lemniscus to the ventral posterolateral nucleus of the thalamus.
   c. **Internal arcuate fibers**
      - arise from the nucleus gracilis and nucleus cuneatus and form the contralateral medial lemniscus.
   d. **Decussation of the medial lemniscus** (see Figure 9-3)
      - is formed by decussating internal arcuate fibers.
   e. **Medial lemniscus**
      - conveys dorsal column modalities to the ventral posterolateral nucleus.
   f. **Spinal lemniscus** (see II B 4 i)
      - contains the lateral and ventral spinothalamic tracts and the spinotectal tract.
2. **Descending motor pathways**
   a. **Pyramidal decussation** (see Figure 9-2)
      - is located at the spinomedullary junction.
      - consists of crossing corticospinal fibers.

133

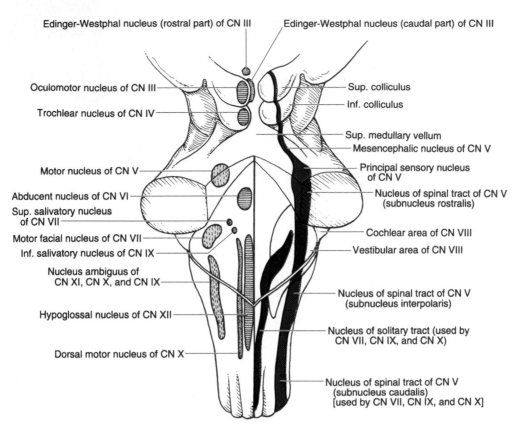

Figure 9-1. Outline of the brainstem showing the location of motor and sensory cranial nerve nuclei. Motor nuclei are shown on the *left* side of the figure, and sensory nuclei are shown on the *right* side.

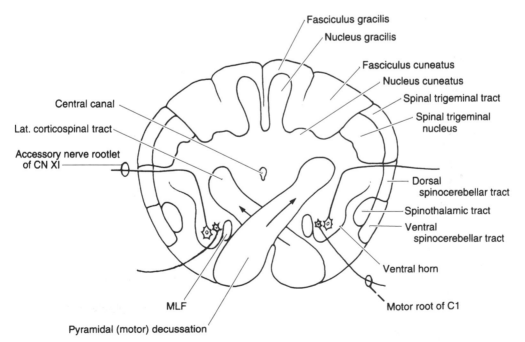

Figure 9-2. Transverse section of the caudal medulla at the level of the pyramidal (motor) decussation. The nucleus of the accessory nerve (CN XI) is located in the ventral horn and gives rise to the spinal root of CN XI. Ventral horn neurons from the spinal nucleus give rise to the ventral roots of C1.

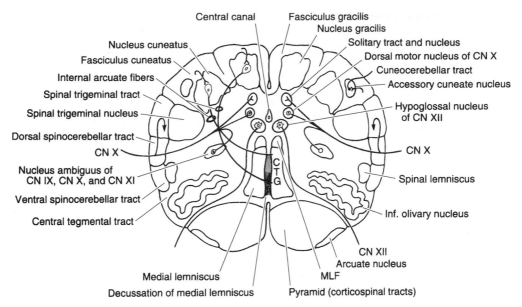

Figure 9-3. Transverse section of the caudal medulla at the level of the decussation of the medial lemniscus. The internal arcuate fibers decussate and form the medial lemniscus. *CTG* = cuneate (arm), trunk, and gracile (leg) components of the medial lemniscus. GSA fibers of the vagal nerve (CN X) enter the spinal trigeminal tract of CN V (*arrow*).

  b. Pyramids (see Figures 9-4 and 9-5)
   • constitute the base of the medulla.
   • contain uncrossed corticospinal fibers.
 3. Cerebellar pathways and relay nuclei
  a. Accessory (lateral) cuneate nucleus
   • contains second-order neurons of the cuneocerebellar tract.
   • projects to the cerebellum via the inferior cerebellar peduncle.

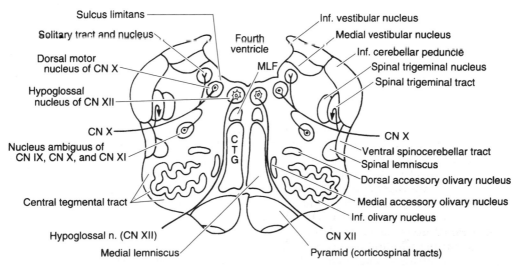

Figure 9-4. Transverse section of the medulla at the midolivary level. The vagal (CN X), hypoglossal (CN XII), and vestibular (CN VIII) nerves are prominent in this section. The nucleus ambiguus gives rise to SVE fibers to CN IX, CN X, and CN XI. The dorsal spinocerebellar tract is in the inferior cerebellar peduncle.

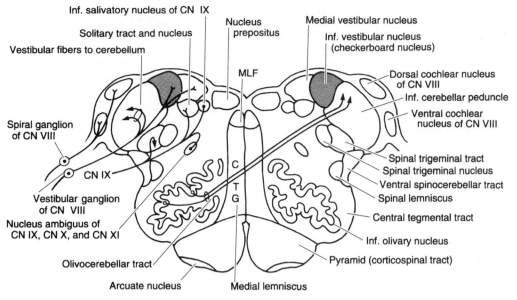

Figure 9-5. Rostral medulla at the level of the dorsal and ventral cochlear nuclei (of CN VIII). The glossopharyngeal nerve (CN IX) is also found at this level. The hypoglossal nucleus (of CN XII) has been replaced by the nucleus prepositus. GSA fibers of the glossopharyngeal nerve (CN IX) enter the spinal trigeminal tract of CN V (*arrow*).

   b. Inferior olivary nucleus
   - underlies the olive.
   - is a cerebellar relay nucleus that projects olivocerebellar fibers via the inferior cerebellar peduncle to the contralateral cerebellar cortex and cerebellar nuclei.
   - receives input from the red nucleus.
   c. Central tegmental tract
   - extends from the midbrain to the inferior olivary nucleus.
   - contains rubro-olivary and reticulothalamic fibers.
   - contains taste fibers.
   d. Lateral reticular nucleus
   - is a cerebellar relay nucleus that projects via the inferior cerebellar peduncle to the cerebellum.
   e. Arcuate nucleus
   - is located on the ventral surface of the pyramids.
   - gives rise to arcuatocerebellar fibers that become the striae medullares of the rhomboid fossa.
   f. Dorsal spinocerebellar tract
   - mediates unconscious proprioception from the lower extremities to the cerebellum via the inferior cerebellar peduncle.
   g. Ventral spinocerebellar tract
   - mediates unconscious proprioception from the lower extremities to the cerebellum via the superior cerebellar peduncle.
   h. Inferior cerebellar peduncle
   - connects the medulla to the cerebellum.
 4. Cranial nerve nuclei and associated tracts
   a. Medial longitudinal fasciculus (MLF)
   - contains vestibular fibers of CN VIII that coordinate eye movements via CN III, IV, and CN VI.
   - mediates nystagmus and lateral conjugate gaze.

b. **Solitary tract**
   - receives general visceral afferent (GVA) input from CN IX and CN X.
   - receives special visceral afferent (SVA) (taste) input from CN VII, CN IX, and CN X.
c. **Solitary nucleus**
   - projects GVA and SVA input ipsilaterally via the central tegmental tract to the parabrachial nucleus of the pons and to the posteromedial nucleus of the thalamus.
d. **Dorsal motor nucleus of CN X** (see Figures 9-1, 9-3, and 9-4)
   - gives rise to vagal preganglionic parasympathetic general visceral efferent (GVE) fibers that synapse in the terminal (intramural) ganglia of the thoracic and abdominal viscera.
e. **Inferior salivary nucleus of CN IX**
   - gives rise to preganglionic parasympathetic (GVE) fibers that synapse in the otic ganglion.
f. **Hypoglossal nucleus of CN XII** (see Figures 9-1, 9-3, and 9-4)
   - gives rise to general somatic efferent (GSE) fibers that innervate the intrinsic and extrinsic muscles of the tongue.
g. **Nucleus ambiguus of CN IX, CN X, and CN XI** (see Figures 9-1 and 9-3 through 9-5)
   - represents a special visceral efferent (SVE) cell column whose axons innervate pharyngeal arch muscles of the larynx and pharynx. These fibers contribute to parts of CN IX, CN X, and CN XI; they exit the medulla via the postolivary sulcus.
h. **Ventral horn of CN XI** (see Figure 9-2)
   - is located at the level of the pyramidal decussation.
   - contains motor neurons of the spinal accessory nerve.
i. **Spinal trigeminal tract** (Figure 9-6; see Figures 9-2 through 9-4)
   - replaces the dorsolateral tract of Lissauer.
   - contains first-order neuron general somatic afferent (GSA) fibers that mediate pain, temperature, and light touch sensations from the face via CN V, CN VII, CN IX, and CN X.

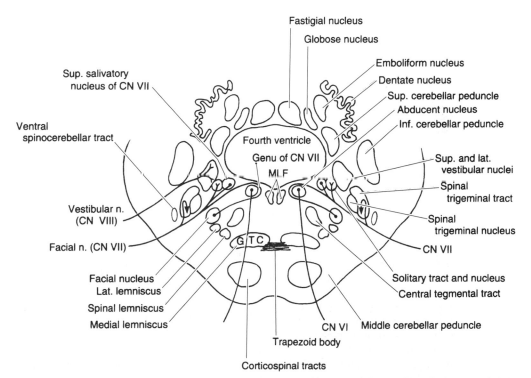

Figure 9-6. Caudal pons at the level of the abducent (CN VI) and facial (CN VII) nuclei. The intra-axial abducent fibers pass through the medial lemniscus and the descending corticospinal fibers. Note the looping course of the intra-axial facial nerve fibers that exit the brainstem in the cerebellopontine angle. The four cerebellar nuclei overlie the fourth ventricle. Note also the looping course of the facial nerve fibers.

> - projects to the spinal trigeminal nucleus.
> **j. Spinal trigeminal nucleus** (see Figures 9-1 through 9-6)
> - replaces the substantia gelatinosa of the spinal cord.
> - gives rise to decussating axons that form the ventral trigeminothalamic tract. This tract terminates in the ventral posteromedial nucleus of the thalamus.
> **k. Inferior and medial vestibular nuclei of CN VIII**
> - receives proprioceptive (special somatic afferent [SSA]) input from the semicircular ducts, utricle, saccule, and cerebellum.
> - project to the cerebellum and MLF.
> **5. Area postrema**
> - lies rostral to the obex in the floor of the fourth ventricle.
> - is a circumventricular organ with no blood–brain barrier.

III. Pons

A. Overview: the pons
- extends from the inferior pontine sulcus to the superior pontine sulcus.
- consists of the **base**, which contains corticobulbar, corticospinal, and corticopontine tracts and pontine nuclei; and the **tegmentum**, which contains cranial nerve nuclei, reticular nuclei, and the major ascending sensory pathways.
- is connected to the cerebellum by the middle cerebellar peduncle.
- contains auditory relay nuclei and vestibular nuclei; the latter regulate postural mechanisms and vestibulo-ocular reflexes.
- contains, in its caudal portion, the facial motor nucleus of CN VII, which innervates the muscles of facial expression.
- contains, in the mid pons, the trigeminal motor nucleus of CN V; its axons innervate the muscles of mastication.
- contains a center for lateral gaze.
- gives rise to CN V to VIII.

B. Internal structures of the pons (Figure 9-7; see Figure 9-6)
1. Ascending sensory pathways and relay nuclei
  a. Dorsal and ventral cochlear nuclei (see Figure 9-5)
   - receive auditory input from the cochlea through SSA fibers via the cochlear branch of CN VIII.
   - are auditory relay nuclei that give rise to the ipsilateral and contralateral lateral lemniscus.
  b. Trapezoid body
   - is formed by decussating fibers of the ventral cochlear nuclei.
   - contains the acoustic striae, medial lemnisci, exiting abducent (CN VI) fibers, and aberrant corticobulbar fibers.
  c. Superior olivary nucleus
   - is an auditory relay nucleus at the level of the trapezoid body.
   - receives input from the cochlear nuclei.
   - contributes bilaterally to the lateral lemniscus.
  d. Lateral lemniscus
   - is a pontine auditory pathway extending from the trapezoid body to the nucleus of the inferior colliculus.
   - conducts a preponderance of contralateral cochlear input.
  e. Medial lemniscus
   - mediates contralateral dorsal column modalities to the ventral posterolateral nucleus of the thalamus.
  f. Spinal lemniscus
   - contains lateral and ventral spinothalamic tracts and the spinotectal tract.
2. Descending motor pathways (base of the pons)
  a. Corticobulbar tract

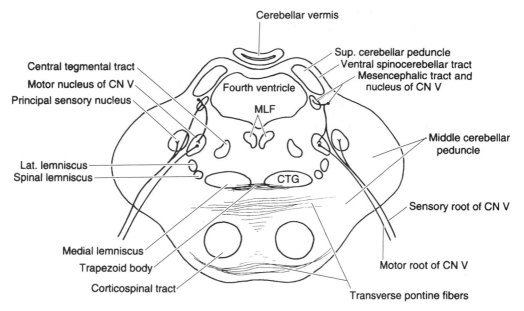

Figure 9-7. Mid pons at the level of the motor and principal sensory nuclei of the trigeminal nerve (CN V). The mesencephalic tract and nucleus provide the afferent limb of the myotatic jaw jerk reflex; the motor trigeminal nucleus is the efferent limb.

- synapses in the motor nuclei of the cranial nerves except in the ocular motor nuclei of CN III, IV, and VI.
  b. **Corticospinal tract (pyramidal tract)**
    - synapses in the ventral horn of the spinal cord.
  c. **Corticopontine tract**
    - synapses in the pontine nuclei.
3. **Cerebellar pathways and relay nuclei**
  a. **Central tegmental tract**
    - extends from the midbrain to the inferior olivary nucleus.
    - contains rubro-olivary and reticulothalamic fibers.
  b. **Juxtarestiform body**
    - forms part of the inferior cerebellar peduncle.
    - contains vestibulocerebellar, cerebellovestibular, and cerebelloreticular fibers.
  c. **Middle cerebellar peduncle**
    - contains pontocerebellar fibers.
    - connects the pons to the cerebellum.
  d. **Superior cerebellar peduncle**
    - connects the cerebellum to the pons and midbrain.
    - contains the dentatorubrothalamic fibers and the ventral spinocerebellar tract.
  e. **Pontine nuclei**
    - are cerebellar relay nuclei in the base of the pons.
    - give rise to pontocerebellar fibers that constitute the middle cerebellar peduncle.
4. **Cranial nerve nuclei and associated tracts**
  a. **Dorsal and ventral cochlear nuclei of CN VIII**
    - are found at the medullopontine junction.
  b. **Medial, lateral, and superior vestibular nuclei of CN VIII** (see Figure 9-6)
    - receive proprioceptive (SSA) input from the semicircular ducts, utricle, saccule, and cerebellum.
    - project to the cerebellum and the MLF.
    - The lateral vestibular nucleus gives rise to the lateral vestibulospinal tract.

  c. **Medial longitudinal fasciculus**
   - contains vestibular fibers of CN VIII that coordinate eye movements via CN III, CN IV, and CN VI.
   - mediates nystagmus and lateral conjugate gaze.
  d. **Abducent nucleus of CN VI** (see Figure 9-6)
   - underlies, in the caudal medial pontine tegmentum, the facial colliculus of the rhomboid fossa.
   - projects exiting fibers through the trapezoid body and through the corticospinal tract of the base of the pons.
   - gives rise to GSE fibers that innervate the lateral rectus muscle.
   - gives rise to fibers that project via the MLF to the contralateral medial rectus subnucleus of the oculomotor nucleus of CN III.
   - is the **pontine center for lateral conjugate gaze**, which receives commands from the contralateral frontal eye field (area 8). It innervates via the MLF the contralateral medial rectus muscle and via abducent fibers the ipsilateral lateral rectus muscle to execute conjugate lateral gaze.
  e. **Facial nucleus of CN VII** (see Figure 9-6)
   - gives rise to SVE fibers that innervate the muscles of facial expression.
   - receives bilateral input for upper facial muscles and contralateral input for lower facial muscles.
   - contains neurons that project axons dorsomedially, encircle the abducent nucleus as a genu, and pass ventrolaterally between the facial nucleus and spinal trigeminal nucleus to exit the brainstem in the cerebellopontine angle.
  f. **Superior salivatory nucleus of CN VII**
   - includes the lacrimal nucleus.
   - gives rise to GVE preganglionic parasympathetic fibers that synapse in the pterygopalatine and submandibular ganglia.
  g. **Spinal trigeminal tract and nucleus of CN V**
  h. **Motor nucleus of CN V**
   - lies in the lateral midpontine tegmentum at the level of entrance of the trigeminal nerve.
   - lies medial to the principal sensory nucleus of the trigeminal nerve.
   - receives bilateral corticobulbar input.
   - gives rise to SVE fibers that innervate muscles of mastication.
  i. **Principal sensory nucleus of CN V**
   - lies lateral to the motor nucleus of CN V.
   - receives discriminative tactile and pressure sensation input from the face.
   - gives rise to trigeminothalamic fibers that join the contralateral ventral trigeminothalamic tract.
   - gives rise to the uncrossed dorsal trigeminothalamic tract, which terminates in the ventral posteromedial nucleus of the thalamus.
  j. **Mesencephalic nucleus and tract of CN V** (Figures 9-8 and 9-9; see Figure 9-7)
   - extend from the upper pons to the upper midbrain.
   - contain pseudounipolar neurons.
   - receive input from muscle spindles and pressure receptors (muscles of mastication and extraocular muscles).
 5. **Locus ceruleus**
   - is a melanin-containing nucleus in the pons and midbrain.
   - is an important nucleus of the monamine system that projects noradrenergic axons to all parts of the central nervous system (CNS).

IV. Mesencephalon (Midbrain) (see Figures 9-8 and 9-9)

A. **Overview: the midbrain**
 - mediates auditory and visual reflexes.
 - contains the oculomotor nerve (CN III) and the trochlear nerve (CN IV), which innervate the extraocular muscles of the eye.

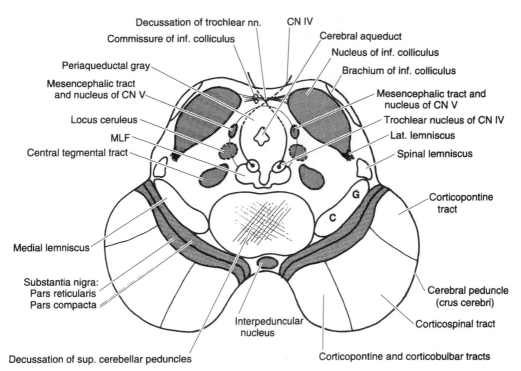

Figure 9-8. Midbrain at the level of the inferior colliculus, the decussation of the superior cerebellar peduncles, and the trochlear nucleus (of CN IV). Trochlear fibers decussate and exit the brainstem of the dorsal surface.

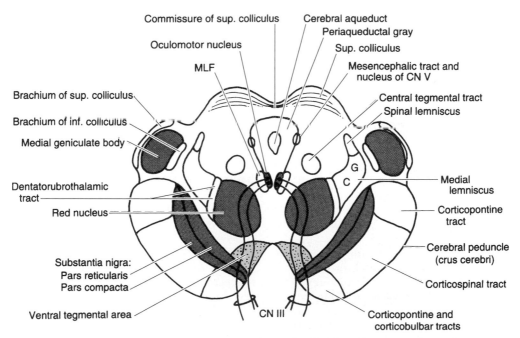

Figure 9-9. Midbrain at the level of the superior colliculus, the oculomotor nucleus (of CN III), and the red nucleus. Oculomotor fibers pass laterally through the red nucleus and basis pedunculi and exit in the interpeduncular fossa.

- contains a center for vertical conjugate gaze in its rostral extent.
- contains the **substantia nigra**, the largest nucleus of the midbrain; degeneration of this extrapyramidal motor nucleus results in Parkinson disease.
- contains the **paramedian reticular formation**; lesions of this formation result in coma.
- extends from the superior medullary velum to the posterior commissure.
- gives rise to two cranial nerves: **CN III** (oculomotor) and **CN IV** (trochlear).
- consists dorsoventrally of three parts: the **tectum**, the **tegmentum**, and the **base** (**basis pedunculi**).

B. **Structures of the midbrain**
   1. **Tectum**
      - is located dorsal to the cerebral aqueduct.
      - forms the roof of the midbrain, including the superior and inferior colliculi.
   2. **Tegmentum**
      - is located between the tectum and the base (basis pedunculi).
      - contains cranial nerve nuclei and sensory pathways.
   3. **Basis pedunculi (crus cerebri)**
      - forms the base of the midbrain and contains corticospinal, corticobulbar, and cortico-pontine tracts.
   4. **Pedunculus cerebri (cerebral peduncle)**
      - includes the tegmentum and basis pedunculi.
   5. **Pretectum (pretectal area)**
      - is located between the superior colliculus and the habenular trigone.

C. **Inferior collicular level of the midbrain** (see Figure 9-8)
   1. **Inferior colliculus**
      - contains the nucleus of the inferior colliculus.
   2. **Nucleus of the inferior colliculus**
      - is an auditory relay nucleus that receives binaural input from the lateral lemniscus.
      - projects to the medial geniculate body via the brachium of the inferior colliculus.
   3. **Lateral lemniscus**
      - projects binaural auditory information to the inferior collicular nucleus.
   4. **Commissure of the inferior colliculus**
      - interconnects the inferior collicular nucleus and its opposite partner.
   5. **Brachium of the inferior colliculus**
      - conducts auditory information from the inferior collicular nucleus to the medial geniculate body.
   6. **Cerebral aqueduct**
      - is located between the tectum and tegmentum.
      - is surrounded by the periaqueductal gray matter.
      - interconnects the third and fourth ventricles.
      - blockage (aqueductal stenosis) results in **hydrocephalus**.
   7. **Periaqueductal gray matter**
      - is the central gray matter that surrounds the cerebral aqueduct.
      - contains several nuclear groups.
        a. **Locus ceruleus**
        b. **Mesencephalic nucleus and tract**
        c. **Dorsal tegmental nucleus**
           - contains enkephalinergic neurons that play a role in endogenous pain control.
        d. **Dorsal nucleus of raphe**
           - contains serotonergic neurons.
   8. **Trochlear nucleus of CN IV** (see Figure 9-8)
      - gives rise to GSE fibers, which encircle the periaqueductal gray matter, decussate in the superior medullary velum, and exit the midbrain from its dorsal aspect to innervate the superior oblique muscle.

9. **Medial longitudinal fasciculus**
   - contains vestibular fibers that coordinate eye movements.
   - interconnects the ocular motor nuclei of CN III, CN IV, and CN VI.
10. **Decussation of the superior cerebellar peduncles** (see Figure 9-8)
    - is most conspicuous structure of this level.
11. **Interpeduncular nucleus**
    - receives input from the habenular nuclei via the habenulointerpeduncular tract (fasciculus retroflexus of Meynert).
12. **Substantia nigra** (see Figures 9-8 and 9-9)
    - is divided into the dorsal **pars compacta**, which contains large pigmented (melanin) cells, and the ventral **pars reticularis**.
    - receives gamma-aminobutyric acid–ergic (GABA-ergic) input from the caudatoputamen (striatonigral fibers).
    - projects dopaminergic fibers to the caudatoputamen (nigrostriatal fibers).
    - projects nondopaminergic fibers to the ventral anterior nucleus, ventral lateral nucleus, and mediodorsal nucleus of the thalamus (nigrothalamic fibers).
13. **Medial lemniscus**
    - mediates dorsal column modalities to the ventral posterolateral nucleus.
14. **Spinal lemniscus**
    - contains the lateral and ventral spinothalamic tracts and the spinotectal tract.
15. **Central tegmental tract**
    - contains rubro-olivary and reticulothalamic fibers.
16. **Basis pedunculi (crus cerebri)** (see Figures 9-8 and 9-9)

D. **Superior collicular level of the midbrain** (see Figure 9-9)
   1. **Superior colliculus**
      - receives visual input from the retina and from frontal (area 8) and occipital (area 19) eye fields.
      - receives auditory input from the inferior colliculus to mediate audiovisual reflexes.
      - is concerned with detection of movement in visual fields, thus facilitating visual orientation, searching, and tracking.
   2. **Commissure of the superior colliculus**
      - interconnects the two superior colliculi.
   3. **Brachium of the superior colliculus**
      - conducts retinal and corticotectal fibers to the superior colliculus and to the pretectum, thus mediating optic and pupillary reflexes.
   4. **Cerebral aqueduct and periaqueductal gray matter**
   5. **Oculomotor nucleus of CN III** (see Figure 9-9)
      - gives rise to GSE fibers that innervate four extraocular muscles (medial, inferior, superior recti, and inferior oblique) and the superior levator palpebrae.
      - projects crossed fibers to the superior rectus.
      - projects crossed and uncrossed fibers to the levator palpebrae.
   6. **Edinger-Westphal nucleus of CN III**
      - gives rise to GVE preganglionic parasympathetic fibers that terminate in the ciliary ganglion.
      - Postganglionic fibers from the ciliary ganglion innervate the ciliary body (accommodation) and the sphincter muscle of the iris (pupillary light reflex).
   7. **Medial longitudinal fasciculus**
      - contains vestibular fibers that coordinate eye movements.
      - interconnects the ocular motor cranial nerves (CN III, CN IV, and CN VI).
   8. **Central tegmental tract**
      - contains rubro-olivary and reticulothalamic fibers.
   9. **Red nucleus** (see Figure 9-9)
      - is located in the tegmentum at the level of the oculomotor nucleus (the level of the superior colliculus).
      - receives bilateral input from the cerebral cortex.
      - receives contralateral input from the cerebellar nuclei.
      - gives rise to the crossed rubrospinal tract.

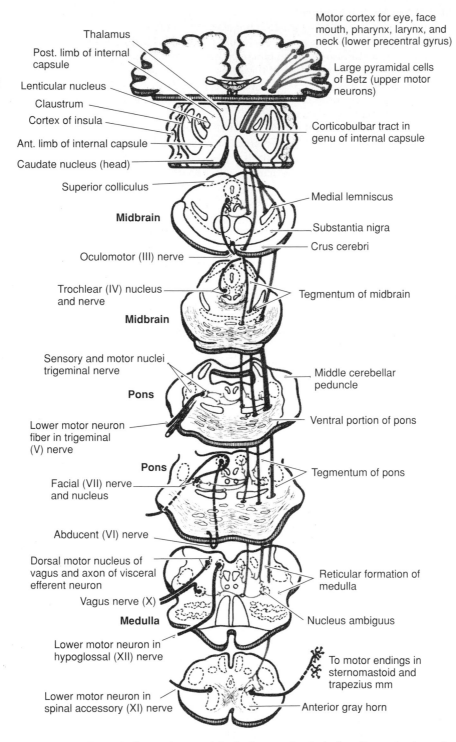

Figure 9-10. Corticobulbar pathways of the brainstem. Corticobulbar fibers arise from the face area of the motor cortex and innervate motor (GSE) and (SVE) cranial nerve nuclei of CN V, CN VII, CN IX, CN X, CN XI, and CN XII. Direct corticobulbar fibers to the ocular motor nerves, CN III, CN IV, and CN VI, have not been demonstrated. Interruption of the corticobulbar fibers results in an UMN lesion. (Reprinted with permission from Carpenter MC: *Core Text of Neuroanatomy*, 3rd ed. Baltimore, Williams & Wilkins, 1985, p 129.)

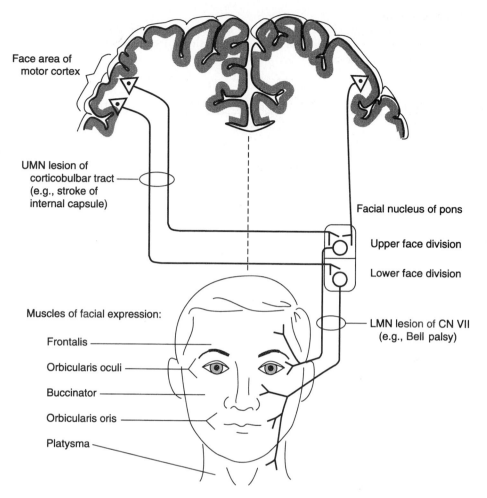

Face area of
motor cortex

UMN lesion of
corticobulbar tract
(e.g., stroke of
internal capsule)

Facial nucleus of pons

Upper face division

Lower face division

Muscles of facial expression:

Frontalis

Orbicularis oculi

Buccinator

Orbicularis oris

Platysma

LMN lesion of CN VII
(e.g., Bell palsy)

Figure 9-11. Corticobulbar innervation of the facial nerve (CN VII) nucleus. An UMN lesion (e.g., a stroke involving the internal capsule) results in contralateral weakness of the lower face and spares in the upper face. A LMN lesion (e.g., Bell palsy) results in paralysis of facial muscles in both the upper and lower face. (Redrawn with permission from DeMyer WE: *Technique of the Neurological Examination; A Programmed Text,* 4th ed. New York, McGraw-Hill, 1994, 6-3, p. 177.)

- gives rise to the uncrossed rubro-olivary tract.
- exerts facilitatory influence on flexor muscles.
10. **Medial lemniscus**
    - mediates dorsal column modalities to the ventral posterolateral nucleus of the thalamus.
11. **Spinal lemniscus**
    - contains the lateral and ventral spinothalamic tracts.
12. **Substantia nigra**
13. **Basis pedunculi (crus cerebri)**

E. **Posterior commissural level (pretectal region)**
   - is a transition area between the mesencephalon and the diencephalon.
   1. **Posterior commissure**
      - marks the caudal extent of the third ventricle.
      - marks the rostral extent of the cerebral aqueduct.
      - interconnects pretectal nuclei, thus mediating consensual pupillary light reflexes.

   2. **Pretectal nucleus**
      - receives retinal input via the brachium of the superior colliculus.
      - projects to the ipsilateral and contralateral Edinger-Westphal nucleus, thus mediating the pupillary light reflexes.

V.   Corticobulbar (Corticonuclear) Fibers (Figure 9-10; see Figure 13-5)

- arise from precentral and postcentral gyri.
- may synapse directly on motor neurons or indirectly via interneurons (corticoreticular fibers).
- innervate sensory relay nuclei (gracile, cuneate, solitary, and trigeminal).
- innervate cranial nerve motor nuclei bilaterally, with the exception of part of the facial nucleus (CN VII). The upper face division of the facial nucleus receives bilateral input; the lower face division of the facial nucleus receives only contralateral input (Figure 9-11).
- innervate the ipsilateral spinal nucleus of CN XI, which supplies the sternocleidomastoid muscle, and the contralateral spinal nucleus of CN XI, which innervates the trapezius muscle.
- The orbicularis oculi muscle receives a variable number of crossed and uncrossed fibers; the paresis therefore varies from patient to patient.

REVIEW TEST

1. A 40-year-old female librarian is brought to the emergency department. Neurologic examination reveals the following: blood pressure 160/90 mm Hg, numbness on the right side of her lower face, no weakness in upper or lower extremities, tongue deviating to right side on protrusion, uvula deviating to the left side when patient says ah. The lesion causing these symptoms is found in which of the following loci?

(A) Anterior limb of internal capsule
(B) Genu of internal capsule, left side
(C) Claustrum
(D) Paracentral lobule, right side
(E) Posterior limb internal capsule

2. The cerebral aqueduct is found in which part of the brain?
(A) Telencephalon
(B) Diencephalon
(C) Mesencephalon
(D) Metencephalon
(E) Myelencephalon

Questions 3 to 10

The response options for items 3 to 10 are the same. Select one answer for each item in the set.

(A) Midbrain, at level of superior colliculus
(B) Midbrain, at level of inferior colliculus
(C) Tegmentum of pons
(D) Base of pons
(E) Lateral medulla
(F) Medial medulla

Match the following structures with the appropriate brainstem division.

3. Decussation of the superior cerebellar peduncle

4. Inferior olivary nucleus

5. Nucleus ambiguus

6. Abducent nucleus

7. Facial nucleus

8. Oculomotor nucleus

9. Red nucleus

10. Trochlear nucleus

ANSWERS AND EXPLANATIONS

1–B. A lesion of the genu of the internal capsule destroys corticobulbar fibers. The facial nucleus receives bilateral corticobulbar input, the upper face division receives bilateral input, and the lower face division receives only contralateral input. The hypoglossal nucleus receives only contralateral corticobulbar input. When the tongue is protruded, it deviates to the weak side due to the unopposed activity of the intact genioglossus muscle. The uvula deviates to the intact side when the patient says ah. The muscles of the uvula and palatal arches are innervated by the vagal nerve (CN X).

2–C. The cerebral aqueduct is found in the mesencephalon; it connects the third ventricle to the fourth ventricle.

3–B. The decussation of the superior cerebellar peduncle is diagnostic of midbrain division at the level of the inferior colliculus.

4–E. The inferior olivary nucleus, a cerebellar relay nucleus, is the most prominent nucleus in the lateral medulla.

5–E. The nucleus ambiguus is found in the lateral medulla; it gives rise to the SVE components of cranial nerves IX, X, and XI.

6–C. The abducent nucleus (CN VI) is located in the dorsomedial tegmentum of the pons. All brainstem cranial nerve nuclei are found in the tegmentum.

7–C. The facial nucleus (CN VII) is located in the lateral tegmentum of the pons.

8–A. The oculomotor nucleus (CN III) lies in the dorsomedial tegmentum of the midbrain at the level of the superior colliculus; it lies medial to the medial longitudinal fasciculus.

9–A. The red nucleus is diagnostic of midbrain division at the level of the superior colliculus; it lies between the oculomotor nucleus (CN III) and the substantia nigra.

10–B. The trochlear nerve (CN IV) is located in the dorsomedial tegmentum of the midbrain at the level of the inferior colliculus.

Trigeminal System

I. Trigeminal Nerve (CN V) (Figure 10-1; see Figures 1-1, 9-1, and 9-7)

- is the largest cranial nerve.
- exits the brainstem from the pons.
- is the nerve of the first branchial arch (mandibular nerve).
- contains sensory (general somatic afferent [GSA]) and motor (special visceral efferent [SVE]) fibers.
- provides sensory innervation to the face and oral cavity.
- innervates the dura of the anterior and middle cranial fossae.
- innervates the muscles of mastication.
- consists of a large ganglion that gives rise to three major divisions: **ophthalmic**, **maxillary**, and **mandibular**.

A. **Trigeminal (or semilunar or gasserian) ganglion**
- is located in the trigeminal fossa of the petrous bone in the middle cranial fossa.
- is enclosed by a duplication of the dura (Meckel cave).
- contains pseudounipolar ganglion cells, which are first-order neurons for the trigemino-thalamic tracts.
- consists of the following divisions:
  1. **Ophthalmic nerve (CN V-1)**
      - lies in the lateral wall of the **cavernous sinus**.
      - enters the orbit via the **superior orbital fissure**.
      - innervates the forehead, dorsum of the nose, upper eyelid, orbit (cornea and conjunctiva), mucous membranes of the nasal vestibule and frontal sinus, and the cranial dura.
      - mediates the afferent limb of the **corneal reflex**.
  2. **Maxillary nerve (CN V-2)**
      - lies in the lateral wall of the **cavernous sinus**.
      - exits the skull via the **foramen rotundum**.
      - innervates the upper lip and cheek, lower eyelid, anterior portion of the temple, paranasal sinuses, oral mucosa of the upper mouth, nose, pharynx, gums, teeth, hard palate, soft palate, and cranial dura.
  3. **Mandibular nerve (CN V-3)**
      - exits the skull via the **foramen ovale**.
      - consists of a motor component that innervates the **muscles of mastication** (i.e., the temporalis, masseter, and lateral and medial pterygoids); two suprahyoid muscles, the **mylohyoid** and the **anterior belly of the digastric**; and the **tensores tympani** and **veli palatini**.
      - consists of a sensory component that innervates the lower lip and chin, posterior portion of the temple, external auditory meatus and tympanic membrane, external ear, teeth of the lower jaw, oral mucosa of the cheeks and the floor of the mouth, anterior two-thirds of the tongue, temporomandibular joint, and cranial dura.

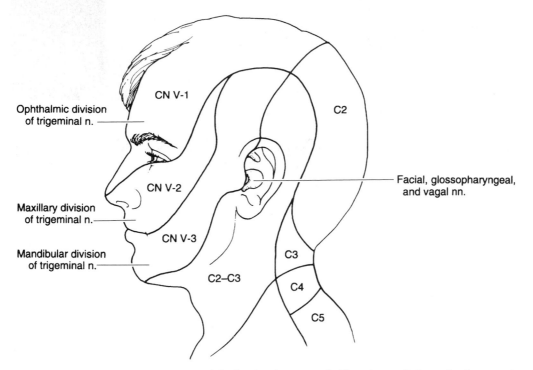

Figure 10-1. The cutaneous innervation of the head and upper neck. There is very little overlap between the three dermatomes of the trigeminal nerve (CN V). The angle of the jaw is innervated by the cervical plexus (C2–C3). CN V-1 is the ophthalmic nerve, CN V-2 is the maxillary nerve, and CN V-3 is the mandibular nerve.

B. Cranial nerves VII, IX, and X
- contribute GSA fibers from the external ear to the trigeminal system.
- use the spinal trigeminal tract and nucleus.

C. Spinal trigeminal tract
- extends from C3 to the level of the trigeminal nerve in the mid pons.
- is a homolog of the dorsolateral tract of Lissauer.
- receives pain, temperature, and light touch input from CN V, CN VII, CN IX, and CN X.
- transection (**tractotomy**) results in ipsilateral facial anesthesia.
- projects to the spinal trigeminal nucleus as follows:
  1. **Pain fibers** terminate in the caudal third of the spinal trigeminal nucleus.
  2. **Corneal reflex fibers** terminate in the rostral two-thirds of the spinal trigeminal nucleus.

II. Ascending Trigeminothalamic Tracts

- convey GSA information from the face, oral cavity, and dura mater to the thalamus.
- consist of chains of three neurons.
- have their first-order neurons, which are pseudounipolar ganglion cells, in the trigeminal ganglion and in the sensory ganglia of CN VII, CN IX, and CN X.

A. Ventral trigeminothalamic tract (Figure 10-2)
- serves as a pain, temperature, and light touch pathway from the face and oral cavity.
- contains GSA fibers from CN VII, CN IX, and CN X (ear and external auditory meatus).
- receives input from free nerve endings and Merkel tactile disks.
- receives discriminative tactile and pressure input from the contralateral principal sensory nucleus of CN V, which terminates in the ventral posteromedial (**VPM**) nucleus of the thalamus.

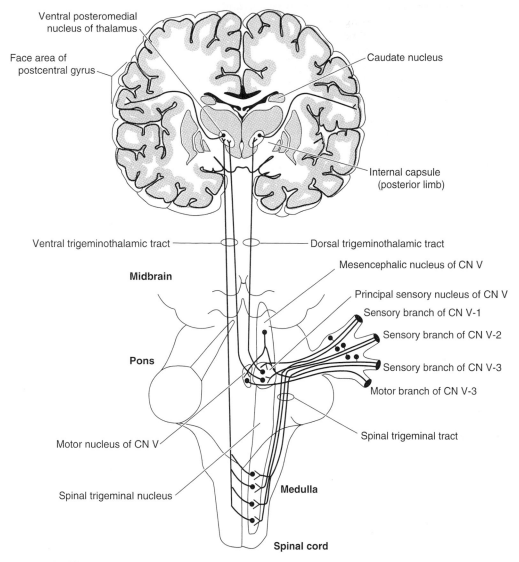

Figure 10-2. The ventral (pain and temperature) and dorsal (discriminative touch) trigeminothalamic pathways. *CN* = cranial nerve. (Reprinted with permission from Fix JD: *High-Yield Neuroanatomy,* 3rd ed. Philadelphia, Lippincott Williams & Wilkins, 2005, p 79.)

- ascends to the contralateral sensory cortex via three neurons:
  1. **First-order neurons**
     - are located in the trigeminal ganglion.
     - mediate pain and temperature sensation and give rise to axons that descend in the spinal trigeminal tract.
     - mediate light touch sensation and give rise to bifurcating axons that ascend and descend in the spinal trigeminal tract.
     - synapse with second-order neurons in the spinal trigeminal nucleus.
  2. **Second-order neurons**
     - are located in the spinal trigeminal nucleus.
     - give rise to decussating axons that terminate in the contralateral VPM nucleus of the thalamus.

- project axons to the reticular formation and to motor cranial nerve nuclei to mediate reflexes (e.g., tearing and corneal reflexes).
- mediate painful stimuli and are found in the caudal third of the spinal trigeminal nucleus.
  3. **Third-order neurons**
     - are located in the VPM nucleus.
     - project via the posterior limb of the internal capsule to the face area of the postcentral gyrus (areas 3, 1, and 2).

B. **Dorsal trigeminothalamic tract** (see Figure 10-2)
  - subserves discriminative tactile and pressure sensation from the face and oral cavity via the GSA fibers of CN V.
  - contains some discriminative **GSA fibers** from CN VII, CN IX, and CN X, which innervate the ear.
  - receives input from Meissner and Pacini corpuscles.
  - is an uncrossed tract.
  - is the rostral equivalent of the dorsal column–medial lemniscus system.
  - ascends to the sensory cortex via three neurons.
    1. **First-order neurons**
       - are located in the trigeminal ganglion.
       - synapse in the principal sensory nucleus of CN V.
    2. **Second-order neurons**
       - are located in the principal sensory nucleus of CN V.
       - project to the ipsilateral VPM nucleus of the thalamus.
    3. **Third-order neurons**
       - are located in the VPM nucleus.
       - project via the posterior limb of the internal capsule to the face area of the postcentral gyrus (areas 3, 1, and 2).

III.   Trigeminal Sensory Nuclei (see Figures 9-1, 9-7 to 9-9, and 10-2)

A. **Principal (or chief) sensory nucleus**
  - is located in the rostral pontine tegmentum at the level of the trigeminal motor nucleus of CN V.
  - receives discriminative tactile input from the face.
  - projects via the uncrossed dorsal trigeminothalamic tract to the VPM nucleus of the thalamus.
  - projects via the crossed ventral trigeminothalamic tract to the VPM nucleus of the thalamus.
  - is a homolog of the dorsal column nuclei of the medulla.

B. **Spinal trigeminal nucleus**
  - is located in the spinal cord (C1–C3), medulla, and pons.
  - receives pain and temperature input from the face and oral cavity.
  - projects via the crossed ventral trigeminothalamic tract to the VPM nucleus of the thalamus.

C. **Mesencephalic nucleus** (see Figures 9-1, 9-7 to 9-9, and 10-2)
  - subserves **GSA proprioception** from the head.
  - consists of large pseudounipolar neurons similar to those found in the trigeminal and dorsal root ganglia.
  - receives input from muscle spindles and pressure and joint receptors.
  - receives input from the muscles of mastication and extraocular muscles, the teeth and hard palate, and the temporomandibular joint.
  - projects to the trigeminal motor nucleus to mediate the muscle stretch (jaw jerk) reflex and regulate the force of bite.

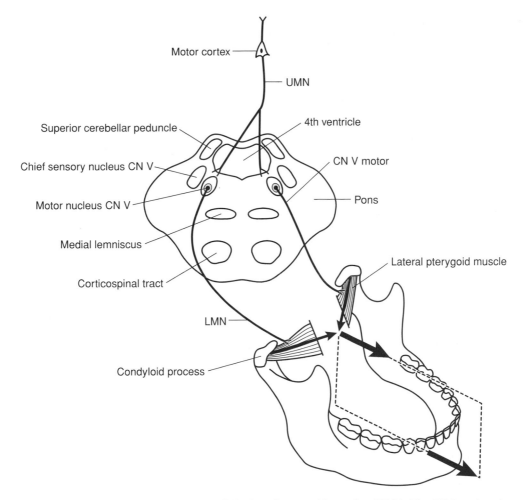

Figure 10-3. Function and innervation of the lateral pterygoid muscles (LPMs). The LPM receives its innervation from the motor nucleus of the trigeminal nerve found in the rostral pons. Bilateral innervation of the LPMs results in protrusion of the tip of the mandible in the midline. The LPMs also open the jaw. Denervation of one LPM results in deviation of the mandible to the ipsilateral, or weak, side. The trigeminal motor nucleus receives bilateral corticobulbar input. *CN* = cranial nerve; *LMN* = lower motor neuron; *UMN* = upper motor neuron. (Modified with permission from DeMyer WE: *Technique of the Neurological Examination; A Programmed Text,* 4th ed. New York, McGraw-Hill, 1994, 6 1, p. 174.)

D. Trigeminal motor nucleus (SVE) (Figure 10-3; see Figures 9-1, 9-7, and 10-2)
  - is located in the rostral pontine tegmentum at the level of the principal sensory nucleus of CN V.
  - innervates the muscles of mastication.
  - receives bilateral corticobulbar input.
  - receives input from the mesencephalic nucleus.

IV. Trigeminocerebellar Fibers

  - project from the mesencephalic nucleus of CN V via the superior cerebellar peduncle to the dentate nucleus.
  - project from the principal sensory and spinal trigeminal nuclei via the inferior cerebellar peduncle to the cerebellar vermis.

V.   Trigeminal Reflexes

A. **Jaw jerk (masseter) reflex** (Figure 10-4)
   - is a monosynaptic myotatic reflex.
     1. The **afferent limb** is the mandibular nerve (**CN V-3**).
     2. The **efferent limb** is the mandibular nerve (**CN V-3**).

B. **Corneal reflex**
   - is a consensual and disynaptic reflex.
   - has its first-order neuron (afferent limb) in the trigeminal ganglion.
   - has its second-order neuron in the rostral two-thirds of the spinal trigeminal nucleus.
   - has its third-order neuron (efferent limb) in the facial nucleus.
     1. The **afferent limb** is the ophthalmic nerve (**CN V-1**).
     2. The **efferent limb** is the facial nerve (**CN VII**).

C. **Lacrimal (tearing) reflex**
   1. The **afferent limb** is the ophthalmic nerve (**CN V-1**); it receives impulses from the cornea and conjunctiva.
   2. The **efferent limb** is the facial nerve (**CN VII**). It transmits impulses via the superior salivatory nucleus, greater petrosal nerve, pterygopalatine ganglion, and the zygomatic (CN V-2) and lacrimal (CN V-1) nerves to the lacrimal gland (see Figure 13-5).

VI.   Clinical Correlations

A. **Trigeminal neuralgia (tic douloureux)**
   - is characterized by recurrent paroxysms of **sharp, stabbing pain** in one or more branches of the trigeminal nerve on one side of the face.
   - usually occurs after 50 years of age and is more common in women than in men.
   - can result from a redundant loop of the superior cerebellar artery that impinges on the trigeminal root. Surgery is the treatment of choice.
   - **Carbamazepine**, a **tricyclic compound** related to **imipramine**, is the drug of choice for treatment of idiopathic trigeminal neuralgia.

B. **Herpes zoster ophthalmicus**
   - is a viral infection affecting the ophthalmic nerve (CN V-1).
   - corneal ulceration with infection may result in blindness.

C. **Paratrigeminal (Raeder) syndrome**
   - is due to lesions of the trigeminal ganglion and sympathetic fibers; the lesion is usually in the parasellar region.
   - results in miosis, ptosis, facial pain (similar to trigeminal neuralgia), and trigeminal palsy.
   - may involve CN III, CN IV, and CN VI.

D. **Central lesions of the spinal trigeminal tract and nucleus**
   - may result in a **loss of sensation**, occurring in an **onion-skin distribution**.
   - The face is represented somatotopically in the spinal trigeminal nucleus as a number of semicircular territories that extend from the perioral region to the ear.
   - Fibers innervating the mouth area terminate near the obex; fibers innervating the back of the head terminate in the upper cervical levels.

E. **Acoustic neuroma (schwannoma)**
   - is an extramedullary tumor of the vestibulocochlear nerve (CN VIII) that is found in the cerebellopontine angle or in the internal acoustic meatus.

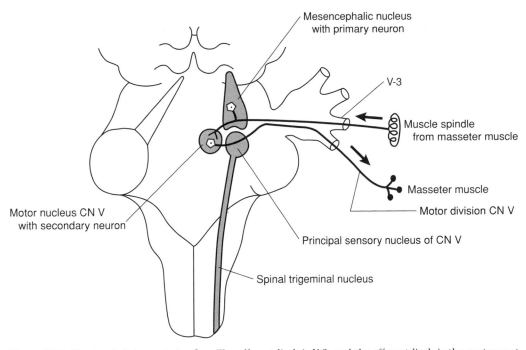

Figure 10-4. The jaw jerk (masseter) reflex. The afferent limb is V-3, and the efferent limb is the motor root that accompanies V-3. First-order sensory neurons are located in the mesencephalic nucleus. The jaw jerk reflex, like all muscle stretch reflexes, is a monosynaptic myotactic reflex. Hyperreflexia indicates an upper motor neuron lesion. *CN* = cranial nerve. (Modified with permission from Fix JD: *High-Yield Neuroanatomy*, 3rd ed. Philadelphia, Lippincott Williams & Wilkins, 2005, p 80.)

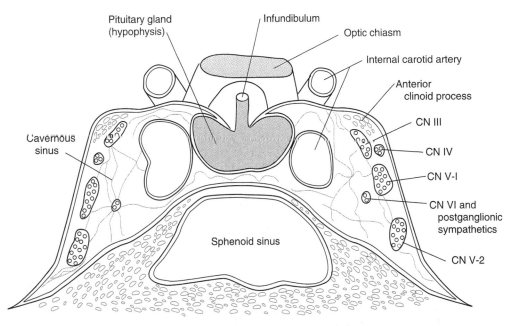

Figure 10-5. Diagram of the contents of the cavernous sinus. The wall of the cavernous sinus contains the ophthalmic (CN V-1) and maxillary (CN V-2) divisions of the trigeminal nerve (CN V) and the trochlear (CN IV) and oculomotor (CN III) nerves. The siphon of the internal carotid artery and the abducent nerve (CN VI) along with postganglionic sympathetic fibers lie within the cavernous sinus. (Modified with permission from Fix JD: *High-Yield Neuroanatomy*, 3rd ed. Philadelphia, Lippincott Williams & Wilkins, 2005, p 81.)

- results in initial symptoms that include unilateral **tinnitus** and unilateral **hearing loss** as a result of a CN VIII lesion.
- results in symptoms that include **facial weakness** and **loss of corneal reflex** (efferent limb) due to facial nerve (CN VII) involvement.
- affects the spinal trigeminal tract as the tumor expands, resulting in ipsilateral **loss of pain and temperature sensation** and **loss of the corneal reflex.**

F. **Cavernous sinus syndrome (Figure 10-5)**
- may be caused by an aneurysm of the cavernous sinus.
- may involve any or all of the following cranial nerves:
    1. **Ocular motor nerves CN III, CN IV, and CN VI**
        - Destruction of CN III results in complete **internal ophthalmoplegia** (parasympathetic paresis).
    2. **Trigeminal nerve branches of CN V-1 and CN V-2**
    3. **Postganglionic sympathetic fibers to the orbit**
        - Interruption results in **Horner syndrome.**

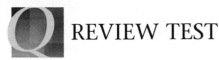

REVIEW TEST

1. A 55-year-old patient with idiopathic trigeminal neuralgia reports sharp, stabbing pain in the upper lip and nose. Which branch of the trigeminal nerve is affected?

(A) Ophthalmic
(B) Maxillary
(C) Mandibular
(D) Lacrimal
(E) Corneal

2. What is the treatment drug of choice for the patient in question 1?

(A) Carbamazepine
(B) Lamotrigine
(C) Clonazepam
(D) Gabapentin
(E) Clobazam

3. The dorsal trigeminothalamic tract is a pathway for which type of sensation?

(A) Light touch
(B) Extreme pain
(C) Discriminative tactile
(D) Hot temperature
(E) Cold temperature

4. Which of the following muscles opens the jaw?

(A) Buccinator
(B) Temporalis
(C) Masseter
(D) Medial pterygoid
(E) Lateral pterygoid

5. The auricle (pinna) of the external ear is innervated by which of the following nerves?

(A) V-3
(B) V-2
(C) V-1
(D) III
(E) VIII

6. An absent lacrimal reflex indicates problems with which two cranial nerves?

(A) V, VII
(B) III, VII
(C) VII, X
(D) II, V
(E) V, VIII

7. Destruction of which cranial nerve results in complete internal ophthalmoplegia?

(A) I
(B) II
(C) III
(D) IV
(E) V

ANSWERS AND EXPLANATIONS

1–B. The maxillary branch of the trigeminal nerve (CN V-2) innervates the upper lip and cheek, lower eyelid, anterior portion of the temple, paranasal sinuses, oral mucosa of the upper mouth, nose, pharynx, gums, teeth hard palate, soft palate, and cranial dura.

2–A. Carbamazepine is the drug of choice for treatment of idiopathic trigeminal neuralgia. It, along with lamotrigine, clonazepam, gabapentin, and clobazam, is also used to treat seizure disorders.

3–C. The dorsal trigeminothalamic tract subserves discriminative tactile and pressure sensation from the face and oral cavity via the GSA fibers of the trigeminal nerve (CN V). Pain, temperature, and light touch sensations are conveyed via the ventral trigeminothalamic tract.

4–E. The lateral pterygoid muscle is one of four muscles of mastication. Unlike the other muscles, it opens the mouth by depressing the jaw. It also helps the medial pterygoid muscles in moving the jaw from side to side. The temporalis, medial pterygoid, and masseter muscles work to close the jaw. The muscles of mastication are innervated by the trigeminal motor nucleus (SVE).

5–A. The mandibular nerve, CN V-3, is a division of the trigeminal nerve (CN V) and innervates the external ear, external auditory meatus and tympanic membrane, lower lip and chin, posterior portion of the temple, teeth of the lower jaw, oral mucosa of the cheeks, floor of the mouth, anterior two-thirds of the tongue, temporomandibular joint and cranial dura.

6–A. The lacrimal reflex involves the first branch of the trigeminal nerve, the ophthalmic nerve (CN V-1), and the facial nerve (CN VII). The afferent limb is CN V-1, receiving impulses from the cornea and conjunctiva. The efferent limb is CN-VII, transmitting impulses via the superior salivatory nucleus, greater petrosal nerve, pterygopalatine ganglion, and the zygomatic and lacrimal nerves to the lacrimal gland (see Figure 13-5).

7-E. Destruction of CN III results in complete internal ophthalmoplegia, which is paralysis of the pupillary sphincter and ciliary muscle.

Auditory System

I. Introduction: The Auditory System

- is an exteroceptive special somatic afferent (SSA) system.
- detects sound frequencies from 20 Hz to 20,000 Hz.
- ordinary conversation ranges between 300 and 3000 Hz.
- functions over an intensity range of 120 decibels (dB) and can discriminate changes in intensity between 1 dB and 2 dB.
- is characterized by tonotopic (pitch) localization at all levels of the neuraxis.
- there is a loss of high-frequency tones with advanced age.

II. Outer, Middle, and Inner Ear

A. Outer ear
- consists of an **auricle** and an external auditory **meatus**.
- is separated from the middle ear by the **tympanic membrane**.
- conducts sound waves to the tympanic membrane.
- Blockage (with wax) causes conduction deafness.

B. Middle ear (tympanic cavity)
- is located within the temporal bone.
- serves as an amplifier and impedance-matching device.
- communicates with the nasopharynx via the auditory tube.
- receives its blood supply from the stylomastoid branch of the occipital or posterior auricular artery.
- receives sensory innervation mediated by the glossopharyngeal nerve (cranial nerve [CN] IX).
- contains the **chorda tympani** of CN VII, which mediates taste sensation and parasympathetic input into the submandibular and sublingual glands.
- Pathology results in conduction deafness.
- contains the following auditory structures:
  1. **Tympanic membrane**
     - receives airborne sound vibrations and transmits energy to the middle ear ossicles.
  2. **Middle ear ossicles**
     - consist of the **malleus, incus**, and **stapes**.
     - Vibration of the tympanic membrane forces the footplate of the stapes into the oval window, creating a traveling wave in the perilymph-filled scala vestibuli.
  3. **Tensor tympani and stapedius muscles**
     - are innervated by the trigeminal and facial nerves (CN V and CN VII), respectively.
     - dampen vibrations of the ossicular chain, thus protecting the cochlea from loud low-frequency sounds (<1000 Hz).

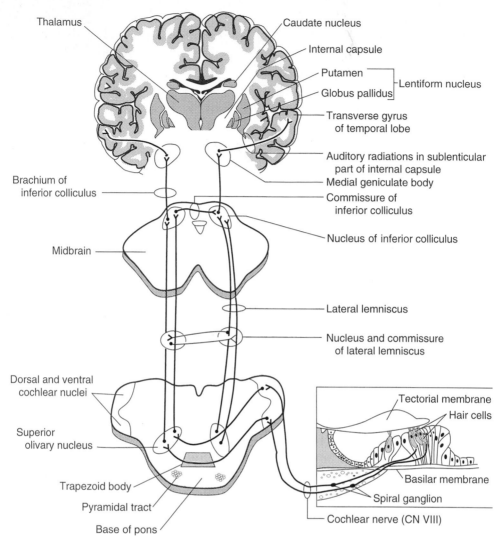

Figure 11-1. Peripheral and central connections of the auditory system. This system arises from the hair cells of the organ Corti and terminates in the transverse temporal gyri of Heschl of the superior temporal gyrus. It is characterized by bilaterally of projections and tonotopic localization of pitch at all levels. For example, high pitch (20,000 Hz) is localized at the base of the cochlea and in the posteromedial part of the transverse temporal gyri. *CN* = cranial nerve. (Modified with permission from Fix JD: *High-Yield Neuroanatomy*, 3rd ed. Philadelphia, Lippincott Williams & Wilkins, 2005, p 83.)

C. **Inner ear (membranous labyrinth)** (Figure 11-1)
- is derived from the otic placode of the rhombencephalon.
- is located within the **bony labyrinth** of the temporal bone.
- receives its blood supply from the labyrinthine artery, usually a branch of the anterior inferior cerebellar artery.
- contains the **cochlea**, which houses the following structures:
  1. **Scala vestibuli**
     - contains **perilymph**.
     - transmits traveling waves toward the **helicotrema**, **scala tympani**, and **round window**. Traveling waves extend to the portion of the basilar membrane that has the same resonant frequency, through the basilar membrane, and via the scala tympani to the round window.

2. **Cochlear duct (scala media)**
   - contains the organ of Corti.
   - contains **endolymph**.
   - lies between the scala vestibuli and scala tympani.
3. **Organ of Corti**
   - contains hair cells and the tectorial membrane.
   - rests on and is supported by the basilar membrane.
   - is a frequency analyzer.
4. **Hair cells**
   - are auditory receptor cells that have **stereocilia** (microvilli) and no kinocilium. The stereocilia are embedded in the overlying tectorial membrane.
   - are mechanoreceptors that transduce mechanical (sound) energy into generator potentials.
   - are stimulated by vibrations of the basilar membrane.
   - are innervated by bipolar neurons of the spiral ganglion.
   - receive efferent input via the olivocochlear bundle.
5. **Basilar membrane**
   - separates the cochlear duct from the scala tympani.
   - has a pitch localization along its length: 20 Hz at the apex and 20,000 Hz at the base of the cochlea.
   - Vibration results in deformation of the hair cell microvilli against the tectorial membrane; this action serves as the adequate stimulus.
6. **Spiral ganglion (of CN VIII)**
   - is located in the **bony modiolus** of the cochlea.
   - consists of bipolar neurons of the cochlear division of the vestibulocochlear nerve (CN VIII).

III. Auditory Pathway (see Figure 11-1)

- is characterized by reciprocal connections throughout its caudorostral extent and by multiple decussations at all levels.
- consists of the following structures:

A. Hair cells of the organ of Corti
- are innervated by peripheral processes of bipolar cells of the spiral ganglion.
- consists of two types:
  1. **Inner hair cells**
     - synapse with numerous afferent fibers, each of which makes contact with only one hair cell; the majority of fibers in the cochlear nerve come from the inner hair cells.
  2. **Outer hair cells**
     - synapse with afferent fibers that contact numerous other outer hair cells.
     - outnumber the inner hair cells three to one.

B. Bipolar cells of the spiral (cochlear) ganglion
- project peripherally to hair cells of the organ of Corti.
- project centrally as the **cochlear nerve** to the dorsal and ventral cochlear nuclei of the medullopontine junction.

C. Cochlear nerve (CN VIII) (see Figures 1-1, 9-5, and 11-1)
- extends from the spiral ganglion to the cerebellopontine angle, where it enters the brainstem.

D. Cochlear nuclei
- are the only auditory nuclei that do not receive binaural input.
- Damage results in unilateral deafness.

   1. **Dorsal cochlear nucleus**
      - underlies the acoustic tubercle of the floor of the fourth ventricle.
      - receives input from the cochlear nerve (CN VIII).
      - projects contralaterally to the lateral lemniscus.
   2. **Ventral cochlear nucleus**
      - receives input from the cochlear nerve (CN VIII).
      - projects bilaterally to the superior olivary nuclei.
      - projects contralaterally to the lateral lemniscus.
      - gives rise to the trapezoid body (ventral acoustic striae).

E. **Superior olivary nucleus**
   - is located in the pons at the level of the facial nucleus.
   - receives input from ventral cochlear nuclei.
   - projects bilaterally to the lateral lemniscus.
   - plays a role in sound localization and binaural processing.
   - gives rise to the efferent olivocochlear bundle, a cochlear feedback pathway.

F. **Trapezoid body**
   - is located in the caudal pontine tegmentum at the level of the abducent nucleus.
   - is transversed by intra-axial abducent fibers of CN VI.
   - contains decussating fibers from the ventral cochlear nucleus.

G. **Lateral lemniscus**
   - receives input from the contralateral cochlear nuclei.
   - receives input from the superior olivary nuclei.
   - is connected to the contralateral lateral lemniscus via commissural fibers.
   - projects to the nucleus of the inferior colliculus.

H. **Nucleus of the inferior colliculus**
   - receives input from the lateral lemniscus.
   - projects via the **brachium of the inferior colliculus** to the medial geniculate body.
   - projects to the superior colliculus to mediate audiovisual reflexes.

I. **Medial geniculate body** (see Figures 1-6 and 11-1)
   - receives input from the nucleus of the inferior colliculus.
   - projects via the **auditory radiation** to the primary auditory cortex, the transverse gyri of Heschl (areas 41 and 42).
   - projects to the amygdala.

J. **Auditory radiation** (see Figures 11-1 and 16-3)
   - extends from the medial geniculate body via the posterior limb of the internal capsule to the transverse gyri of Heschl.

K. **Transverse temporal gyri of Heschl** (see Figure 11-1)
   - contain the primary auditory cortex (areas 41 and 42).
   - are located in the depths of the lateral sulcus.
   - receive auditory input via the auditory radiation.
   - project to the auditory association cortex (area 22).

IV.   Efferent Cochlear (Olivocochlear) Bundle

- is a crossed and uncrossed tract that arises from the superior olivary nucleus and projects to the hair cells of the organ of Corti.
- suppresses auditory nerve activity when stimulated.
- plays a role, through inhibition, in "auditory sharpening."

V. Hearing Defects

- may be classified as:

A. Conduction deafness
- is caused by interruption of the passage of sound waves through the external or middle ear.
- includes the following causes:
    1. **Obstruction by wax (cerumen) or a foreign body** in the external auditory meatus
    2. **Otosclerosis**
        - is produced by neogenesis of the labyrinthine spongy bone around the oval window, resulting in fixation of the stapes.
        - is the most frequent cause of progressive conduction deafness.
    3. **Otitis media**
        - is an **inflammation of the middle ear.**
        - is the most common cause of meningitis (excluding meningococcus) and the most common cause of brain abscesses.

B. Nerve deafness (sensorineural or perceptive deafness)
- is due to **disease** of the cochlea, cochlear nerve, or central auditory connections (acoustic neuroma).
- may result from the **action of drugs and toxins** (e.g., quinine, aspirin, streptomycin).
- may result from **prolonged exposure to loud noise** (industrial noise or rock music [high-frequency loss]).
- may result from **rubella infection in utero**, cytomegalovirus, and syphilis.
- includes the following:
    1. **Presbycusis**
        - is **hearing loss occurring with aging**. It results from degenerative disease of the organ of Corti in the first few millimeters of the basal coil of the cochlea (high-frequency loss of 4000–8000 Hz).
        - is the most common cause of hearing loss.
    2. **Acoustic neuroma** (schwannoma or neurilemoma) (see Figure 14-4)
        - consists of a peripheral nerve tumor of the vestibulocochlear nerve (CN VIII).
        - is located in the internal auditory meatus or in the cerebellopontine angle of the posterior cranial fossa.
        - includes symptoms such as **unilateral deafness** and **tinnitus** (ear ringing).

VI. Tuning Fork Tests

- are used to distinguish between conduction deafness and nerve deafness (sensorineural deafness).
- compare air conduction with bone conduction.

A. Weber test (Table 11-1)
- is performed by placing a vibrating tuning fork on the vertex of the skull.
- Normal subject hears equally on both sides.
- Patient with unilateral conduction deafness hears the vibration louder in the diseased ear.
- Patient with unilateral partial nerve deafness hears the vibration louder in the normal ear.

B. Rinne test (see Table 11-1)
- compares air and bone conduction.
- is performed by placing a vibrating tuning fork on the mastoid process until it is no longer heard; then it is held in front of the ear.
- Normal subject hears vibration in the air after bone conduction is gone.

TABLE 11–1	*Tuning Fork Test Results*	
Otologic Finding	**Weber Test**	**Rinne Test**
Conduction deafness (left ear)	Lateralizes to left ear	BC > AC on left AC > BC on right
Conduction deafness (right ear)	Lateralizes to right ear	BC > AC on right AC > BC on left
Nerve deafness (left ear)	Lateralizes to right ear	AC > BC, both ears
Nerve deafness (right ear)	Lateralizes to left ear	AC > BC, both ears
Normal ears	No lateralization	AC > BC, both ears

Conduction deafness = middle ear deafness (e.g., otosclerosis, otitis media); nerve deafness = sensorineural deafness (e.g., presbycusis); AC = air conduction; BC = bone conduction.

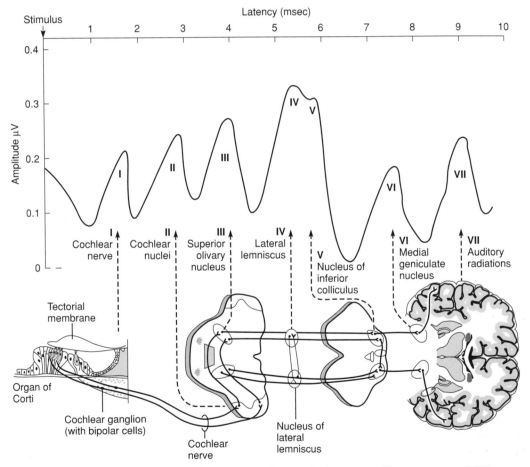

Figure 11-2. Graphic representation of brainstem auditory evoked responses. The seven waves (I–VII) correspond to way stations in the auditory pathway. (Adapted with permission from Stockard JJ, Stockard JE, Sharbrough FW: Detection and localization of occult lesions with brainstem auditory responses. *Mayo Clin Proc* 52:761–769, 1977. Modified from original drawing by Ellen Grass.)

- Patient with unilateral conduction deafness fails to hear vibrations in the air after bone conduction is gone.
- Patient with unilateral partial nerve deafness hears vibrations in the air after bone conduction is gone.

C. **Schwabach test**
- compares bone conduction of a patient with that of a person with normal hearing.
- demonstrates bone conduction to be better than normal in cases of conduction deafness.
- demonstrates bone conduction to be less than normal in cases of nerve deafness.

VII.   Brainstem Auditory Evoked Response (BAER) (Figure 11-2)

- is a noninvasive method used to evaluate the integrity of the auditory pathways.
- Clicks are delivered to the ear and recorded via scalp electrodes.
- Seven waves (I–VII) correspond to the auditory nerve, cochlear nuclei, superior olivary nucleus, lateral lemniscus, inferior colliculus, medial geniculate body, and auditory radiations.
- is used to assess hearing in young children and to diagnose brainstem lesions (multiple sclerosis) and acoustic neuromas of the posterior fossa.

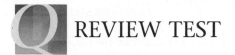

1. A 70-year-old woman has the following Weber and Rinne test results:

Test	Left Ear	Right Ear
Weber	No lateralization	Lateralization
Rinne	AC > BC	BC > AC

AC = air conduction; BC = bone conduction.

The patient's otologic findings are most consistent with which of the following conditions?

(A) Otosclerosis involving the right ear
(B) Otosclerosis involving the left ear
(C) Presbycusis involving the right ear
(D) Presbycusis involving the left ear
(E) A normal examination

2. Frequency is analyzed in the inner ear by the

(A) Stapes
(B) Tensor tympani
(C) Scala vestibuli
(D) Organ of Corti
(E) Spiral ganglion

3. Abnormal latency of wave V of a BAER test corresponds to a problem in sound transmission at what level of the auditory pathway?

(A) Nucleus of inferior colliculus
(B) Lateral lemniscus
(C) Cochlear nuclei
(D) Superior olivary nucleus
(E) Medial geniculate nucleus

4. A 2-year-old girl presents at the doctor's office with congestion and a fever of 102ºF. Her mother reports that she has been coughing and occasionally pulls at her right ear. What is the most likely diagnosis?

(A) Presbycusis
(B) Acoustic neuroma
(C) Otitis media
(D) Wax obstruction
(E) Otosclerosis

5. A 35-year-old male drummer of a heavy metal band complains of hearing loss. He reports hearing the vibration from the Weber test louder in his right ear, and his Rinne test is normal. The most likely explanation for his hearing loss is

(A) Conduction deafness caused by obstruction
(B) Nerve deafness caused by cochlear nerve disease
(C) Nerve deafness caused by prolonged exposure to noise
(D) Conduction deafness caused by otosclerosis
(E) Conduction deafness caused by exposure to heavy-metal drums

6. Presbycusis results from degeneration of the

(A) Organ of Corti
(B) Bipolar cells of the cochlear ganglion
(C) Cochlear nerve
(D) Dorsal cochlear nucleus
(E) Ventral cochlear nucleus

7. One component of the inner ear is the

(A) Organ of Corti
(B) Auricle
(C) Incus
(D) Scala vestibuli
(E) Meatus

ANSWERS AND EXPLANATIONS

1–A. The woman has otosclerosis involving the right ear. A patient with unilateral conduction deafness hears the vibration more loudly in the affected ear, and bone conduction is greater than air conduction. Otosclerosis is a conduction defect that involves the ossicles of the middle ear. The most common type of hearing loss in adults, it has a strong autosomal dominant inheritance pattern. Presbycusis, the most common cause of sensorineural hearing loss in adults, affects the cochlea or the cochlear nerve (CN VIII).

2–D. The organ of Corti, or spiral organ, is a frequency analyzer of the inner ear. It contains hair cells and the tectorial membrane; it rests on and is supported by the basilar membrane. The organ of Corti is contained within the cochlear duct.

3–A. Wave V corresponds to the nucleus of the inferior colliculus. Wave I, cochlear nerve; wave II, cochlear nuclei; wave III, superior olivary nucleus; wave IV, lateral lemniscus; wave VI, medial geniculate nucleus; and wave VII, auditory radiations.

4–C. The most likely diagnosis is otitis media, commonly known as an ear infection. Acute otitis media is often associated with upper respiratory tract infections. Children are more prone to ear infections because their eustachian tubes are shorter and more horizontal than those of adults and are therefore more easily blocked.

5–C. The most likely cause of nerve deafness, or sensorineural hearing loss, in this patient is prolonged exposure to loud noise. Because the Rinne test was normal and the Weber test lateralized to his right ear, this patient has nerve deafness in his left ear. Conduction deafness is caused by interruption of the passage of sounds waves through the external or middle ear, such as wax obstruction, otosclerosis or otitis media.

6–A. Presbycusis results from degenerative disease of the organ of Corti in the first few millimeters of the basal coil of the cochlea (high-frequency loss of 4000 to 8000 Hz). Presbycusis is hearing loss that occurs as a natural process of aging.

7–C. The middle ear contains the incus, or anvil, which together with the stapes and malleus make up the three middle ear ossicles. The middle ear also consists of the tympanic membrane, tensor tympani muscle and stapedius muscle.

Vestibular System

I. Introduction: The Vestibular System

- is a special somatic afferent (**SSA**) proprioceptive system.
- maintains **posture** and **equilibrium** and coordinates **head and eye movements**.
- functions in concert with the cerebellum and the visual system.
- contains receptors (hair cells) in the labyrinth of the temporal bone.

II. Labyrinth (Figure 12-1)

- constitutes the inner ear (**auris interna**) of the temporal bone.

A. **Structure**
   1. **Bony labyrinth**
      - is a series of cavities (cochlea, vestibule, and semicircular canals) that house the membranous labyrinth.
      - contains **perilymph**, which fills the space between the bony labyrinth and the membranous labyrinth.
   2. **Membranous labyrinth**
      - is suspended within the bony labyrinth.
      - is filled with **endolymph**.
      - is a closed system; endolymph and perilymph do not mix.
      - contains receptor (or hair) cells that are bathed in endolymph.

B. **Function**
   1. **Semicircular canal system (kinetic labyrinth)**
      - detects and responds to angular acceleration and deceleration of the head.
      - consists of **three semicircular canals**.
      - includes the following structures:
         a. **Three semicircular ducts**
            - consist of anterior, posterior, and lateral structures that lie in perpendicular planes; each semicircular duct lies within a semicircular canal.
            - contain hair cells.
         b. **Hair cells**
            - are embedded in the **cupulae of the cristae ampullares**.
            - are bathed in endolymph.
            - contain one **kinocilium** and many **stereocilia**.
            - are innervated by bipolar cells of the vestibular ganglion (Scarpa ganglion).
            - receive inhibitory input from vestibular nuclei.
            - are stimulated by endolymphatic flow. Flow toward the kinocilium and the utricle is excitatory; flow away from the kinocilium is inhibitory.

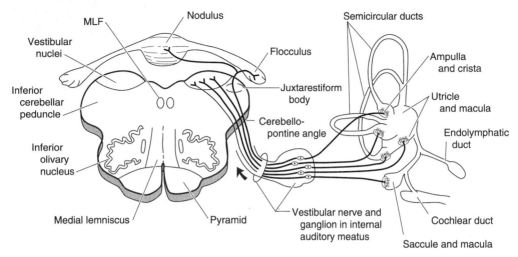

Figure 12-1. Peripheral connections of the vestibular system. The hair cells of the cristae ampullares and the maculae of the utricle and saccule project through the vestibular nerve to the vestibular nuclei of the medulla and pons and the flocculonodular lobe of the cerebellum (vestibulocerebellum). *MLF* = medial longitudinal fasciculus. (Modified with permission from Fix JD: *High-Yield Neuroanatomy,* 3rd ed. Philadelphia: Lippincott Williams & Wilkins, 2005, p 85.)

2. **Utricle and saccule (static labyrinth)**
   - detect and respond to the position of the head with respect to **linear acceleration** and pull of **gravity**.
   - are endolymph-containing dilations of the membranous labyrinth.
   - are located within the vestibule of the bony labyrinth.
   - contain hair cells in the maculae of the utricle and the saccule; they both respond to **head tilt**.
     a. **Maculae of the utricle and saccule** ("otolith organ")
        - are two patches of sensory epithelium.
        - consist of supporting cells and hair cells.
        - exert a tonic influence on the body musculature, reinforce muscle tone, and excite the muscle contractions necessary for the maintenance of equilibrium.
        - are essential to the static, postural, tonic neck, and righting reflexes.
        - The utricular macula is disposed in the horizontal plane. It is maximally stimulated when the head is bent forward or backward.
        - The saccular macula is disposed in the vertical plane. It is maximally stimulated when the head is bent to the side.
     b. **Hair cells**
        - are structurally similar to those of the cristae ampullares.
        - are embedded in the gelatinous **otolithic membrane**, which contains calcareous otolith crystals.
        - are stimulated by the shearing effect of the otolithic membrane during head movements.
        - receive an efferent innervation from the vestibular nuclei of the brainstem.

C. **Fluids of the labyrinth**
   1. **Perilymph**
      - resembles extracellular fluid and surrounds the membranous labyrinth (in the perilymphatic space).
      - communicates with the subarachnoid space via the **perilymphatic duct of the cochlear canaliculus**.
      - has an unknown site of production and absorption.

2. Endolymph
- resembles intracellular fluid and is found within the membranous labyrinth (endolymphatic space).
- is secreted by the **stria vascularis** of the cochlear duct.
- is thought to be absorbed by the **endolymphatic sac.**

III.   Vestibular Pathways (Figure 12-2; see Figure 12-1)

A. Hair cells (see II B)

B. Bipolar neurons of the vestibular ganglion (see Figure 12-1)
- are located in the fundus of the **internal auditory meatus.**
- project, via their peripheral processes, to hair cells.
- project their central processes, as the **vestibular nerve**, to the **vestibular nuclei** of the medulla and pons and via the **juxtarestiform body** to the **flocculonodular lobe** of the cerebellum (vestibulocerebellum).

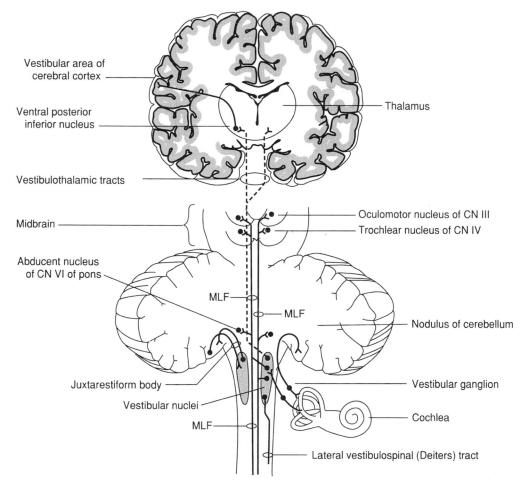

Figure 12-2.   Major central connections of the vestibular system. Vestibular nuclei project through the ascending MLFs to the ocular motor nuclei and subserve vestibulo-ocular reflexes. Vestibular nuclei also project through the descending MLFs and the lateral vestibulospinal tracts to the ventral horn motor neurons of the spinal cord and mediate postural reflexes. *CN* = cranial nerve. (Modified with permission from Fix JD: *High-Yield Neuroanatomy,* 3rd ed. Philadelphia: Lippincott Williams & Wilkins, 2005, p 86.)

C. **Vestibular nuclei** (see Figures 9-4 through 9-6)
- include the inferior, medial, superior, and lateral nuclei.
    1. **Receive input from the following structures:**
       a. Bipolar neurons of the vestibular ganglion
       b. Flocculonodular lobe and uvula of the cerebellum
       c. Vermis of the anterior lobe of the cerebellum
       d. Vestibular nuclei of the contralateral side
       e. Fastigial nuclei of the cerebellum
    2. **Project fibers to the following structures:**
       a. **Flocculonodular lobe and uvula of the cerebellum**
       b. **Vestibular nuclei of the contralateral side**
       c. **Inferior olivary nucleus**
           - receives input via the vestibulo-olivary tract.
           - mediates vestibular influence to the caudal vermis of the cerebellum.
       d. **Abducent, trochlear, and oculomotor nuclei**
           - receive input via the medial longitudinal fasciculus (**MLF**).
       e. **Ventral horn motor neurons**
           - receive vestibular input from two descending pathways:
             (1) **MLF**
                 - contains fibers from the medial vestibular nucleus that terminate in cervical and upper thoracic levels.
                 - coordinates head, neck, and eye movements.
             (2) **Vestibulospinal tract**
                 - contains fibers from the ipsilateral lateral vestibular nucleus and is found at all spinal cord levels.
                 - facilitates extensor muscle tone in the antigravity muscles, thus maintaining upright posture.
       f. **Ventral posteroinferior (VPI) and ventral posterolateral (VPL) nuclei of the thalamus**
           - receive bilateral input from the vestibular nuclei.

D. **VPI and VPL nuclei of the thalamus**
- project to the primary vestibular cortex of the parietal lobe (VPI to area 2v; VPL to area 3a).

IV. Efferent Vestibular Connections

- arise from neurons found in the vestibular nuclei.
- exit the brainstem with the vestibular nerve and innervate hair cells in the cristae ampullares and maculae of the utricle and saccule.
- are thought to modulate the spontaneous firing rate of vestibular nerve fibers.

V. Medial Longitudinal Fasciculus

- extends from the spinal cord to the rostral midbrain.
- contains ascending vestibulo-ocular fibers to the ocular motor nuclei of cranial nerve (CN) III, CN IV, and CN VI.
- contains a descending medial vestibulospinal tract that coordinates head and eye movements.
- mediates adduction of the eyeball in lateral conjugate gaze on command.
- mediates vestibular nystagmus.
- Transection results in medial rectus palsy on attempted lateral gaze; convergence is unaffected.

VI. Vestibulo-ocular Reflexes

- may be tested in conscious or unconscious subjects by stimulating the kinetic labyrinth.

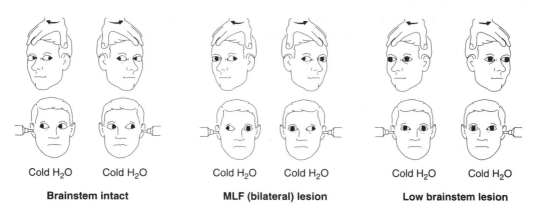

Figure 12-3. Ocular reflexes in comatose patients. The upper head shows doll's head eye movements. The external auditory meatus of the lower head is irrigated with cold water. If the brainstem is intact, the eyes deviate toward the irrigated side. If the MLFs are transected, the eyes deviate toward the side of the abducted eye only. With lower brainstem damage, the eyes do not deviate from the midline. (Adapted with permission from Plum F, Posner GB: *The Diagnosis of Stupor and Coma*, 3rd ed. Philadelphia, FA Davis, 1982, p 55.)

A. **Doll's head eye phenomenon (oculocephalic reflex)** (Figure 12-3)
   - is not present in normal alert people unless they voluntarily fix vision.
   1. **Test method**
      - consists of rapid movement of the head in horizontal or vertical planes.
   2. **Test results**
      - With intact proprioception and brainstem (vestibular nuclei), the eyes move conjugately in the opposite direction.
      - Doll's head eye movements are absent or abnormal when lesions of the vestibular nuclei and MLFs are present.

B. **Vestibular nystagmus**
   - consists of involuntary to-and-fro, up-and-down, or rotary movements of one or both eyes.
   - consists of a slow component, opposite the direction of rotation, and a fast compensatory component, in the direction of rotation.
   - is named after the fast component.
   - results from the stimulation of hair cells within the semicircular ducts on rotation or after irrigation of the external auditory meatus with hot or cold water.

C. **Postrotational nystagmus**
   1. **Test method**
      a. The subject sits in a Bárány chair with head erect and inclined 30° forward (to place horizontal canals in the plane of rotation).
      b. The subject is rotated to the right 10 turns within 20 seconds and then is suddenly stopped.
   2. **Test results in normal subjects**
      a. The subject with normal labyrinths will have a horizontal nystagmus to the left (fast phase).
      b. The subject will past-point (show dysmetria), and tend to fall to the right, and experience a sensation of turning (vertigo) to the left.
      c. The induced nystagmus usually lasts 15 to 40 seconds.

D. **Caloric nystagmus** (see Figure 12-3)
   - may be induced with cold- or hot-water irrigation of the external auditory meatus.
   - may be used to stimulate each labyrinth separately.
   - may be used to evaluate unconscious patients.
   - may be used to stimulate individual semicircular canals.

1. **Test method used to stimulate the horizontal semicircular canal**
   a. While sitting erect, the subject tilts the head back 60°, or the recumbent subject elevates the head 30° from a horizontal position.
   b. Cold or hot water is syringed into the external ear canal.
2. **Test results in normal subjects**
   a. Cold-water irrigation results in nystagmus to the opposite side and past-pointing and falling to the same side.
   b. Hot water irrigation results in the reverse reactions.
   c. Remember the mnemonic **COWS** = Cold, Opposite; Warm, Same.
3. **Test results in comatose subjects**
   a. No nystagmus is seen.
   b. With the brainstem intact, the eyes deviate to the side of cold irrigation.
   c. With bilateral MLF transection, the abducting eye deviates to the side of cold irrigation.
   d. With lower brainstem damage to vestibular nuclei, the eyes do not deviate.

VII. Decerebrate and Decorticate Rigidity

- Descending vestibulospinal and pontoreticulospinal pathways play an important role in the control of extensor muscle tone.
- Transection of the brainstem or decortication results in a tremendous increase in antigravity tone.

A. **Decerebrate rigidity (posturing)**
   - results from a lesion that transects the brainstem between the red nucleus and the vestibular nuclei.
   - results from the tonic activity of the pontine reticular formation and the lateral vestibular nucleus, which activate alpha and gamma motor neurons that innervate extensor muscles.
   - is characterized by **opisthotonos**, which is extension, adduction, and hyperpronation of the arms and extension of the feet with plantarflexion.
   - is also known as **gamma rigidity** in its classic form.
   - can be abolished by section of the vestibular nerve, destruction of vestibular nuclei or the vestibulospinal tract, and dorsal or ventral rhizotomy.

B. **Decorticate rigidity (posturing)**
   - usually results from lesions of the internal capsule or the cerebral hemisphere.
   - results in posture that consists of flexion of the arm, wrist, and fingers with adduction in the upper extremity; and with extension, internal rotation, and plantarflexion in the lower extremity.
   - is characterized by a motor pattern that is typical of chronic spastic hemiplegia.
   - is known as **bilateral spastic hemiplegia**, in the form of bilateral decorticate rigidity.

VIII. Clinical Correlations

A. **Vertigo**
   - is a sensation of irregular or whirling motion; it is an **illusion of movement**.

B. **Ménière disease**
   - is an inner ear disease associated with an **increase in endolymphatic fluid pressure**.
   - is characterized by episodic attacks of vertigo, tinnitus, hearing loss, nausea, vomiting, and a sensation of fullness and pressure in the ear.
   - is characterized by the presence of horizontal nystagmus during the attack. The fast phase is to the opposite ear; past-pointing and falling occur to the affected side.

C. **Labyrinthitis**
- is characterized by **inflammation of the labyrinth**, which may result from bacterial, viral, or toxic (e.g., alcohol, quinine, salicylates) causes.
- exhibits the same symptoms seen in Ménière disease (see VIII B).

D. **Labyrinthectomy**
1. **Unilateral labyrinthectomy**
   - results in predominantly horizontal nystagmus directed to the opposite side.
2. **Bilateral simultaneous labyrinthectomy**
   - does not give rise to nystagmus.

E. **Benign positional vertigo**
- is the most common cause of recurrent vertigo.
- is elicited by certain head positions; the paroxysm of vertigo is accompanied by nystagmus.
- is not associated with hearing loss or tinnitus.
- is due presumably to **cuprolithiasis** of the posterior semicircular duct (dislocation of the utricular macular otoliths).

F. **MLF syndrome (internuclear ophthalmoplegia [INO])**
- consists of medial rectus paresis on attempted lateral gaze.
- is associated with monocular horizontal nystagmus in the abducting eye and intact convergence (this is diagnostically important).
- is usually the result of a demyelinating plaque.
- is most commonly seen in **multiple sclerosis**.

G. **Acoustic schwannoma (vestibular schwannoma)**
- arises from the vestibular nerve of CN VIII within the internal auditory canal.
- usually involves CN V, CN VII, and CN VIII.
- is found in the cerebellopontine (CP) angle.
- causes symptoms such as unilateral loss of hearing, tinnitus, and vertigo.
- is marked by a lack of response to caloric stimulation—"dead labyrinth."
- Incidence is highest in individuals 40 to 50 years of age.

REVIEW TEST

1. A 40-year-old dentist complains of headaches and inability to control his walking (gait). His physician refers him to a neurologist for further evaluation. The man remembers that 10 years ago he noticed a noise in his right ear that sounded like frying bacon. Neurologic examination reveals the following: loss of hearing on the right side; tinnitus, vertigo, and nausea; wide-based ataxic gait with lurching to the right side; dysphagia; facial weakness on the right side; sensory loss over the face on the right side; loss of the corneal reflex on the right side; absent gag reflex; and diplopia. The lesion site responsible for these neurologic deficits is the

(A) lateral medulla
(B) medial medulla
(C) lateral pons
(D) medial pons
(E) CP angle

2. Tilting the head forward would maximally stimulate the hair cells in the

(A) crista ampullaris of the anterior semicircular duct
(B) crista ampullaris of the lateral semicircular duct
(C) crista ampullaris of the posterior semicircular duct
(D) macula of the utricle
(E) macula of the saccule

3. A comatose patient's head is elevated 30° from the horizontal. Cold water is injected into the left external auditory meatus. If the brainstem is intact, which one of the following ocular reflexes do you expect to see?

(A) Horizontal nystagmus to the left
(B) Vertical upper nystagmus
(C) Horizontal nystagmus to the right
(D) Deviation of the eyes to the left
(E) Deviation of the eyes to the right

Questions 4 to 8

The response options for items 4 to 8 are the same. Select one answer for each item in the set.

(A) Ménière disease
(B) Benign positional vertigo
(C) Acoustic schwannoma
(D) MLF syndrome
(E) Multiple sclerosis

Match each characteristic with the condition it best describes.

4. Causes the symptoms of CN V, CN VII, and CN VIII

5. Is an inner ear disease associated with increased endolymphatic fluid pressure

6. Is the most common cause of INO

7. Results in cuprolithiasis of the posterior semicircular duct

8. Consists of lateral gaze palsy and monocular nystagmus

ANSWERS AND EXPLANATIONS

1–E. The acoustic neuroma (acoustic schwannoma), which represents 8% of primary intracranial neoplasms, is found in the CP angle. Each of the examination findings is evidence of a particular condition. The loss of hearing on the right side and the tinnitus indicate damage to cochlear nerve. The vertigo and nausea indicate damage to the vestibular nerve. The wide-based ataxic gait with lurching to the right indicates damage to the cerebellum. The dysphagia indicates damage to the glossopharyngeal and vagal nerves. The facial weakness on the right side indicates damage to the facial nerve. The sensory loss over the face on the right side indicates damage to the spinal trigeminal tract of CN V. The loss of the corneal reflex on the right side indicates damage to trigeminal (afferent limb) and to facial (efferent limb) nerves. The absent gag reflex indicates damage to glossopharyngeal (afferent limb) and vagal (efferent limb) nerves. The diplopia indicates damage to the abducent nerve. A large tumor can damage the pyramidal tract and the abducent nerve. The differential diagnosis should include other tumors of the CP angle (**S**chwannoma, **A**rachnoid, **M**eningioma, **E**pidermoid; remember SAME).

2–D. Tilting the head forward would maximally stimulate the hair cells in the utricle. Tilting the head to the side would maximally stimulate the hair cells in the saccule. The utricle and saccule both respond to linear acceleration and the force of gravity.

3–D. Nystagmus is not seen in comatose patients. In this case, the patient's eyes will deviate toward the side of cold water injection.

4–C. The acoustic schwannoma, which is found in the CP angle of the posterior cranial fossa, impinges on CN V, CN VII, and CN VIII. CN V lesions result in loss of pain and temperature sensation on the ipsilateral face and loss of the corneal reflex. CN VII lesions result in a lower motor neuron paralysis of the ipsilateral muscles of facial expression and loss of the corneal reflex. CN VIII lesions result in loss of hearing, nystagmus, tinnitus, nausea, vertigo, and vomiting. (See Chapter 13, Cranial Nerves.)

5–A. Ménière disease (labyrinthine vertigo) is the most common cause of true vertigo. It is characterized by abrupt attacks of vertigo, nystagmus, nausea, vomiting, tinnitus, fullness in the ear, and hearing loss. This disease is caused by a distention of the endolymphatic system (labyrinthine hydrops). Drugs used to treat motion sickness may be helpful. Destruction (decompression) of the vestibule and an endolymphatic-subarachnoid shunt have proved useful.

6–E. The most common cause of INO is multiple sclerosis. Other causes of INO are vascular insults and intraparenchymal tumors (pontine gliomas). Multiple sclerosis, a demyelinating disease of the central nervous system is characterized by the following deficits: Ocular signs (retrobulbar neuritis and INO); brainstem and cerebellar signs (deafness, vertigo, ataxia, and intention tremor); pyramidal tract signs (spastic paresis with Babinski sign); sensory disturbances (paresthesias or dysesthesias); and bladder and rectal incontinence.

7–B. Benign positional vertigo, which is more common than Ménière disease, is characterized by paroxysmal vertigo, oscillopsia, and nystagmus. It occurs as the result of assumption of certain positions of the head (i.e., lying down or rolling over in bed). Such vertigo is due to cuprolithiasis of the posterior semicircular duct—a dislocation of the otoliths that move freely with movement of the head.

The following procedure is diagnostic. The patient is moved from a sitting to a recumbent position (on an examination table), and the head is tilted 30° down over the edge of the table, then 30° to one side, and then 30° to the other side. The patient has a paroxysm of vertigo (Hallpike maneuver).

8–D. MLF syndrome (INO) consists of medial rectus palsy on attempted lateral gaze. Nystagmus in the abducting eye is evident. Convergence is intact. This syndrome is seen frequently in multiple sclerosis.

CHAPTER

13

Cranial Nerves

I. Introduction: Cranial Nerves

- are the 12 pairs of nerves that arise from the brain and supply the structures of the head and neck (Figures 13-1 through 13-3; see Figures 1-1 and 1-7).

II. Olfactory Nerve (CN I) (see Chapter 20 I and Appendix)

A. General characteristics of CN I
- is a special visceral afferent (**SVA**) nerve that mediates the **sense of smell** (olfaction).
- consists of unmyelinated axons of bipolar neurons located in the nasal mucosa, the olfactory epithelium.
- enters the skull via the foramina of the cribriform plate of the ethmoid bone.
- projects directly to the telencephalon.
- synapses with mitral and tufted cells found in the olfactory bulb, an outgrowth of the telencephalon.
- is the only cranial nerve that projects directly to the forebrain.

B. Clinical correlation: CN I damage
- results in **anosmia**, loss of olfactory sensation (e.g., ethmoid bone fracture).

III. Optic Nerve (CN II) (see Figures 1-2, 17-2, and 17-4; see Chapter 17 III B)

A. General characteristics of CN II
- is a special somatic afferent (**SSA**) nerve that subserves **vision** and **pupillary light reflexes** (the afferent limb).
- consists of axons of neurons located in the ganglion cell layer of the retina.
- enters the skull via the optic canal of the sphenoid bone.
- has axons that continue via the optic chiasm and optic tracts to the lateral geniculate body, a thalamic relay nucleus that projects to the visual cortex (area 17) of the occipital lobe.
- is **not a true peripheral nerve** but a tract of the diencephalon.
- contains fibers from the nasal retina that decussate in the optic chiasm.
- contains fibers from the temporal retina that continue ipsilaterally through the optic chiasm.
- contains axons that are myelinated by oligodendrocytes.
- is invested by the dura and pia–arachnoid membranes and lies within the subarachnoid space.

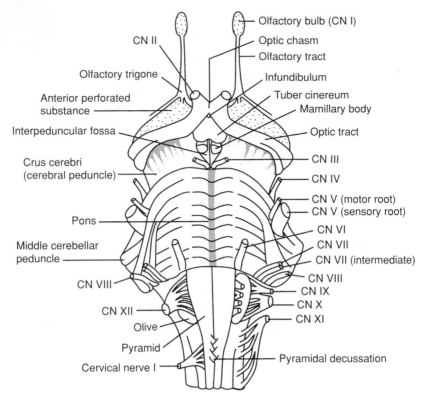

Figure 13-1. The base of the brain with attached cranial nerves (*CN*). (Reprinted with permission from Truex RC, Kellner CE: *Detailed Atlas of the Head and Neck.* New York, Oxford University Press, 1958, p 34.)

B. Clinical correlations: CN II
- When it is transected, **ipsilateral blindness** and **loss of direct pupillary light reflex** result; regeneration of the optic nerve does not occur.
- When it is subjected to increased intracranial pressure (e.g., tumor), **papilledema**, a choked optic disk results.
- When it is constricted, **optic atrophy** (i.e., axonal degeneration) results.

IV. Oculomotor Nerve (CN III) (see Figures 1-1, 1-7, and 13-3; Chapter 17)

A. General characteristics of CN III
- contains general somatic efferent (**GSE**) and general visceral efferent (**GVE**) fibers.
- is a pure motor nerve that **moves the eye, constricts the pupil, accommodates**, and con-verges.
- exits the brainstem from the interpeduncular fossa of the midbrain, passes through the lateral wall of the cavernous sinus, and enters the orbit via the superior orbital fissure.
  1. **GSE component**
     - arises from the oculomotor nucleus of the midbrain.
     - innervates four extraocular muscles and the levator palpebrae muscle. (Remember the mnemonic: **SIN, S**uperior muscles are **IN**torters of the globe.)
     a. **Medial rectus muscle**
        - adducts the eye.
        - with its opposite partner, converges the eyes.

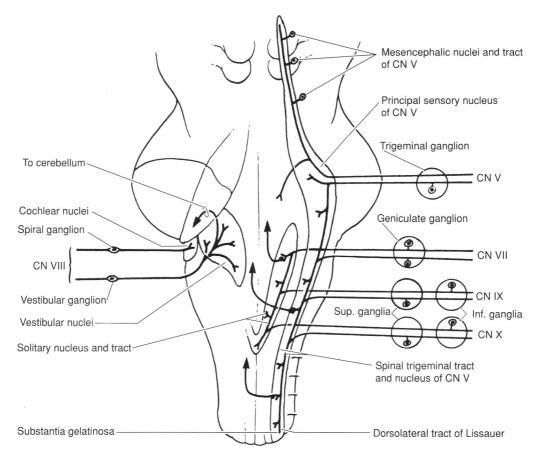

Figure 13-2. Location of the sensory cranial nerve nuclei within the brainstem. Phantom view of the brainstem from the dorsal aspect. The spinal trigeminal tract and nucleus extend into the cervical cord (C3). Three sensory areas are prominent: the special somatic afferent (SSA) area, including the cochlear and vestibular nuclei of CN VIII; the combined general visceral afferent (GVA) and SVA column, the solitary nucleus of CN VII, CN IX, and CN X; and the GSA column, including the spinal trigeminal, principal, sensory, and mesencephalic nuclei of CN V, CN VII, CN IX, and CN X. (Modified with permission from Noback CR, Demarest RJ: *The Human Nervous System.* Baltimore, Williams & Wilkins, 1991, p 222.)

      b. **Superior rectus muscle**
         • elevates, intorts, and adducts the eye.
      c. **Inferior rectus muscle**
         • depresses, extorts, and adducts the eye.
      d. **Inferior oblique muscle**
         • elevates, extorts, and abducts the eye.
      e. **Levator palpebrae muscle**
         • elevates the upper lid.
    2. **GVE component**
      a. **Composition**
         • consists of preganglionic parasympathetic fibers.
      b. **Pathway**
         • arises from the Edinger-Westphal nucleus (accessory oculomotor nucleus) of the midbrain.
         (1) **Edinger-Westphal nucleus**
            • projects to the ciliary ganglion of the orbit via CN III.

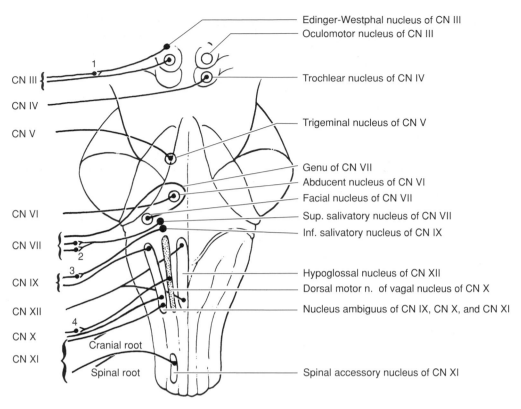

Figure 13-3. Location of motor cranial nerve nuclei within the brainstem. Three functional cell columns are visible from medial to lateral; the GSE column of CN III, CN IV, CN VI, and CN XII; the GVE column of CN III, CN VII, CN IX, and CN X; and the SVE column of CN V, CN VII, CN IX, CN X, and CN XI. Parasympathetic ganglia are indicated as *1* = ciliary ganglion; *2* = pterygopalatine and submandibular ganglia; *3* = otic ganglion; and *4* = terminal (intramural) ganglia. (Modified with permission from Noback CR, Demarest RJ: *The Human Nervous System.* Baltimore, Williams & Wilkins, 1991, p 223.)

       (2) Ciliary ganglion
- projects postganglionic parasympathetic fibers to the sphincter muscle of the iris (miosis) and to the ciliary muscle (accommodation).

B. **Clinical correlations: CN III**
   1. **Oculomotor paralysis**
- is seen frequently with **transtentorial herniation** (subdural or epidural hematoma).
- results in **diplopia** (double vision) when the patient looks in the direction of the paretic muscle.
- Denervation of the levator palpebrae muscle results in **ptosis** (drooping of the upper eyelid).
- Denervation of the extraocular muscles causes the affected eye to **look down and out** because the action of the lateral rectus and superior oblique muscles is unopposed. The superior oblique and lateral rectus muscles are innervated by CN IV and CN VI.
- Interruption of parasympathetic innervation results in a **dilated and fixed pupil** and **paralysis of accommodation (cycloplegia).**
   2. **Other conditions associated with CN III impairment**
      a. **Transtentorial (uncal) herniation**
- Increased supratentorial pressure (tumor) forces the hippocampal uncus through the tentorial notch and compresses the oculomotor nerve. Pupilloconstrictor fibers are affected first, resulting in a dilated and fixed pupil; somatic efferent fibers are affected later, resulting in an external strabismus (exotropia).

b. **Aneurysms (carotid and posterior communicating arteries)**
  • frequently compress the oculomotor nerve within the cavernous sinus or the interpeduncular cistern.
  • usually affect the peripheral pupilloconstrictor fibers first, as in uncal herniation.
c. **Diabetes mellitus (diabetic oculomotor palsy)**
  • frequently affects the oculomotor nerve, damaging the central fibers and sparing the pupilloconstrictor fibers.

V. Trochlear nerve (CN IV) (see Figures 1-7 and 13-3)

A. **General characteristics of CN IV**
  • is a pure **GSE** nerve that **innervates the superior oblique muscle**, which **depresses**, **intorts**, and **abducts** the eye.
  • arises from the contralateral trochlear nucleus of the midbrain.
  • decussates within the midbrain and exits the brainstem on its dorsal surface, caudal to the inferior colliculus.
  • encircles the midbrain in the subarachnoid space, passes through the lateral wall of the cavernous sinus, and enters the orbit via the superior orbital fissure.

B. **Clinical correlations: CN IV paralysis** (Figure 13-4)
  • results in the following conditions:
   1. **Extorsion of the eye and weakness of downward gaze**
   2. **Vertical diplopia**, which increases when looking down
   3. **Head tilting**, to compensate for extorsion

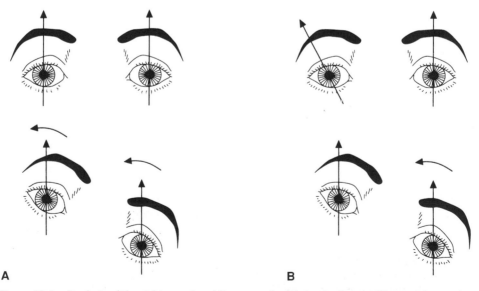

Figure 13-4. Paralysis of the right superior oblique muscle. **(A)** A pair of eyes with normal extorsion and intorsion movements. Tilting the chin to the right side results in compensatory intorsion of the left eye and extorsion of the right eye. **(B)** Paralysis of the right superior oblique muscle results in extorsion of the right eye, causing diplopia. Tilting the chin to the right side results in compensatory intorsion of the left eye, thus permitting binocular alignment.

VI. Trigeminal Nerve (CN V) (see Figures 1-1, 1-7, 10-4, 13-2, and 13-3; see Chapter 10)

A. **General characteristics of CN V**
- contains general somatic afferent (**GSA**) and special visceral efferent (**SVE**) fibers.
- innervates the **muscles of mastication** and mediates **general sensation** from the face, eye, and nasal and oral cavities.
- is the nerve of the first pharyngeal arch (mandibular).
- exits the brainstem from the pons.
- contains first-order sensory neurons in the trigeminal ganglion and in the mesencephalic nucleus.
- contains motor neurons in the motor trigeminal nucleus of the rostral pons.
- has three divisions: **ophthalmic** (CN V-1), **maxillary** (CN VI-2), and **mandibular** (CN V-3) (see Figures 10-1 and 10-2; see Chapter 10 I A 1–3).
  1. **GSA component** (see Figure 10-1)
     - provides **sensory innervation** to the face, mucous membranes of the nasal and oral cavities and frontal sinus, teeth, hard palate, soft palate, and deep structures of the head (proprioception from muscles and the temporomandibular joint).
     - innervates the dura of the anterior and middle cranial fossae.
     - innervates the external ear with CN VII, CN IX, and CN X.
  2. **SVE component**
     - innervates the **muscles of mastication** (temporalis, masseter, lateral and medial pterygoids), the **tensores tympani** and **veli palatini**, the **mylohyoid**, and the **anterior belly of the digastric muscles**.

B. **Clinical correlations: lesions of CN V**
- result in the following conditions:
  1. **Loss of general sensation** from the face and mucous membranes of the oral and nasal cavities
  2. **Loss of the corneal reflex** (afferent limb, CN V-1)
  3. **Flaccid paralysis of the muscles of mastication**
  4. **Deviation of the jaw to the weak side** due to the unopposed action of the opposite lateral pterygoid muscle
  5. **Paralysis of the tensor tympani**, leading to hypacusis (partial deafness to low-pitched sounds)

VII. Abducent Nerve (CN VI) (see Figures 1-1, 1-7, and 13-3)

A. **General characteristics of CN VI**
- is a pure **GSE** nerve that innervates the lateral rectus muscle, which **abducts the eye**.
- arises from the abducent nucleus of the caudal pons.
- exits the brainstem from the inferior pontine sulcus.
- passes through the Dorello canal and cavernous sinus and enters the orbit via the superior orbital fissure.

B. **Clinical correlations: CN VI paralysis**
- is the most common isolated muscle palsy.
- results in the following conditions:
  1. **Convergent strabismus** (**esotropia**), with inability to abduct the eye because of the unopposed action of the medial rectus muscle
  2. **Horizontal diplopia**, with maximum separation of the double images when looking toward the paretic lateral rectus muscle

VIII. Facial Nerve (CN VII) (see Figures 1-1, 1-7, 13-2, 13-3, and 13-5)

A. **General characteristics of CN VII**
- contains **GSA, SVA, SVE,** and **GVE** fibers.
- mediates **facial movements, taste, salivation,** and **lacrimation**.
- is the nerve of the second pharyngeal arch (hyoid).
- includes the **facial nerve proper** (motor division), which contains the SVE fibers that innervate the muscles of facial expression.
- includes the **intermediate nerve** (sensory division), which contains GSA, SVA, and GVE fibers. All first-order sensory neurons are found in the geniculate ganglion within the temporal bone.
- exits the brainstem in the cerebellopontine (CP) angle.
- enters the internal auditory meatus and facial canal.
- exits the facial canal and skull via the **stylomastoid foramen**.
  1. **GSA component**
     - has cell bodies in the geniculate ganglion.
     - innervates the **posterior surface of the external ear** via the posterior auricular branch of the facial nerve.
     - projects centrally to the spinal trigeminal tract and nucleus.
  2. **SVA component**
     - has cell bodies in the geniculate ganglion.
     - projects centrally to the solitary tract and nucleus.
     - innervates the **taste buds** from the anterior two-thirds of the tongue via:
     a. **Intermediate nerve**
     b. **Chorda tympani** (Figure 13-6)
        - is located in the tympanic cavity medial to the tympanic membrane and lateral to the malleus.
        - contains **SVA** and **GVA** fibers.
     c. **Lingual nerve** (a branch of CN V-3)

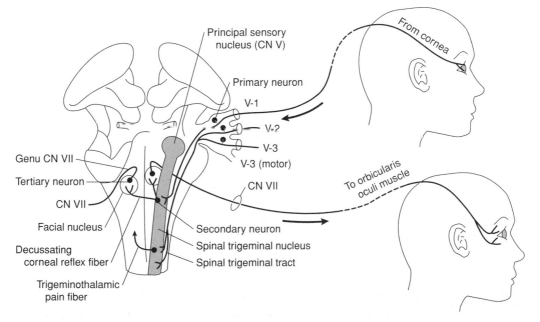

Figure 13-5. The corneal reflex pathway showing the three neurons and decussation. This reflex is consensual, like the pupillary light reflex. Second-order pain neurons are found in the caudal division of the spinal trigeminal nucleus. Second-order corneal reflex neurons are found at more rostral levels. (Reprinted with permission from Fix JD: *High-Yield Neuroanatomy,* 3rd ed. Philadelphia: Lippincott Williams & Wilkins, 2005, p 93.)

3. **GVA component**
   - has cell bodies in the geniculate ganglion.
   - innervates the soft palate and adjacent pharyngeal wall.
   - has no clinical relevance.
4. **GVE component**
   - is a parasympathetic component that innervates the **lacrimal, submandibular,** and **sublingual glands**.
   - contains preganglionic neurons in the superior salivatory nucleus of the caudal pons.
   a. **Lacrimal pathway** (see Figure 13-6)
      - begins in the superior salivatory nucleus, which projects via the intermediate nerve, the greater petrosal nerve, and the nerve of the pterygoid canal to the pterygopalatine ganglion.
      - continues as the postganglionic neurons of the pterygopalatine ganglion project through the inferior orbital fissure and via the zygomatic nerve (a branch of CN V-2) and the lacrimal nerve (a branch of CN V-1) to innervate the lacrimal gland.
   b. **Submandibular pathway** (see Figure 13-6)
      - begins in the superior salivatory nucleus, which projects via the intermediate nerve and chorda tympani to the submandibular ganglion.
      - continues as the postganglionic neurons of the submandibular ganglion, which project to and innervate the submandibular and sublingual glands.

[Au: Okay?]

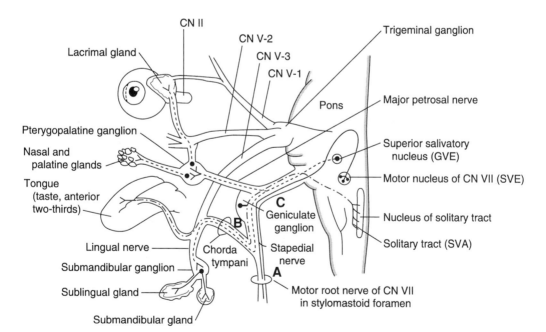

Figure 13-6. Functional components of the facial nerve (CN VII). The intermediate nerve is the sensory and visceromotor division of the seventh nerve. A, B, and C indicate three lesions of the nerve. Lesion A is at the stylomastoid foramen and spares lacrimation, nasal and palatine secretion, taste to the anterior two-thirds of the tongue, salivation, and the stapedial reflex; the patient has a lower motor neuron lesion involving the muscles of facial expression. Lesion B is between the geniculate ganglion and the chords tympani and spares lacrimation and secretion from the nasal palatine glands. Lesion C is proximal to the geniculate ganglion and is total. *GVE* = general visceral efferent; *SVA* = special visceral afferent; *SVE* = special visceral efferent.

5. **SVE component**
- arises from the facial nucleus of the caudal pons and exits the brainstem in the CP angle.
- enters the internal auditory meatus, traverses the facial canal, sends a branch to the stapedius muscle of the middle ear, and exits the skull via the stylomastoid foramen.
- innervates the **muscles of facial expression**, the **stylohyoid muscle**, the **posterior belly of the digastric muscle**, and the **stapedius muscle**.

B. **Clinical correlations: lesions of CN VII** (see Figure 13-6)
- result in the following conditions:
  1. **Flaccid paralysis** of the muscles of facial expression (upper and lower face)
  2. **Loss of the corneal (blink) reflex** (efferent limb), which may lead to corneal ulceration (keratitis paralytica)
  3. **Loss of taste** (ageusia) from the anterior two-thirds of the tongue
  4. **Hyperacusis** (increased acuity to sounds), due to stapedius paralysis
  5. **Bell palsy** (see Figure 9-11)
     - is caused by trauma to the nerve within the facial canal.
     - is a lower motor neuron (LMN) lesion with paralysis of all muscles of facial expression.
  6. **Bell phenomenon**
     - is seen in Bell palsy.
     - occurs when trying to close the eyes—the affected eye looks up and out.
  7. **Central facial palsy** (supranuclear palsy)
     - results from transection of corticobulbar fibers in the internal capsule.
     - results in contralateral facial weakness below the orbit.
     - is an upper motor neuron (UMN) lesion affecting the muscles of the lower face.
  8. **Crocodile tears syndrome** (lacrimation during eating)
     - is caused by a facial nerve lesion proximal to the geniculate ganglion. Regenerating preganglionic salivatory fibers are misdirected to the pterygopalatine ganglion, which projects to the lacrimal gland.
  9. **Möbius syndrome** (congenital oculofacial paralysis)
     - consists of a congenital facial diplegia (CN VII) and a convergent strabismus (CN VI).

IX. Vestibulocochlear Nerve (CN VIII) (see Figures 1-1, 1-7, and 13-2)

- **maintains balance** and **mediates hearing.**
- **consists of two** functional divisions: the **vestibular nerve** and the **cochlear nerve.**
- is a pure **SSA** nerve.
- exits the brainstem at the CP angle.
- enters the internal auditory meatus and is confined to the temporal bone.

A. **Vestibular nerve** (see Chapters 11 II C 6 and 12 I)
  1. **General characteristics of the vestibular nerve**
     - plays a role in **equilibrium** and **balance**.
     - is associated functionally with the cerebellum (flocculonodular lobe).
     - regulates **compensatory eye movements**.
     - has first-order sensory bipolar neurons in the vestibular ganglion of the internal auditory meatus.
     - projects peripheral processes to the hair cells of the cristae ampullares of the semicircular ducts and to hair cells of the utricular and saccular maculae.
     - projects central processes to the four vestibular nuclei of the brainstem and to the flocculonodular lobe of the cerebellum.
     - conducts efferent fibers to hair cells from the brainstem.
  2. **Clinical correlation: lesions of the vestibular nerve**
     - result in **disequilibrium**, **vertigo**, and **nystagmus**.

B. Cochlear nerve (see Chapter 11 III C)

1. **General characteristics of the cochlear nerve**
   - serves **audition** (hearing).
   - has first-order sensory bipolar neurons in the spiral (cochlear) ganglion of the modiolus of the cochlea, within the temporal bone.
   - projects peripheral processes to the hair cells of the organ of Corti.
   - projects central processes to the dorsal and ventral cochlear nuclei of the brainstem.
   - conducts efferent fibers to the hair cells from the brainstem.

2. **Clinical correlations: lesions of the cochlear nerve** (see Chapter 11 V B 2)
   - result in **hearing loss** (sensorineural deafness) (destructive lesions).
   - cause **tinnitus** (irritative lesions).

X. Glossopharyngeal Nerve (CN IX) (see Figures 1-1, 1-7, 13-2, and 13-3)

A. General characteristics of CN IX
- contains GSA, GVA (general visceral afferent), SVA, SVE, and GVE components.
- mediates **taste** (gustation), **salivation**, and (with CN X and CN XII) **swallowing**.
- mediates **input from the carotid sinus**, which contains baroreceptors that monitor arterial blood pressure.
- mediates **input from the carotid body**, which contains chemoreceptors that monitor the carbon dioxide and oxygen concentration of the blood.
- is the nerve of the third pharyngeal arch.
- is predominantly a sensory nerve.
- exits the brainstem (medulla) from the postolivary sulcus with CN X and CN XI.
- exits the skull via the jugular foramen with CN X and CN XI.

1. **GSA component**
   - innervates **part of the external ear** and the **external auditory meatus** via the auricular branch of the vagus nerve.
   - has cell bodies in the superior ganglion.
   - projects its central processes to the spinal trigeminal tract and nucleus.

2. **GVA component**
   - innervates **structures derived from the endoderm** (e.g., pharynx [foregut]).
   - innervates the **mucous membranes of the posterior third of the tongue, tonsil, upper pharynx** (soft palate), **tympanic cavity**, and **auditory tube**.
   - innervates the **carotid sinus** (baroreceptors) and the **carotid body** (chemoreceptors) via the sinus nerve.
   - has cell bodies in the inferior (petrosal) ganglion.
   - is the afferent limb of the gag reflex and the carotid sinus reflex.

3. **SVA component**
   - innervates the **taste buds** of the posterior third of the tongue.
   - has cell bodies in the inferior (petrosal) ganglion.
   - projects its central processes to the solitary tract and nucleus.
   - is the most important nerve for taste sensation.

4. **SVE component**
   - innervates the **stylopharyngeus muscle**.
   - arises from the nucleus ambiguus of the lateral medulla.

5. **GVE component**
   - is a parasympathetic component that innervates the **parotid gland**.
   - consists of preganglionic neurons in the inferior salivatory nucleus of the medulla that project, via the tympanic nerve and via the lesser petrosal nerve, through the innominate canal to the otic ganglion; postganglionic fibers from the otic ganglion project to the parotid gland via the auriculotemporal nerve (CN V-3).

B. **Clinical correlations: lesions of CN IX**
1. **Loss of the gag (pharyngeal) reflex** (interruption of afferent limb)
2. **Loss of the carotid sinus reflex** (interruption of the sinus nerve)
3. **Loss of taste from the posterior third of the tongue**
4. **Glossopharyngeal neuralgia**

XI. Vagal Nerve (CN X) (see Figures 1-1, 1-7, 13-2, and 13-3)

A. **General characteristics of CN X**
- contains **GSA, GVA, SVA, SVE,** and **GVE** components.
- mediates **phonation, swallowing** (with CN IX and CN XII), **elevation of the palate,** and **taste.**
- innervates **viscera of the neck, thorax,** and **abdomen.**
- is the nerve of the fourth and sixth branchial arches.
- exits the brainstem (medulla) from the postolivary sulcus.
- exits the skull via the jugular foramen with CN IX and CN XI.
  1. **GSA component**
     - innervates the **infratentorial dura** (with C2 and C3) **posterior surface of the external ear, external auditory meatus,** and **tympanic membrane.**
     - has cell bodies in the superior (jugular) ganglion.
     - projects its central processes to the spinal trigeminal tract and nucleus.
  2. **GVA component**
     - innervates the **mucous membranes** of the **pharynx, larynx, esophagus, trachea,** and **thoracic and abdominal viscera** (to the left colic flexure).
     - has cell bodies in the inferior (nodose) ganglion.
     - projects its central processes to the solitary tract and nucleus.
  3. **SVA component**
     - innervates the **taste buds** in the **epiglottis.**
     - has cell bodies in the inferior (nodose) ganglion.
     - projects its central processes to the solitary tract and nucleus.
  4. **SVE component**
     - innervates the **pharyngeal arch muscles of the larynx and pharynx, striated muscle of the upper esophagus, muscle of the uvula,** and **levator veli palatini** and **palatoglossus muscles.**
     - receives SVE input from the cranial division of the spinal accessory nerve (CN XI).
     - arises from the nucleus ambiguus in the lateral medulla.
     - provides the efferent limb of the gag reflex.
  5. **GVE component** (see Figure 18-2)
     - innervates the **viscera of the neck** and the **thoracic and abdominal cavities** as far as the left colic flexure.
     - consists of preganglionic parasympathetic neurons in the dorsal motor nucleus of the medulla, which project to the intramural ganglia of the visceral organs.
     - consists of preganglionic parasympathetic neurons in the **nucleus ambiguus** of the medulla, which project to the intramural ganglia of the heart.

B. **Clinical correlations: lesions of CN X** (Figure 13-7)
- result in the following conditions:
  1. **Ipsilateral paralysis** of the soft palate, pharynx, and larynx leading to **dysphonia** (hoarseness), **dyspnea, dysarthria,** and **dysphagia**
  2. **Loss of the gag (palatal) reflex** (efferent limb)
  3. **Anesthesia of the pharynx and larynx,** leading to unilateral loss of the cough reflex
  4. **Aortic aneurysms and tumors of the neck and thorax**
     - frequently compress the vagal nerve.

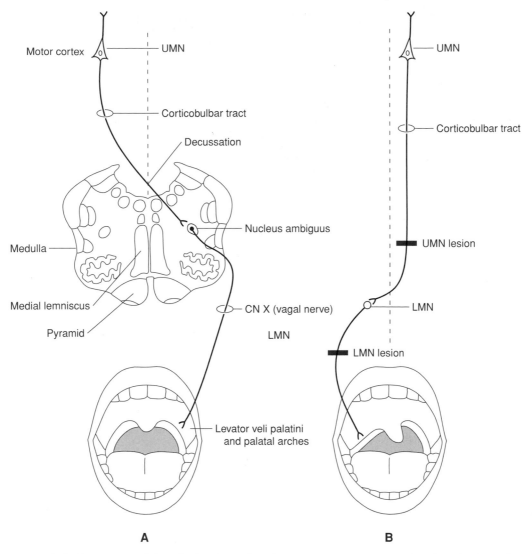

Figure 13-7. Innervation of the palatal arches and uvula. Sensory innervation is mediated by the glossopharyngeal nerve (CN IX). Motor innervation of the palatal arches and uvula is mediated by the vagus nerve (CN X). **(A)** A normal palate and uvula in a person who is saying "ah." **(B)** A patient with an upper motor neuron (*UMN*) lesion (*left*) and a lower motor neuron (*LMN*) lesion (*right*). When this patient says "ah," the palatal arches sag. The uvula deviates toward the intact (left) side. (Modified with permission from DeMyer WE: *Technique of the Neurological Examination; A Programmed Text,* 4th ed. New York, McGraw-Hill, 1994, 6–9, p. 191.)

XII. Accessory Nerve (CN XI) (Figure 13-8; see Figures 1-1, 1-7, and 13-3)

A. **General characteristics of CN XI**
- contains the **SVE** component.
- mediates **head and shoulder movement** and innervates **laryngeal muscles**.
- includes the following divisions:
  1. **Cranial division**
     - arises from the **nucleus ambiguus** of the medulla.
     - exits the medulla from the postolivary sulcus and joins the vagal nerve (CN X).

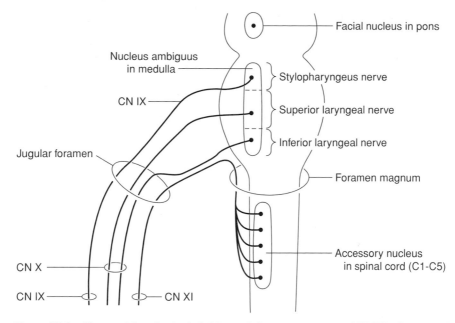

Figure 13-8. The cranial and spinal divisions of the accessory nerve (CN IX). The cranial division hitchhikes a ride with the accessory nerve, then joins the vagal nerve to become the inferior (recurrent) laryngeal nerve. The recurrent laryngeal nerve innervates the intrinsic muscles of the larynx, except for the cricothyroid muscle. The spinal division innervates the trapezoid and sternocleidomastoid muscles. Three nerves pass through the jugular foramen (glomus jugulare tumor). (Reprinted with permission from Fix JD: *High-Yield Neuroanatomy,* 3rd ed. Philadelphia: Lippincott Williams & Wilkins, 2005, p 101.)

- exits the skull via the jugular foramen with CN IX and CN X.
- innervates the **intrinsic muscles of the larynx** via the inferior (recurrent) laryngeal nerve, with the exception of the cricothyroid muscle.
2. **Spinal division**
  - arises from the ventral horn of cervical segments C1 to C6.
  - Spinal roots exit the spinal cord laterally between the ventral and dorsal spinal roots, ascend through the foramen magnum, and exit the skull via the jugular foramen.
  - innervates the **sternocleidomastoid** (with C2) and **trapezius muscles** (with C3 and C4).

B. **Clinical correlations: lesions of CN XI**
  - result in the following conditions:
    1. **Paralysis of the sternocleidomastoid muscle**
      - results in difficulty in turning the head to the side opposite the lesion.
    2. **Paralysis of the trapezius muscle**
      - results in a shoulder droop.
      - results in the inability to shrug the ipsilateral shoulder.
    3. **Paralysis of the larynx** occurs if the cranial root is involved.

XIII. Hypoglossal Nerve (CN XII) (see Figures 1-1, 1-7, and 13-3)

A. **General characteristics of CN XII**
  - mediates **tongue movement**.
  - is a pure **GSE** nerve.
  - arises from the hypoglossal nucleus of the medulla.

- exits the medulla in the preolivary sulcus.
- exits the skull via the hypoglossal canal.
- innervates **intrinsic and extrinsic muscles of the tongue**.
- has three extrinsic muscles: the genioglossus, styloglossus, and hyoglossus.

B. **Clinical correlations: CN XII** (Figure 13-9)
   - When it is transected, **hemiparalysis of the tongue** results.
   - When it is protruded, the tongue points toward the weak side due to the unopposed action of the opposite genioglossus muscle.

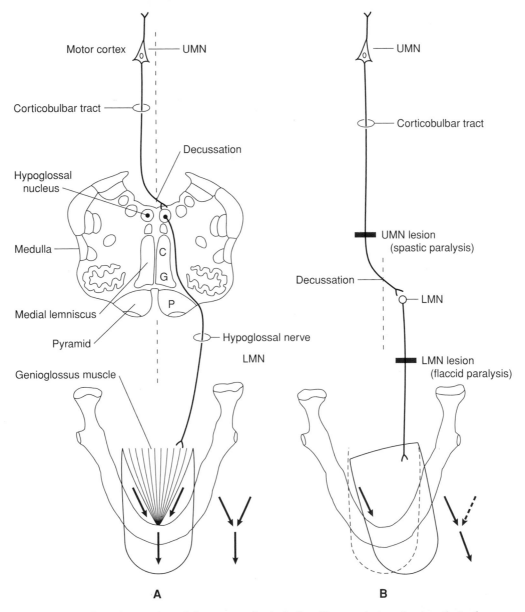

Figure 13-9. Motor innervation of the tongue. Corticobulbar fibers project predominantly to the contralateral hypoglossal nucleus. An upper motor neuron (*UMN*) lesion causes deviation of the protruded tongue to the weak (contralateral) side. A lower motor neuron (*LMN*) lesion causes deviation of the protruded tongue to the weak (ipsilateral) side. **(A)** Normal tongue. **(B)** Tongue with UMN and LMN lesions. (Modified with permission from DeMyer WE. *Technique of the Neurological Examination; A Programmed Text,* 4th ed. New York, McGraw-Hill, 1994, 6–11, p. 195.)

1. A 50-year-old family physician has vertical diplopia; the man feels unsure when descending stairs. He can eliminate the double vision by tilting his chin toward the paretic side. Which of the following extraocular muscles is responsible for the ocular malalignment?

(A) Superior rectus
(B) Inferior rectus
(C) Inferior oblique
(D) Lateral rectus
(E) Superior oblique

2. Anosmia results from damage to which cranial nerve?

(A) CN I
(B) CN II
(C) CN III
(D) CN IV
(E) CN V

3. A 50-year old retired army major complained of severe pain in the ear and throat. Pain was episodic and triggered by swallowing, chewing, coughing, and laughing. Symptoms included loss of gag (pharyngeal) reflex; analgesia and anesthesia in the region of the tonsils; and dysphagia. A lesion of which cranial nerve would produce these neurologic deficits?

(A) Facial nerve
(B) Glossopharyngeal nerve
(C) Hypoglossal nerve
(D) Trigeminal nerve
(E) Vagal nerve

4. Which cranial nerve's fibers are myelinated by oligodendrocytes?

(A) CN I
(B) CN II
(C) CN III
(D) CN VII
(E) CN X

5. A 25-year-old woman's a neck was injured in an automobile accident. At examination, she reports difficulty in turning her head away from the side of her neck that was injured. She also has a visible shoulder droop. Which nerve was likely damaged?

(A) CN VIII
(B) CN IX
(C) CN X
(D) CN XI
(E) CN XII

Questions 6 to 10

The response options for items 6 to 10 are the same. Select one answer for each item in the set.

(A) Glossopharyngeal nerve
(B) Accessory nerve
(C) Trigeminal nerve
(D) Facial nerve
(E) Vagal nerve

Match each description with the appropriate nerve.

6. Innervates the parotid gland

7. Is the efferent limb of the corneal reflex

8. Is the efferent limb of the gag reflex

9. Innervates the infratentorial dura

10. Is a pure motor nerve

Questions 11 to 16

The response options for items 11 to 16 are the same. Select one answer for each item in the set.

(A) Foramen jugular
(B) Innominate canal
(C) Foramen magnum
(D) Foramen ovale
(E) Foramen rotundum
(F) Foramen spinosum
(G) Foramen stylomastoideum
(H) Superior orbital fissure

Match the anatomic structure(s) below with the foramen or fissure through which it passes.

11. A branch of the maxillary artery

12. The nerve that innervates the buccinator muscle

13. The nerve that innervates the skin of the upper lip

14. CN IX, CN X, and CN XI

15. The nerve that projects to the otic ganglion

16. Four cranial nerves traverse this orifice

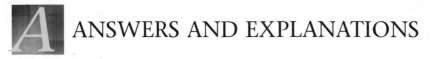

1–E. The superior oblique muscle depresses, abducts, and intorts the eye. Paralysis of this muscle results in extorsion and weakness of downward gaze. Head tilting compensates for extorsion.

2–A. Anosmia, a loss of olfactory sensation, results from damage to the olfactory nerve, or CN I.

3–B. Glossopharyngeal neuralgia has the following neurologic deficits: Excruciating, paroxysmal pain that comes from the tonsillar area and radiates into the ear; loss of taste sensation from the posterior third of the tongue; and loss of palatal and gag reflexes. Potential causes of glossopharyngeal impairment include fractures of the skull base, thrombosis of the sigmoid sinus, tumors, and aneurysms of the posterior fossa. Pain may be triggered by a blood vessel pressing on the nonmyelinated root of the glossopharyngeal nerve, and relocation of the vessel may alleviate symptoms. Treatment is with carbamazepine and other antiepileptic drugs.

4–B. The fibers of the optic nerve (CN II) are myelinated by oligodendrocytes. This is an important distinction from the other cranial nerves, whose fibers are myelinated by Schwann cells, because the optic nerve is considered a tract of the central nervous system and thus incapable of regeneration.

5–D. The accessory nerve (CN XI) mediates head and shoulder movement and innervates laryngeal muscles. Lesions result in paralysis of the sternocleidomastoid muscle, making it difficult to turn the head to the side opposite the lesion, and paralysis of the trapezius muscle, resulting in a shoulder droop and inability to shrug the shoulder on the side of the lesion.

6–A. The glossopharyngeal nerve (CN IX) innervates the parotid gland via the tympanic and lesser petrosal nerves, the otic ganglion, and the auriculotemporal nerve.

7–D. The facial nerve (CN VII) provides the efferent limb of the corneal reflex (orbicularis oculi muscle).

8–E. The vagal nerve (CN X) provides the efferent limb of the gag reflex (muscles of the soft palate). The glossopharyngeal nerve provides the afferent limb of the gag reflex.

9–E. The vagal nerve (CN X) innervates, via the recurrent meningeal ramus, the infratentorial dura (the dura of the posterior cranial fossa).

10–B. The accessory nerve (CN XI) is a pure SVE motor nerve. The cranial division innervates, via the recurrent laryngeal nerve, the intrinsic muscles of the larynx; the spinal division innervates, via motor branches, the sternocleidomastoid muscle and upper parts of the trapezius muscle.

11–F. The middle meningeal artery, a branch of the maxillary artery, traverses the foramen spinosum.

12–G. The facial nerve (CN VII) exits the base of the skull via the stylomastoid foramen; CN VII innervates the muscles of facial expression, including the buccinator muscle.

13–E. The maxillary nerve (CN V-2) exits the skull via the foramen rotundum.

14–A. CN IX, CN X, and CN XI exit the posterior cranial fossa via the jugular foramen.

15–B. The lesser petrosal nerve of CN IX passes through the innominate canal to synapse with postganglionic neurons of the otic ganglion. The innominate canal lies between the foramen ovale and the foramen spinosum.

16–H. CN III, CN IV, CN VI, and CN V-1 pass through the superior orbital fissure.

Lesions of the Brainstem

I. Introduction: Lesions of the Brainstem

- are most frequently syndromes of arterial occlusion or circulatory insufficiency that involve the vertebrobasilar system.

II. Vascular Lesions of the Medulla

- result from occlusion of the vertebral artery or its branches (i.e., the anterior and posterior spinal arteries and the posterior inferior cerebellar artery [PICA]).

A. **Medial medullary syndrome** (Figure 14-1A)
  - results from occlusion of the anterior spinal artery.
  - includes the following affected **structures** and resultant **deficits**:
    1. **Corticospinal tract**
       - contralateral hemiparesis of the trunk and extremities
    2. **Medial lemniscus**
       - contralateral loss of proprioception, discriminative tactile sensation, and vibration sensation from the trunk and extremities
    3. **Hypoglossal nerve roots (intra-axial fibers)**
       - ipsilateral flaccid paralysis of the tongue

B. **Lateral medullary syndrome (PICA syndrome)** (see Figure 14-1B)
  - is also called Wallenberg syndrome.
  - results from occlusion of the vertebral artery or one of its medullary branches (e.g., PICA).
  - includes the following affected **structures** and resultant **deficits**:
    1. **Vestibular nuclei (medial and inferior)**
       - nystagmus, nausea, vomiting, and vertigo
    2. **Inferior cerebellar peduncle**
       - ipsilateral cerebellar signs (dystaxia, dysmetria, dysdiadochokinesia)
    3. **Nucleus ambiguus of cranial nerve (CN) IX, CN X, and CN XI (somatic visceral efferent [SVE])**
       - ipsilateral laryngeal, pharyngeal, and palatal paralysis (loss of the gag reflex [efferent limb], dysarthria, dysphagia, and dysphonia [hoarseness])
    4. **Glossopharyngeal nerve roots (intra-axial fibers)**
       - loss of the gag reflex (afferent limb)
    5. **Vagal nerve roots (intra-axial fibers)**
       - neurologic deficits same as those seen in lesion of the nucleus ambiguus
    6. **Spinothalamic tracts**
       - contralateral loss of pain and temperature sensation from the trunk and extremities

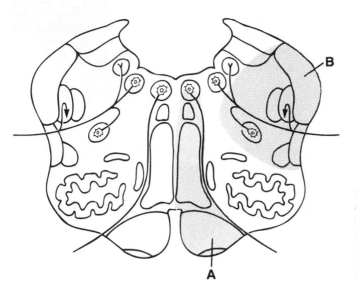

Figure 14-1. Vascular lesions of the caudal medulla at the level of the hypoglossal nucleus of CN XII and the dorsal motor nucleus of CN X. **(A)** Medial medullary syndrome (anterior spinal artery). **(B)** Lateral medullary syndrome (PICA syndrome).

7. **Spinal trigeminal nucleus and tract**
   - ipsilateral loss of pain and temperature sensation from the face
8. **Descending sympathetic tract**
   - ipsilateral Horner syndrome (ptosis, miosis, hemianhidrosis, vasodilation, and apparent enophthalmos)

III. Vascular Lesions of the Pons

- result from occlusion of the basilar artery or its branches (the anterior inferior cerebellar artery [AICA], transverse pontine arteries, and superior cerebellar artery).

A. Medial inferior pontine syndrome (Figure 14-2A)
   - results from occlusion of the paramedian branches of the basilar artery.

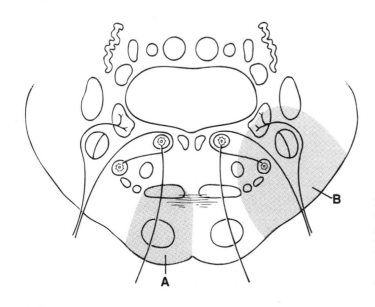

Figure 14-2. Vascular lesions of the caudal pons at the level of the abducent nucleus of CN VI and the facial nucleus of CN VII. **(A)** Medial inferior pontine syndrome. **(B)** Lateral inferior pontine syndrome (AICA syndrome).

- includes the following affected **structures** and resultant **deficits**:
    1. **Abducent nerve roots (intra-axial fibers)**
        - ipsilateral lateral rectus paralysis
    2. **Corticobulbar tracts**
        - contralateral weakness of the lower face
    3. **Corticospinal tracts**
        - contralateral hemiparesis of the trunk and extremities
    4. **Base of the pons (middle cerebellar peduncle)**
        - ipsilateral limb and gait ataxia
    5. **Medial lemniscus**
        - contralateral loss of proprioception, discriminative tactile sensation, and vibration sensation from the trunk and extremities

B. Lateral inferior pontine syndrome (AICA syndrome) (see Figure 14-2B)
- results from occlusion of a long circumferential branch of the basilar artery, AICA.
- includes the following affected **structures** and resultant **deficits**:
    1. **Facial nucleus and intra-axial nerve fibers**
        - ipsilateral facial nerve paralysis
        - loss of taste from the anterior two-thirds of the tongue
        - loss of the corneal and stapedial reflexes
    2. **Cochlear nuclei and intra-axial nerve fibers**
        - unilateral central nerve deafness
    3. **Vestibular nuclei and intra-axial nerve fibers**
        - nystagmus, nausea, vomiting, and vertigo
    4. **Spinal trigeminal nucleus and tract**
        - ipsilateral loss of pain and temperature sensation from the face
    5. **Middle and inferior cerebellar peduncles**
        - ipsilateral limb and gait dystaxia
    6. **Spinothalamic tracts**
        - contralateral loss of pain and temperature sensation from the trunk and extremities
    7. **Descending sympathetic tract**
        - ipsilateral Horner syndrome (ptosis, miosis, hemianhidrosis, vasodilation, and apparent enophthalmos)

C. Lateral midpontine syndrome
- results from occlusion of a short circumferential branch of the basilar artery.
- includes the following affected **structures** and resultant **deficits**:
    1. **Trigeminal nuclei and nerve root (motor and principal sensory nuclei)**
        - complete ipsilateral trigeminal paralysis, including:
            a. **Paralysis of the muscles of mastication**
            b. **Jaw deviation to the paretic side** (due to unopposed action of the intact lateral pterygoid muscle)
            c. **Facial hemianesthesia** (pain, temperature, touch, and proprioception)
            d. **Loss of the corneal reflex** (afferent limb of CN V-1)
    2. **Middle cerebellar peduncle (base of the pons)**
        - ipsilateral limb and gait dystaxia

D. Lateral superior pontine syndrome
- results from occlusion of a long circumferential branch of the basilar artery, the **superior cerebellar artery.**
- includes the following affected **structures** and resultant **deficits**:
    1. **Superior and middle cerebellar peduncles**
        - ipsilateral limb and trunk dystaxia
    2. **Dentate nucleus**
        - signs similar to those seen with damage to the superior cerebellar peduncle (dystaxia, dysmetria, and intention tremor)

3. **Spinothalamic and trigeminothalamic tracts**
   - contralateral loss of pain and temperature sensation from the trunk, extremities, and face
4. **Descending sympathetic tract**
   - ipsilateral Horner syndrome (ptosis, miosis, hemihidrosis, and apparent enophthalmos)
5. **Medial lemniscus (lateral division [gracilis])**
   - contralateral loss of proprioception, discriminative tactile sensation, and vibration sensation from the trunk and lower extremity

E. **Locked-in syndrome (pseudocoma)**
   - results from infarction of the base of the superior pons; infarcted structures include the corticobulbar and corticospinal tracts, resulting in quadriplegia and paralysis of the lower cranial nerves.
   - also may result from **central pontine myelinolysis.**
   - Communication occurs only by blinking or moving the eyes vertically.

IV. Lesions of the Midbrain

- result from vascular occlusion of the mesencephalic branches of the posterior cerebral artery.
- may result from aneurysms of the posterior circle of Willis.
- may result from tumors of the pineal region.
- may result from hydrocephalus.

A. **Dorsal midbrain (Parinaud) syndrome** (Figure 14-3A)
   - is frequently the result of a **pinealoma** or **germinoma** of the pineal region.
   - includes the following affected **structures** and resultant **deficits:**
     1. **Superior colliculus and pretectal area**
        - paralysis of upward and downward gaze, pupillary disturbances, and absence of convergence
     2. **Cerebral aqueduct**
        - noncommunicating hydrocephalus (as a result of compression from a pineal tumor)

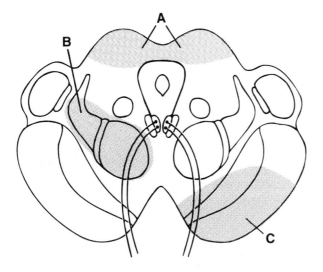

Figure 14-3. Lesions of the rostral midbrain at the level of the superior colliculus and oculomotor nucleus of CN III. **(A)** Dorsal midbrain (Parinaud) syndrome. **(B)** Paramedian midbrain (Benedikt) syndrome. **(C)** Medial midbrain (Weber) syndrome.

B. **Paramedian midbrain (Benedikt) syndrome** (see Figure 14-3B)
- results from occlusion or hemorrhage of the paramedian midbrain branches of the posterior cerebral artery.
- includes the following affected **structures** and resultant **deficits**:
  1. **Oculomotor nerve roots (intra-axial fibers)**
     - complete **ipsilateral oculomotor nerve paralysis**
     - **eye abduction and depression** because of the unopposed action of the lateral rectus (CN VI) and the superior oblique (CN IV) muscles
     - severe **ptosis** (paralysis of the levator palpebrae muscle)
     - ipsilateral **fixed and dilated pupil** (complete internal ophthalmoplegia)
  2. **Red nucleus and dentatorubrothalamic tract**
     - contralateral cerebellar dystaxia with intention tremor
  3. **Medial lemniscus**
     - contralateral loss of proprioception, discriminative tactile sensation, and vibration sensation from trunk and extremities

C. **Medial midbrain (Weber) syndrome** (see Figure 14-3C)
- results from occlusion of midbrain branches of the posterior cerebral artery and aneurysms of the circle of Willis.
- includes the following **structures** and resultant **deficits**:
  1. **Oculomotor nerve roots (intra-axial fibers)** (see IV B 1)
  2. **Corticobulbar tracts**
     - contralateral weakness of the lower face (CN VII), tongue (CN XII), and palate (CN X)
  3. **Corticospinal tracts**
     - contralateral hemiparesis of the trunk and extremities

V.   Acoustic Neuroma (Schwannoma) (Figure 14-4)

- is a benign tumor of the Schwann cells affecting the vestibulocochlear nerve (CN VIII).
- is a posterior fossa tumor of the internal auditory meatus and the cerebellopontine (CP) angle.
- frequently compresses the facial nerve (CN VII), which accompanies CN VIII in the CP angle and internal auditory meatus.
- may impinge on the pons and affect the spinal trigeminal tract (CN V).
- includes the following affected **structures** and resultant **deficits**:

A. **Cochlear nerve of CN VIII**
- unilateral nerve deafness and tinnitus

B. **Vestibular nerve of CN VIII**
- vertigo, nystagmus, nausea, vomiting, and unsteadiness of gait

C. **Facial nerve (CN VII)**
- facial weakness and loss of corneal reflex (efferent limb)

D. **Spinal trigeminal tract (CN V)**
- paresthesias and anesthesia of ipsilateral face
- loss of the corneal reflex (afferent limb)

E. **Abducent nerve (CN VI)** (in advanced cases with large tumors)
- diplopia

F. **Corticospinal tract** [in advanced cases with large tumors]
- contralateral spastic paresis

VI. Internuclear Ophthalmoplegia (INO)

- is also known as medial longitudinal fasciculus (MLF) syndrome, which results from a lesion of the MLF. Lesions occur in the dorsomedial pontine tegmentum and may affect one or both MLFs.
- is a frequent sign of multiple sclerosis.
- results in medial rectus palsy on attempted lateral gaze and monocular nystagmus in the abducting eye with normal convergence.
- Lesions of the abducent nucleus of CN VI result in all MLF signs and a lateral rectus paralysis with internal strabismus.

VII. Jugular Foramen (Vernet) Syndrome

- affects CN IX, CN X, and CN XI.
- includes the following affected **structures** and resultant **deficits**:

A. Glossopharyngeal nerve (CN IX)
  - loss of the gag reflex (afferent limb)
  - loss of taste sensation in the posterior third of the tongue
  - unilateral loss of the carotid sinus reflex

B. Vagal nerve (CN X)
  - laryngeal paralysis with dysarthria, dysphagia, and dysphonia (hoarseness)
  - palatal paralysis with loss of the gag reflex (efferent limb)

C. Accessory nerve (CN XI)
  - weakness of the sternocleidomastoid and upper trapezius muscles (the shoulder droops)

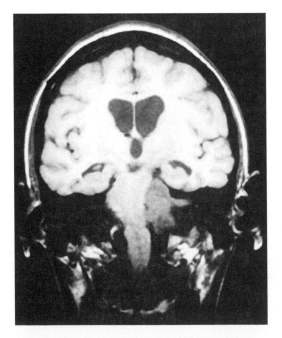

Figure 14-4. Magnetic resonance image of an acoustic neuroma. This coronal section shows dilation of the ventricles. The vestibulocochlear nerve is visible in the left internal auditory meatus. The tumor indents the lateral pons. Cranial nerve palsies include CN V, VII, and VIII. Symptoms include unilateral deafness, facial anesthesia and weakness, and an absent coronal reflex. This is a T_1-weighted image. (Reprinted with permission from Fix JD: High-Yield Neuroanatomy, 3rd ed. Philadelphia, Lippincott Williams & Wilkins, 2005, p 108.)

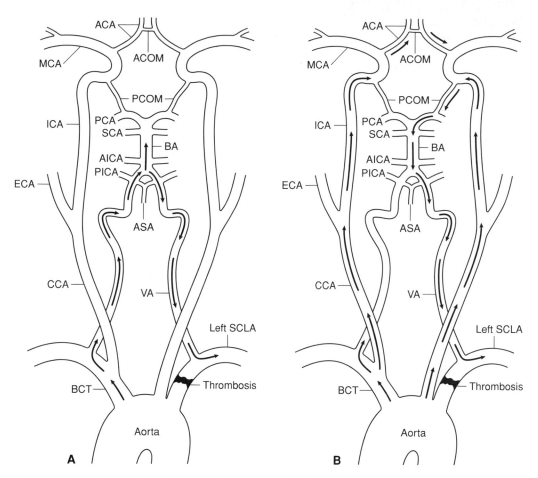

Figure 14-5.   Anatomy of subclavian steal syndrome. Thrombosis of the proximal part of the subclavian artery on the left side results in retrograde blood flow through the ipsilateral vertebral artery and into the left subclavian artery. Blood can be shunted from the right vertebral artery and down the left vertebral artery (**A**). Blood may also reach the left vertebral artery via the carotid circulation (**B**). *ACA* = anterior cerebral artery; *ACOM* = anterior communicating artery; *AICA* = anterior inferior cerebellar artery; *ASA* = anterior spinal artery; *BA* = basilar artery; *BCT* = brachiocephalic trunk; *CCA* = common carotid artery; *ECA* = external carotid artery; *ICA* = internal carotid artery; *MCA* = middle cerebral artery; *PCA* = posterior cerebral artery; *PCOM* = posterior communicating artery; *PICA* = posterior inferior cerebellar artery; *SCA* = superior cerebellar artery; *SCLA* = subclavian artery; *VA* = vertebral artery. (Reprinted with permission from Fix JD: *High-Yield Neuroanatomy,* 3rd ed. Philadelphia: Lippincott Williams & Wilkins, 2005, p 109.)

VIII. Subclavian Steal Syndrome (Figure 14-5)

- results from thrombosis of the left subclavian artery proximal to the vertebral artery. Blood is shunted retrograde down the vertebral artery and into the left subclavian artery.
- leads to the following clinical signs: transient weakness and claudication of the left arm on exercise and vertebrobasilar insufficiency (vertigo, dizziness).

REVIEW TEST

1. During a gang fight, a 16-year-old male is shot with a 22-caliber short bullet in the occiput. Computed tomography (CT) shows that the bullet is lodged in the left medullary pyramid. The most prominent neurologic deficit is

(A) Apallesthesia, right side
(B) Exaggerated muscle stretch reflexes, left side
(C) Plantar reflex extensor, right side
(D) Fasciculations, right side
(E) Hyperreflexia, left side

2. A 70-year-old retired army colonel has right-sided hemiparesis. Which of the following signs best localizes the lesion to the brainstem?

(A) Loss of kinesthetic and pallesthetic sensation, right side
(B) Lower facial weakness (numbness), right side
(C) Exaggerated muscle stretch reflexes, right side
(D) Tonic deviation of eyes to the right
(E) Lateral strabismus

3. A 10-year-old boy has right arm and leg dystaxia, nystagmus, hoarseness, along with miosis and ptosis on the right. Bronchoscopy reveals a paretic vocal cord on the right. The lesion site responsible is most likely the

(A) right dorsal motor nucleus of CN X
(B) left red nucleus
(C) dorsolateral medulla
(D) dorsolateral pons
(E) internal capsule

4. Neurologic examination reveals miosis, ptosis, hemianhidrosis, left side; laryngeal and palatal paralysis, left side; facial anesthesia, left side; and loss of pain and temperature sensation from the trunk and extremities, right side. The lesion is in the

(A) caudal medulla, ventral median zone, right side
(B) rostral medulla, lateral zone, left side
(C) rostral pontine base, left side
(D) caudal pontine tegmentum, lateral zone, right side
(E) rostral pontine tegmentum, dorsal median zone, left side

5. Neurologic examination reveals severe ptosis, eye looks down and out, right side; fixed, dilated pupil, right side; spastic hemiparesis, left side; and lower facial weakness, left side. The lesion is in the

(A) caudal pontine tegmentum, dorsal median zone, left side
(B) rostral pontine tegmentum, dorsal lateral zone, right side
(C) pontine isthmus, dorsal lateral tegmentum, left side
(D) rostral midbrain, medial basis pedunculi, right side
(E) rostral midbrain, medial tegmentum, left side

6. Neurologic examination reveals sixth nerve palsy, right side; facial weakness, left side; hemiparesis, left side; and limb and gait dystaxia, right side. The lesion is in the

(A) caudal pontine tegmentum, lateral zone, right side
(B) caudal pontine tegmentum, dorsal median zone, left side
(C) caudal medulla, ventral median zone, right side
(D) rostral pontine tegmentum, lateral zone, left side
(E) caudal pontine base, median zone, right side

7. Neurologic examination reveals paralysis of upward and downward gaze, absence of convergence, and absence of pupillary reaction to light. The lesion is in the

(A) rostral midbrain tectum
(B) caudal midbrain tectum
(C) rostral pontine tegmentum
(D) caudal pontine tegmentum
(E) caudal midbrain tegmentum

8. Neurologic examination reveals bilateral medial rectus paresis on attempted lateral gaze, monocular horizontal nystagmus in the abducting eye, and unimpaired convergence. The lesion is in the

(A) midpontine tegmentum, dorsomedial zones, bilateral
(B) rostral midbrain tectum
(C) caudal midbrain tectum
(D) caudal pontine base
(E) rostral midbrain, bases pedunculorum

9. Neurologic examination reveals ptosis, miosis, and hemianhidrosis, left side; loss of vibration sensation in the right leg; loss of pain and temperature sensation from the trunk, extremities,

and face, right side; and severe dystaxia and intention tremor, left arm. The lesion is in the

(A) rostral midbrain tegmentum, right side
(B) rostral pontine tegmentum, dorsal medial zone, left side
(C) pontine isthmus, dorsal lateral zone, left side
(D) rostral medulla, lateral zone, left side
(E) caudal medulla, lateral zone, right side

10. Neurologic examination reveals weakness of the pterygoid and masseter muscles, left side; corneal reflex absent, left side; and facial hemianesthesia, left side. The lesion is in the

(A) midpontine tegmentum, lateral zone, left side
(B) midpontine base, medial zone, left side
(C) caudal pontine tegmentum, lateral zone, left side
(D) caudal pontine tegmentum, dorsal medial zone, left side
(E) foramen ovale, left side

11. Neurologic examination reveals loss of the stapedial reflex, loss of the corneal reflex, inability to purse the lips, and loss of taste sensation on the apex of the tongue. The lesion is in the

(A) stylomastoid foramen
(B) basis pedunculi of the midbrain
(C) rostral lateral pontine tegmentum
(D) caudal lateral pontine tegmentum
(E) rostral medulla

12. Paramedian infarction of the base of the pons involves which of the following structures?

(A) Trapezoid body
(B) Descending trigeminal tract
(C) Rubrospinal tract
(D) Pyramidal tract
(E) Ventral spinocerebellar tract

Questions 13 to 20

Match the description in items 13 to 20 with the appropriate lettered structure shown in the figure.

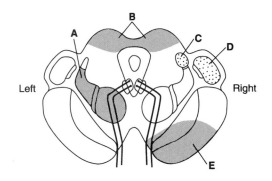

13. Paralysis of upward gaze

14. Loss of pain and temperature on the left side of the body

15. Deviation of the tongue to the left side and the uvula to the right side

16. Intention tremor on the right side

17. Complete third nerve palsy on the right side

18. Loss of vibration sensation in the right extremities

19. Babinski sign on the left side

20. Lesion leads to terminal axonal degeneration in the right transverse gyrus of Heschl

ANSWERS AND EXPLANATIONS

1–C. The bullet transected the left medullary pyramid, which contains the uncrossed corticospinal tract. This UMN lesion has produced a right contralateral spastic paresis with all pyramidal signs.

2–E. Lateral strabismus (exotropia) is seen in midbrain lesions (e.g., Weber syndrome) that transect intra-axial fibers of the oculomotor nerve. The intact lateral rectus pulls the globe laterally.

3–C. The lateral medullary syndrome is also called PICA syndrome. The dorsolateral medulla contains the nucleus ambiguus (larynx), hypothalamospinal tract (Horner syndrome), inferior cerebellar peduncle (dystaxia), and vestibular nuclei (nystagmus).

4–B. The lesion is a classic Wallenberg syndrome (PICA syndrome) of the lateral medullary zone. Interruption of the descending sympathetic tract produces ipsilateral Horner syndrome. Involvement of the nucleus ambiguus or its exiting intra-axial fibers accounts for LMN paralysis of the larynx and soft palate. The ipsilateral facial anesthesia is due to interruption of the spinal trigeminal tract; the contralateral loss of pain and temperature sensation from the trunk and extremities is due to transection of the spinothalamic tracts. The combination of ipsilateral and contralateral sensory loss is called alternating hemianesthesia. Singultus (hiccup) is frequently seen in this syndrome and is thought to result from irritation of the reticulophrenic pathway.

5–D. This constellation of deficits constitutes Weber syndrome, which affects the basis pedunculi and the exiting intra-axial oculomotor fibers. Severe ptosis (compare mild ptosis of Horner syndrome), the abducted and depressed eyeball, and the internal ophthalmoplegia (fixed, dilated pupil) are third nerve signs. The contralateral hemiparesis results from interruption of the corticospinal tracts; lower facial weakness is due to interruption of the corticobulbar tracts. The combination of ipsilateral and contralateral motor deficits is called alternating hemiplegia.

The corticospinal tract is closely related to three cranial nerves (CN III, CN VI, and CN XII); third nerve signs put the lesion in the midbrain, sixth nerve signs put the lesion in the pons, and twelfth nerve signs put the lesion in the medulla. With the exception of the trochlear nerve, all cranial nerves have ipsilateral signs. Transection of the corticospinal tract rostral to the decussation results in a contralateral spastic hemiparesis. The trochlear nucleus, an exception, gives rise to intra-axial axons that cross the midline and exit just caudal to the frenulum of the superior medullary velum. A lesion of the trochlear nucleus results in a contralateral superior oblique palsy.

6–E. These signs point to the base of the pons (medial inferior pontine syndrome) on the right side and include involvement of the exiting intra-axial abducent fibers that pass through the uncrossed corticospinal fibers; this results in an ipsilateral lateral rectus paralysis (LMN lesion) and contralateral hemiparesis. Contralateral facial weakness results from damage to the corticobulbar fibers prior to their decussation. Involvement of the transverse pontine fibers destined for the middle cerebellar peduncle results in cerebellar signs. Again, the involved cranial nerve and pyramidal tract indicate where the lesion must be to account for the deficits. An ipsilateral sixth nerve paralysis and crossed hemiplegia is called the Millard-Gubler syndrome.

7–A. These deficits indicate the Parinaud syndrome, dorsal midbrain syndrome. This condition frequently is the result of a tumor in the pineal region (e.g., germinoma or pinealoma); a pinealoma compresses the superior colliculus and the underlying accessory oculomotor nuclei that are responsible for upward and downward vertical conjugate gaze. Patients usually have pupillary disturbances and absence of convergence.

8–A. The MLF is located in the dorsomedial midpontine tegmentum. MLF syndrome is frequently seen in multiple sclerosis and less often in vascular lesions. Another pontine lesion results in one-and-a-half syndrome; it includes the MLF syndrome and a lesion of the abducent nucleus (CN VI). See Chapter 17:.

9–C. These deficits correspond to a lesion in the dorsolateral zone of the pontine isthmus, lateral superior pontine syndrome. Interruption of the descending sympathetic pathway to the ciliospinal center of Budge (T1–T2) results in Horner syndrome (always ipsilateral). Involvement of the lateral aspect (includes the leg fibers) of the medial lemniscus results in a loss of vibration sensation and other dorsal column modalities. Damage to the trigeminothalamic and spinothalamic tracts at this level results in contralateral hemianesthesia of the face and body. Infarction of the superior cerebellar peduncle leads to severe cerebellar dystaxia on the same side.

10–A. These signs indicate the lateral midpontine syndrome. This lesion involves the motor and principal trigeminal nuclei and the intra-axial root fibers of the trigeminal nerve as it passes through the base of the pons. All signs are ipsilateral and refer to CN V. The afferent limb of the corneal reflex has been interrupted. This syndrome results from occlusion of the trigeminal artery, a short circumferential branch of the basilar artery.

11–D. These signs constitute the lateral inferior pontine syndrome (AICA syndrome). The neurologic findings are all signs of a lesion involving the facial nerve (CN VII). The facial nerve nucleus and intra-axial fibers are found in the caudal lateral pontine tegmentum. A lesion of the stylomastoid foramen would not include the absence of the stapedial reflex or the loss of taste sensation from the anterior two-thirds of the tongue. The stapedial nerve and the chorda tympani exit the facial canal proximal to the stylomastoid foramen.

12–D. The base of the pons includes the corticospinal (pyramidal), corticobulbar, and corticopontine tracts, pontine nuclei, and transverse pontine fibers. At caudal levels, intra-axial abducent fibers of CN VI pass through the lateral pyramidal fascicles.

13–B. Paralysis of upward gaze results from compression of the mesencephalic tectum by a tumor in the pineal region; this is called Parinaud syndrome.

14–C. Loss of pain and temperature on the left side of the body is due to a lesion on the right side of the lateral spinothalamic tract.

15–E. Deviation of the tongue to the left side results from transection of the right corticobulbar fibers (CN XII) in the medial aspect of the crus cerebri. Deviation of the uvula to the right side results from transection of the right corticobulbar fibers (CN X) in the medial aspect of the crus cerebri.

16–A. Transection of the left dentatothalamic tract results in an intention tremor on the right side. The dentatothalamic tract decussates in the caudal midbrain, below the level of this lesion.

17–E. Complete third nerve palsy on the right side results from transection of the oculomotor nerve fibers as they pass through the right side of the crus cerebri.

18–A. A loss of vibration sensation in the right extremities results from destruction of the left medial lemniscus.

19–E. A Babinski sign on the left side results from transection of the corticospinal tract within the middle three-fifths of the crus cerebri.

20–D. Destruction of the right medial geniculate body results in terminal axonal degeneration of the auditory radiation in the right transverse gyrus of Heschl.

Cerebellum

I.   Overview: The Cerebellum

- develops from the alar plates (rhombic lips) of the metencephalon.
- is located infratentorially within the posterior fossa and lies between the temporal and occipital lobes and the brainstem.
- has three primary functions: the **maintenance of posture and balance**, the **maintenance of muscle tone**, and the **coordination of voluntary motor activity**.

II.   Major Divisions of the Cerebellum

- consists of a midline **vermis** and two lateral **hemispheres**.
- is covered by a three-layered **cortex**, which contains folia and fissures.
- contains a central medullary core, which is the **white matter** that contains myelinated axons and the four cerebellar nuclei (dentate, emboliform, globose, and fastigial nuclei). The emboliform and globose nuclei are called the interposed nucleus.

A. **Cerebellar lobes** (Figure 15-1)
- are phylogenetic and functional divisions.
  1. **Anterior lobe**
     - lies anterior to the primary fissure.
     - receives input from stretch receptors (muscle spindles) and Golgi tendon organs (GTOs) via the spinocerebellar tracts.
     - plays a role in the regulation of muscle tone.
  2. **Posterior lobe**
     - lies between the primary fissure and the posterolateral fissure.
     - receives massive input from the neocortex via the corticopontocerebellar fibers.
     - plays a role in the coordination of voluntary motor activity.
  3. **Flocculonodular lobe (vestibulocerebellum)**
     - consists of the nodulus (of the vermis) and the flocculus.
     - receives input from the vestibular system.
     - plays a role in the maintenance of posture and balance.

B. **Longitudinal organization of the cerebellum** (see Figure 15-1)
- includes three functional longitudinal zones that are associated with specific cerebellar nuclei and pathways.
  1. **Median (vermal) zone of the hemisphere**
     - contains the vermal cortex, which projects to the fastigial nucleus.
  2. **Paramedian (paravermal) zone of the hemisphere**
     - contains the paravermal cortex, which projects to the interposed nuclei (emboliform and globose nuclei).

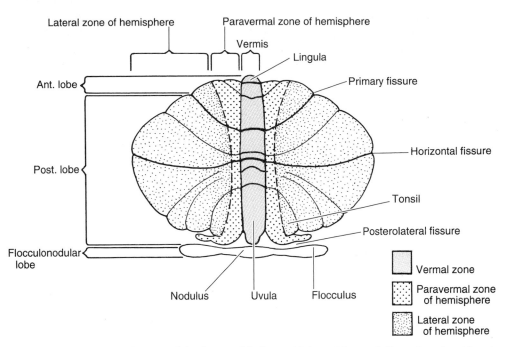

Figure 15-1. Schematic diagram of the fissures, lobules, and lobes of the cerebellum. Functional longitudinal zones of the cerebellum are associated with cerebellar nuclei. The vermal (median) zone projects to the fastigial nucleus, the paravermal (paramedian) zone projects to the interposed nucleus, and the lateral zone projects to the dentate nucleus.

3. **Lateral zone of the hemisphere**
   - contains the hemispheric cortex, which projects to the dentate nucleus.

C. **Cerebellar peduncles** (see Figure 1-7)
   1. **Inferior cerebellar peduncle**
      - connects the cerebellum to the medulla.
      - consists of two divisions:
         a. **Restiform body**
            - is an afferent fiber system containing:
               (1) **Dorsal spinocerebellar tract**
               (2) **Cuneocerebellar tract**
               (3) **Olivocerebellar tract**
         b. **Juxtarestiform body**
            - contains afferent and efferent fibers:
               (1) **Vestibulocerebellar fibers (afferent)**
               (2) **Cerebellovestibular fibers (efferent)**
   2. **Middle cerebellar peduncle**
      - connects the cerebellum to the pons.
      - is an afferent fiber system containing **pontocerebellar fibers** to the neocerebellum.
   3. **Superior cerebellar peduncle**
      - connects the cerebellum to the pons and midbrain.
      - represents the major output from the cerebellum.
         a. **Efferent pathways**
            (1) **Dentatorubrothalamic tract**
            (2) **Interpositorubrothalamic tract**
            (3) **Fastigiothalamic tract**
            (4) **Fastigiovestibular tract**

 b. **Afferent pathways**
  (1) **Ventral spinocerebellar tract**
  (2) **Trigeminocerebellar fibers**
  (3) **Ceruleocerebellar fibers**

III. Cerebellar Cortex

A. **Three-layered cerebellar cortex** (Figure 15-2)
 1. **Molecular layer**
  • is the outer cell-sparse layer that underlies the pia mater.
  • contains dendritic arborizations of Purkinje cells and the parallel fibers of the granule cells.
  • contains stellate (outer) cells and basket (inner stellate) cells.
 2. **Purkinje cell layer**
  • is found between the molecular layer and the granule cell layer.

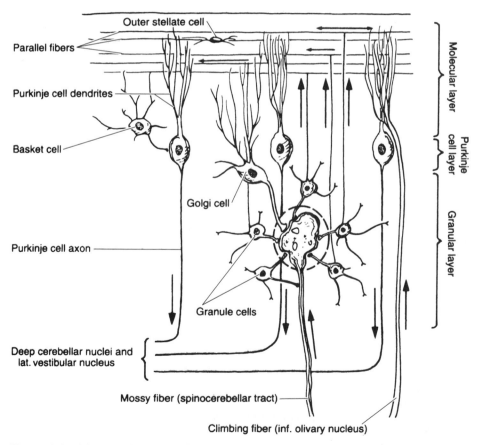

Figure 15-2. Schematic diagram of the three-layered cerebellar cortex, showing the neuronal elements and their connections. The *circular broken line* contains a cerebellar glomerulus. Climbing and mossy fibers represent excitatory input. Purkinje cell axons provide the sole output from the cerebellar cortex, which is inhibitory.

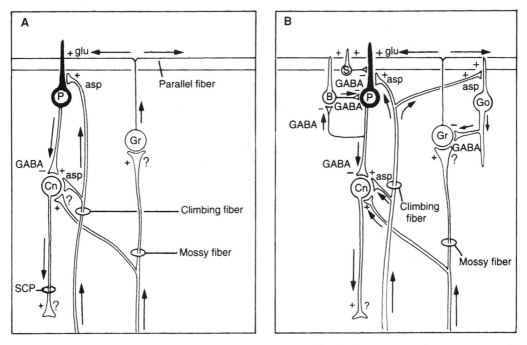

Figure 15-3. The basic connections of the cerebellar cortex. **(A)** The basic input and output circuit. **(B)** Connections of the inhibitory interneurons of the cerebellar cortex. *asp* = aspartate; *B* = basket cell; *Cn* = neuron of the cerebellar nuclei; *Gr* = granule cell; *GABA* = gamma-aminobutyric acid; *glu* = glutamate; *Go* = Golgi cell; *P* = Purkinje cell; *S* = stellate cell; *SCP* = superior cerebellar peduncle. Inhibitory neurons of the cerebellum use GABA. Glutamate is the transmitter for granule cells. Aspartate is thought to be the transmitter of the climbing fibers. Excitatory synapses are indicated by a plus sign (+); inhibitory synapses are indicated by a minus sign (−); the question mark (?) indicates that the neurotransmitter is not known.

   3. **Granule cell layer**
- is found between the Purkinje cell layer and the cerebellar white matter.
- contains granule cells, Golgi cells, and cerebellar glomeruli.

B. Neurons and fibers of the cerebellum (Figure 15-3; see Figure 15-2)
   1. **Purkinje cell**
- conveys the only output from the cerebellar cortex.
- projects inhibitory output (gamma-aminobutyric acid [GABA]) to the cerebellar and vestibular nuclei.
- is excited by parallel and climbing fibers.
- is inhibited (by GABA) by basket and stellate cells.

   2. **Granule cell**
- excites (by glutamate) Purkinje, basket, stellate, and Golgi cells via parallel fibers.
- is inhibited by Golgi cells.
- is excited by mossy fibers.

   3. **Mossy fibers**
- are the afferent excitatory fibers of the **spinocerebellar and pontocerebellar tracts**.
- terminate as mossy fiber rosettes on granule cells.
- excite granule cells to discharge via their parallel fibers.

   4. **Climbing fibers**
- are the afferent excitatory fibers of the **olivocerebellar tract**.
- terminate on neurons of the cerebellar nuclei and on dendrites of Purkinje cells.

IV. Major Cerebellar Pathways (Figure 15-4)

A. **Vestibulocerebellar pathway**
- plays a role in the maintenance of posture, balance, and the coordination of eye movements.
- receives its major input from the vestibular receptors of the kinetic and static labyrinths.
    1. **Semicircular ducts and otolith organs**
        - project to the flocculonodular lobe and the vestibular nuclei.
    2. **Flocculonodular lobe**
        - receives visual input from the superior colliculus and the striate cortex.
        - projects to the vestibular nuclei.
    3. **Vestibular nuclei**
        - project via the medial longitudinal fasciculi (MLFs) to the ocular motor nuclei of CN III, CN IV, and CN VI to coordinate eye movements.
        - project via the medial and lateral vestibulospinal tracts to the spinal cord to regulate neck and antigravity muscles, respectively.

B. **Vermal spinocerebellar pathway**
- maintains muscle tone and postural control over truncal (axial) and proximal (limb girdle) muscles.

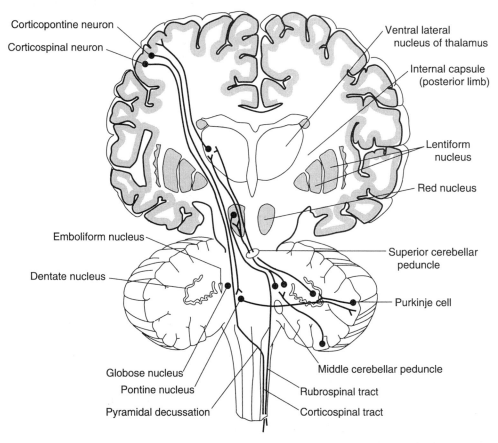

Figure 15-4. The principal cerebellar connections. The major efferent pathway is the dentatothalamocortical tract. The cerebellum receives input from the cerebral cortex through the corticopontocerebellar tract. (Modified with permission from Fix JD: High-Yield Neuroanatomy, 3rd ed. Philadelphia, Lippincott Williams & Wilkins, 2005, p 112.)

1. **Vermis**
   - receives spinocerebellar and labyrinthine input.
   - projects to the fastigial nucleus.
2. **Fastigial nucleus**
   - has excitatory output.
   - projects via the vestibular nuclei to the spinal cord.
   - projects to the ventral lateral nucleus of the thalamus.
3. **Ventral lateral nucleus of the thalamus**
   - receives input from the fastigial nucleus.
   - projects to the trunk area of the precentral gyrus.
4. **Precentral gyrus**
   - gives rise to the **ventral corticospinal tract**, which regulates muscle tone of the truncal and proximal muscles.

C. **Paravermal spinocerebellar pathway**
   - maintains muscle tone and postural control over distal muscle groups.
   1. **Paravermis**
      - receives spinocerebellar input from distal muscles.
      - projects to the interposed nuclei.
   2. **Interposed nuclei (emboliform and globose)**
      - have excitatory output.
      - project to:
        a. **Ventral lateral nucleus**
           - projects to the extremities area of the precentral gyrus. The precentral gyrus gives rise to the **lateral corticospinal tract**, which regulates the distal muscle groups.
        b. **Red nucleus**
           - gives rise to the crossed **rubrospinal tract**, which mediates control over distal muscles.
           - receives input from the contralateral nucleus interpositus and bilateral input from the motor and premotor cortices.

D. **Lateral hemispheric cerebellar pathway** (see Figure 15-4)
   - is also called the **neocerebellar** or **pontocerebellar pathway**.
   - regulates the initiation, planning, and timing of volitional motor activity.
   1. **Cerebellar hemisphere**
      - receives input from the contralateral motor and sensory cortex via the **corticopontocerebellar tract**.
      - projects via Purkinje cell axons to the dentate nucleus.
   2. **Dentate nucleus**
      - has excitatory output.
      - projects via the superior cerebellar peduncle to the contralateral red nucleus, ventral lateral nucleus of the thalamus, and the inferior olivary nucleus.
        a. **Red nucleus pathway**
           (1) The **red nucleus** projects to the inferior olivary nucleus.
           (2) The **inferior olivary nucleus** projects via the contralateral inferior cerebellar peduncle to the cerebellum.
        b. **Ventral lateral nucleus pathway**
           (1) The **ventral lateral nucleus of the thalamus** projects to the motor (4) and premotor (6) cortices.
           (2) The **motor and premotor cortices** give rise to the following tracts:
               (a) **Corticobulbar tract**
                   - innervates cranial nerve nuclei.
               (b) **Lateral corticospinal tract**
                   - regulates volitional synergistic motor activity.
               (c) **Corticopontocerebellar tracts**
                   - regulate the output of the neocerebellum.

   c. **Inferior olivary nucleus pathway**
     (1) The inferior olivary nucleus **receives direct input from the dentate nucleus** via the crossed descending fibers of the superior cerebellar peduncle.
     (2) The inferior olivary nucleus **projects directly to the dentate nucleus** via the contralateral inferior cerebellar peduncle.

V.   Cerebellar Dysfunction (Figure 15-5)

- is characterized by the **triad hypotonia, disequilibrium,** and **dyssynergia.**

A. Hypotonia
- is a loss of the resistance normally offered by muscles to palpation or to passive manipulation.
- results from the loss of cerebellar facilitation of the motor cortex via tonic firing of the cerebellar nuclei.
- results in a floppy, loose-jointed, rag-doll appearance with pendular reflexes; the patient appears inebriated.

B. Disequilibrium
- refers to loss of balance, characterized by gait and trunk dystaxia.

C. Dyssynergia
- is a loss of coordinated muscle activity and includes:
  1. **Dysarthria**
     - is slurred or scanning speech.
  2. **Dystaxia**
     - is a lack of coordination in the execution of voluntary movement (e.g., gait, trunk, leg, and arm dystaxia).
  3. **Dysmetria**
     - is the inability to arrest muscular movement at the desired point (past-pointing).
  4. **Intention tremor**
     - is a type of dysmetria that occurs during a voluntary movement.
  5. **Dysdiadochokinesia**
     - is the inability to perform rapid alternating movements (e.g., rapid supination and pronation of the hands).
  6. **Nystagmus**
     - is a form of dystaxia consisting of to-and-fro eye movements (ocular dysmetria).
  7. **Decomposition of movement (by-the-numbers phenomenon)**
     - consists of breaking down a smooth muscle act into a number of jerky awkward component parts.
  8. **Rebound or lack of check**
     - results from the inability to adjust to changes in muscle tension.
     - is caused by loss of the cerebellar component of the stretch reflex.
     - may be tested for by having the patient flex the forearm at the elbow against resistance; sudden release results in the forearm striking the patient's chest.

VI.   Cerebellar Lesions (Figure 15-6)

A. **Anterior vermis syndrome** (see Figure 15-6)
- involves the leg region of the anterior lobe.
- results from atrophy of the rostral vermis, most commonly caused by alcohol abuse.
- results in gait, trunk, and leg dystaxia.

(*text continues on page 213*)

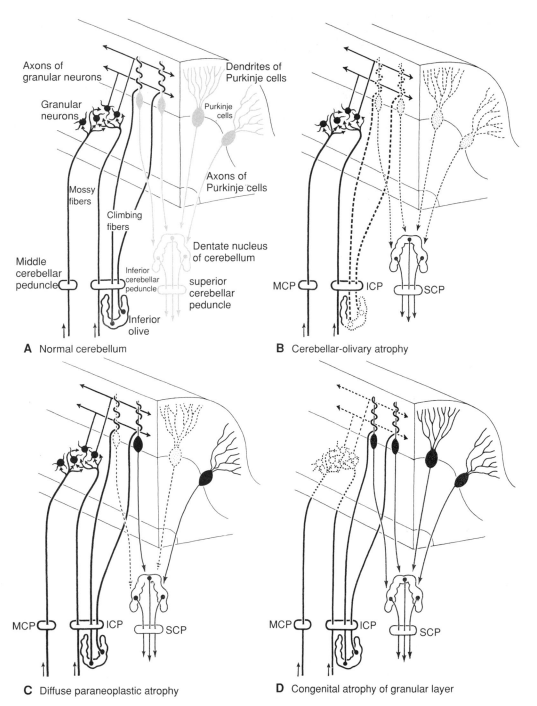

Figure 15-5. Various forms of cerebellar atrophy. MCP = middle cerebellar peduncle; ICP = inferior cerebellar peduncle; SCP = superior cerebellar peduncle. (Reprinted with permission from Poirier J, Gray F, Escourolle R: *Manual of Basic Neuropathy,* 3rd ed. Philadelphia, WB Saunders, 1990, p 155.)

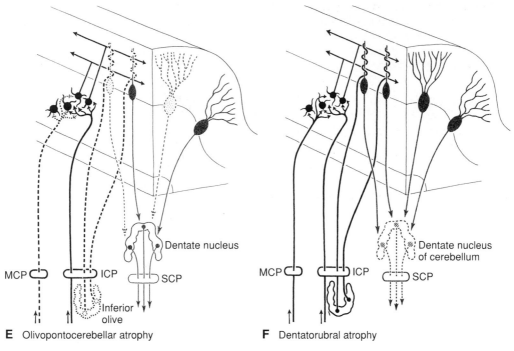

E   Olivopontocerebellar atrophy

F   Dentatorubral atrophy

Figure 15-5.   *(continued)*

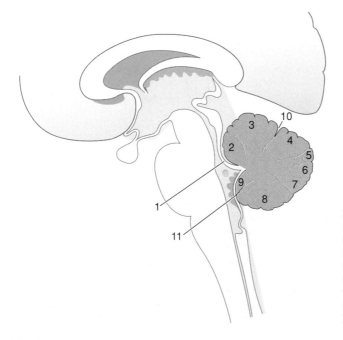

Figure 15-6.   Cerebellar vermis is divided into nine segments: lingula (1), centralis (2), culmen (3), declive (4), folium (5), tuber (6), pyramis (7), uvula (8), nodulus (9). The primary fissure (10) separates the anterior lobe from the posterior lobe. The posterolateral fissure (11) separates the posterior lobe from the flocculonodular lobe.

B. **Posterior vermis syndrome** (see Figure 15-6)
- involves the flocculonodular lobe.
- is usually the result of brain tumors in children.
- is most frequently caused by medulloblastomas or ependymomas.
- results in truncal dystaxia.

C. **Hemispheric syndrome**
- usually involves one cerebellar hemisphere.
- is frequently the result of a brain tumor or an abscess.
- results in arm, leg, trunk, and gait dystaxia.
- results in cerebellar signs that are ipsilateral to the lesion.

D. **Phenytoin (antiepileptic drug) intoxication**
- may cause ataxia, nystagmus, gait disturbances, and dysarthric speech.

E. **Tumors of the cerebellum**
1. **Astrocytomas**
   - constitute 30% of all brain tumors in children.
   - occur most frequently in the cerebellar hemisphere.
   - After surgical removal, survival for many years is common.
2. **Medulloblastomas**
   - are malignant tumors and constitute 20% of all brain tumors in children.
   - occur most frequently in the cerebellar vermis.
   - are thought to originate from the superficial granular layer of the cerebellar cortex.
   - usually obstruct passage of cerebrospinal fluid (CSF) and cause hydrocephalus.
   - often disseminate throughout the CSF tract.
3. **Ependymomas**
   - constitute 10% of all brain tumors in children.
   - are the most common spinal cord tumors in all ages.
   - occur most frequently in the fourth ventricle.
   - usually obstruct passage of CSF and cause hydrocephalus.

F. **Cerebellar atrophies** (see Figure 15-5)
- are inherited disorders.
1. **Friedreich ataxia**
   - is the most common hereditary ataxia, with an autosomal recessive mode of inheritance.
   - involves the dorsal columns, corticospinal tracts, spinocerebellar tracts, and dentate nuclei.
   - has the same spinal cord pathology as **subacute combined degeneration** (see Chapter 8 VII G).
   - is frequently associated with chronic myocarditis.
2. **Cerebello-olivary degeneration (Holmes disease)** (see Figure 15-5B)
   - has an autosomal dominant mode of inheritance.
   - results in a loss of Purkinje and granule cells, followed by a loss of neurons in the inferior olivary nuclei.
   - results in gait ataxia, dysarthria, and intention tremor.
3. **Olivopontocerebellar degeneration (Dejerine-Thomas syndrome)** (see Figure 15-5E)
   - has an autosomal dominant mode of inheritance.
   - results in a loss of Purkinje cells, neurons of the inferior olivary nucleus, and neurons in the pontine nuclei; results in demyelination of the dorsal columns and the spinocerebellar tracts.
   - frequently results in a loss of neurons in the substantia nigra and basal ganglia.
   - results in gait ataxia, dysarthria, and intention tremor; may show parkinsonian signs (rigidity and akinesia).

1. A 30-year-old woman complains of unsteadiness while standing or walking. She tends to deviate to the right. Neurologic examination reveals the following signs: dysmetria on the right, dysdiadochokinesia, and a nystagmus that is more marked when she looks to the right side. The lesion is most likely found in the

(A) cerebellar hemisphere, left side
(B) cerebellar hemisphere, right side
(C) medial medulla, left side
(D) medial medulla, right side
(E) globus pallidus, left side

2. Purkinje cells of the cerebellum project inhibitory axons to which of the following nuclei?

(A) Fastigial nucleus
(B) Superior olivary nucleus
(C) Inferior olivary nucleus
(D) Arcuate nucleus
(E) Ventral lateral nucleus

3. The most common cause of the anterior vermis syndrome is

(A) alcohol abuse
(B) an abscess
(C) a tumor
(D) vascular occlusion
(E) lead intoxication

4. The most common cerebellar tumor in children is

(A) astrocytoma
(B) ependymoma
(C) glioblastoma multiforme
(D) oligodendrocytoma
(E) medulloblastoma

5. A tumor that is derived from the external granular layer of the cerebellar cortex is an

(A) astrocytoma
(B) chordoma
(C) ependymoma
(D) germinoma
(E) medulloblastoma

6. A 10-year-old boy has headache, early-morning vomiting, staggering gait, adiadochokinesia, finger-to-nose sign, heel-to-shin sign, bilateral Babinski signs, choked disk, abducent palsy, and scanning speech, as in "I DID not GIVE any TOYSTO my son for CHRISTmas." What is the most likely diagnosis?

(A) Tabes dorsalis
(B) Olivopontocerebellar degeneration
(C) Posterior vermis syndrome
(D) Sturge-Weber syndrome
(E) Brown-Séquard syndrome

7. An 8-year-old girl is examined by a neurologist who finds the followings deficits: ataxia, marked sensory hypesthesias, kyphoscoliosis, pes cavus, myocarditis, and retinitis pigmentosa inherited as autosomal recessive trait. What is the name of this disease?

(A) Werdnig-Hoffmann
(B) Subacute combined degeneration
(C) Friedrich ataxia
(D) Amyotrophic lateral sclerosis
(E) Brown-Séquard syndrome

ANSWERS AND EXPLANATIONS

1–B. Dysmetria, dysdiadochokinesia, intention tremor, and nystagmus are classic cerebellar signs. In the finger-to-nose test, the patient past-points on the side of the lesion. The medial medulla has no cerebellar pathways. In contrast, the lateral medulla has cerebellar pathways; lesions result in cerebellar ataxia and could be misdiagnosed as a cerebellar hemispheric lesion. The globus pallidus, a basal ganglion, is atrophied in Huntington disease and in Wilson disease, and it is damaged bilaterally by carbon monoxide intoxication.

2–A. Purkinje cells project inhibitory axons to all cerebellar nuclei: fastigial, globose, emboliform, and dentate. In addition, they project to all vestibular nuclei: lateral, superior, medial, and inferior. The superior olivary nucleus is an auditory relay nucleus, and the inferior olivary nucleus is a cerebellar relay nucleus. The arcuate nucleus is an ectopic pontine nucleus that lies next to the pyramidal tract; its function is unknown. The ventral lateral thalamic nucleus receives input from the dentate nucleus.

3–A. Anterior vermis syndrome is a result of chronic alcohol abuse. Patients have dystaxia of the lower limb and trunk. Posterior vermis syndrome involves the flocculonodular lobe; it is most frequently caused by an ependymoma or a medulloblastoma. Patients have truncal dystaxia. Hemispheric syndrome usually is the result of a tumor (astrocytoma) or abscess; patients have arm, leg, trunk, and gait dystaxia.

4–A. Astrocytomas (30%) are the most common cerebellar tumors in children; they are followed by medulloblastomas (20%) and ependymomas (10%).

5–E. Medulloblastomas are derived from the external granular layer of the cerebellar cortex. Medulloblastomas give rise to posterior vermis syndrome.

6–C. Posterior vermis syndrome is generally indicative of brain tumors in children, frequently a medulloblastoma. Symptoms include vomiting, a morning headache, a stumbling gait, frequent falls, diplopia, papilledema, and sixth nerve palsy. Tabes dorsalis is dorsal column syndrome that results from untreated syphilis. Olivopontocerebellar degeneration has an autosomal dominant mode of inheritance and results in gait ataxia, dysarthria, intention tremor, and possibly parkinsonian signs (rigidity and akinesia). Sturge-Weber syndrome is neurocutaneous congenital disorder caused by an arteriovenous malformation in the telencephalon. Brown-Séquard syndrome is paralysis, ataxia, and loss of sensation as a result of a spinal cord hemisection.

7–C. Friedreich ataxia is the most common hereditary ataxia, with an autosomal recessive mode of inheritance. It is often associated with chronic myocarditis; other symptoms include muscle weakness, loss of coordination, vision impairment, hearing loss, slurred speech, and curvature of the spine (kyphoscoliosis). Friedreich ataxia has the same spinal cord pathology (dorsal column syndrome) as subacute combined degeneration, which is caused by a vitamin B_{12} deficiency. Symptoms include loss of tactile discrimination; loss of joint and vibratory sensation; stereoanesthesia; sensory dystaxia; paresthesias and pain; hyporeflexia or areflexia; urinary incontinence, constipation, and impotence; and Romberg sign. Subacute combined degeneration includes both sensory and motor deficits; amyotrophic lateral sclerosis is a pure motor syndrome; Werdnig-Hoffmann disease is a heredofamilial degenerative disease of infants that affects only lower motor neurons; and Brown-Séquard syndrome is paralysis, ataxia, and loss of sensation as a result of spinal cord hemisection (see Chapter 8).

Thalamus

I. Introduction: The Thalamus

- is the largest division of the diencephalon.
- receives precortical input from all sensory systems except the olfactory system.
- receives its largest input from the cerebral cortex.
- projects primarily to the cerebral cortex and to a lesser degree to the basal ganglia and hypothalamus.
- plays an important role in sensory and motor systems integration.

II. Boundaries of the Thalamus

A. **Anterior:** interventricular foramen

B. **Posterior:** free pole of the pulvinar

C. **Dorsal:** free surface underlying the fornix and the lateral ventricle

D. **Ventral:** plane connecting the hypothalamic sulci

E. **Medial:** third ventricle

F. **Lateral:** posterior limb of the internal capsule

III. Primary Thalamic Nuclei and Their Major Connections (Figures 16-1 and 16-2)

A. **Anterior nucleus**
- receives hypothalamic input from the mamillary nucleus via the mamillothalamic tract.
- receives hippocampal input via the fornix.
- projects to the cingulate gyrus.
- is part of the Papez circuit of emotion (the limbic system).

B. **Mediodorsal nucleus (dorsomedial nucleus)**
- is reciprocally connected to the prefrontal cortex.
- has abundant connections with the intralaminar nuclei.
- receives input from the amygdaloid nucleus, the temporal neocortex, and the substantia nigra.

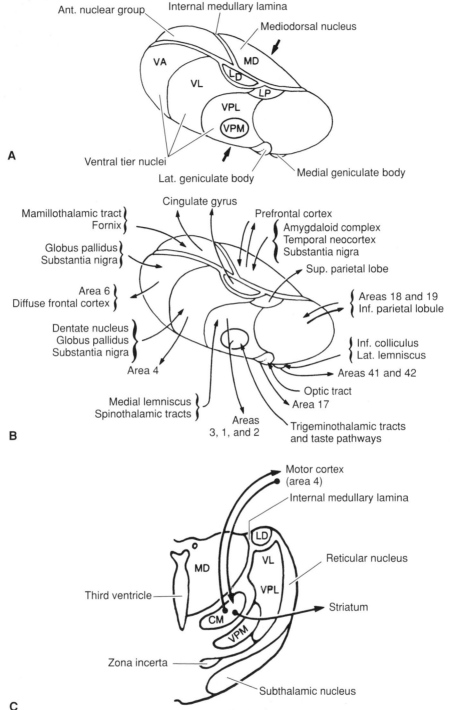

Figure 16-1. Major thalamic nuclei and their afferent connections. **(A)** Oblique dorsolateral aspect of the thalamus and major nuclei. **(B)** The major afferent and efferent connections of the thalamus. **(C)** The transverse section of the thalamus at the level of the *arrows* in **(A)**, showing the major connections of the centromedian nucleus. *CM* = centromedian nucleus; *MD* = mediodorsal nucleus; *LD* = lateral dorsal nucleus; *LP* = lateral posterior nucleus; *VA* = ventral anterior nucleus; *VL* = ventral lateral nucleus; *VPL* = ventral posterolateral nucleus; *VPM* = ventral posteromedial nucleus.

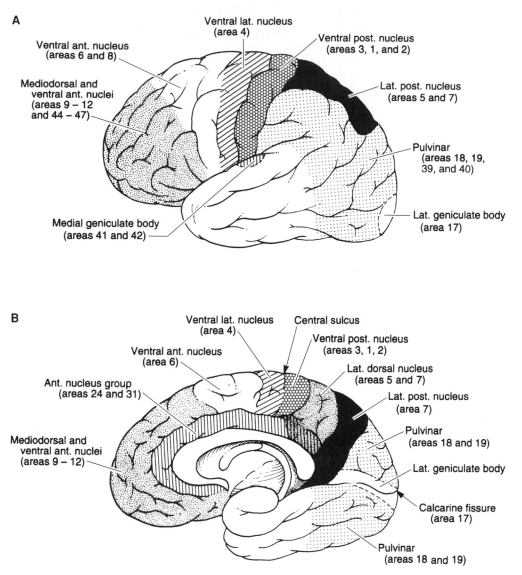

Figure 16-2. (A) Lateral and (B) medial views of the cerebral hemisphere showing the cortical projection areas of the major thalamic nuclei.

- is part of the limbic system and striatal system.
- when destroyed, causes memory loss (Wernicke-Korsakoff syndrome).
- plays a role in the expression of affect, emotion, and behavior (limbic function).

C. Intralaminar nuclei
- receive input from the brainstem reticular formation, the ascending reticular system, and other thalamic nuclei.
- receive spinothalamic and trigeminothalamic input.
- project diffusely to the entire neocortex.
- projects to the mediodorsal nucleus.

1. **Centromedian nucleus**
   - is the largest of the intralaminar nuclei.
   - is reciprocally connected to the motor cortex (area 4).
   - receives input from the globus pallidus.
   - projects to the striatum (caudate nucleus and putamen).
   - projects diffusely to the entire neocortex.
2. **Parafascicular nucleus**
   - projects to the striatum and the supplementary motor cortex (area 6).

D. **Dorsal tier nuclei**
   1. **Lateral dorsal nucleus**
      - is a posterior extension of the anterior nuclear complex.
      - receives mamillothalamic input.
      - projects to the cingulate gyrus.
      - is a part of the limbic system.
   2. **Lateral posterior nucleus**
      - is located between the lateral dorsal nucleus and the pulvinar.
      - has reciprocal connections with the superior parietal cortex (areas 5 and 7).
   3. **Pulvinar**
      - is the largest thalamic nucleus.
      - has reciprocal connections with the association cortex of the occipital, parietal, and posterior temporal lobes.
      - receives input from the lateral and medial geniculate bodies and the superior colliculus.
      - is concerned with the integration of visual, auditory, and somesthetic input.
      - Lesions of the dominant side may result in sensory aphasia.

E. **Ventral tier nuclei**
   - include primarily specific relay nuclei:
   1. **Ventral anterior nucleus**
      - receives input from the globus pallidus (via the thalamic and lenticular fasciculi, H_1 and H_2) and the substantia nigra (motor function).
      - projects diffusely to the prefrontal and orbital cortices.
      - projects to the premotor cortex (area 6).
   2. **Ventral lateral nucleus**
      - receives input from the globus pallidus (via the thalamic and lenticular fasciculi, H_1 and H_2), substantia nigra, and the cerebellum (dentate nucleus).
      - projects to the motor cortex (area 4) and to the supplementary motor area (area 6).
      - influences somatic motor mechanisms via the striatal motor system and the cerebellum.
      - Stereotactic destruction reduces parkinsonian tremor.
   3. **Ventral posterior nucleus**
      - is the nucleus of termination of general somatic afferent (GSA; pain and temperature) and special visceral afferent (SVA; taste) pathways.
      - contains **three subnuclei**:
      a. **Ventral posterolateral (VPL) nucleus**
         - receives the spinothalamic tracts and the medial lemniscus.
         - projects to the somesthetic (sensory) cortex (areas 3, 1, and 2).
         - Lesion results in contralateral loss of pain and temperature sensation as well as loss of tactile discrimination in the trunk and extremities.
      b. **Ventral posteromedial (VPM) nucleus**
         - receives the trigeminothalamic tracts.
         - receives the taste pathway via the solitary nucleus and the parabrachial nucleus.
         - projects to the somesthetic cortex (areas 3, 1, and 2).
         - Lesion results in contralateral loss of pain and temperature sensation, and loss of tactile discrimination in the head; results in ipsilateral loss of taste.

   c. **Ventral posteroinferior (VPI) nucleus**
      • receives vestibulothalamic fibers from the vestibular nuclei.
      • projects to the vestibular area of the somesthetic cortex.

F. **Lateral geniculate body (LGB)**
   • is a visual relay nucleus.
   • receives retinal input via the optic tract.
   • projects to the primary visual cortex (area 17, the lingual gyrus and the cuneus) via the optic radiation.

G. **Medial geniculate body (MGB)**
   • is an auditory relay nucleus.
   • receives auditory input via the brachium of the inferior colliculus.
   • projects to the primary auditory cortex (areas 41 and 42) via the auditory radiation.

IV. Blood Supply of the Thalamus

A. **Posterior communicating artery**
   • gives rise to the anterior thalamoperforating arteries.

B. **Posterior cerebral artery**
   • gives rise to the posterior choroidal arteries.
   • gives rise to the posterior thalamoperforating arteries.

C. **Anterior choroidal artery (LGB)**

V. Internal Capsule (Figure 16-3; see Figures 1-14 through 1-16)

• is a layer of white matter (myelinated axons) that separates the caudate nucleus and thalamus medially from the lentiform nucleus laterally.
• consists of three divisions:

A. **Anterior limb**
   • is located between the caudate nucleus and the lentiform nucleus (the globus pallidus and the putamen).

B. **Genu**
   • contains corticobulbar fibers.

C. **Posterior limb**
   • is located between the thalamus and the lentiform nucleus.
   • contains the sensory radiations (pain, temperature, and touch).
   • contains the corticospinal fibers.
   • contains the visual and auditory radiations.

VI. Blood Supply of the Internal Capsule (see Figure 3-6)

A. **Anterior limb**
   • is irrigated by the medial striate branches of the anterior cerebral artery and by the lateral striate branches (lenticulostriate) of the middle cerebral artery.

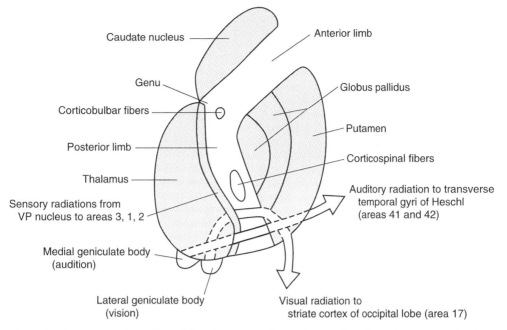

Figure 16-3. Horizontal section of the right internal capsule showing the major fiber projections. Clinically important tracts lie in the genu and in the posterior limb. Lesions of the internal capsule result in contralateral hemiparesis and contralateral hemianopia. (Reprinted with permission from Fix JD: *High-Yield Neuroanatomy,* 3rd ed. Philadelphia, Lippincott Williams & Wilkins, 2005, p 118.)

B. Genu
  • is perfused either by direct branches from the internal carotid artery or by pallidal branches of the anterior choroidal artery.

C. Posterior limb
  • is supplied by branches of the anterior choroidal artery and lenticulostriate branches of the middle cerebral arteries.
  • Ligation of the anterior choroidal artery (in a parkinsonian patient) results in infarction of the corticospinal tract and destruction of the inner segment of the globus pallidus. The patient will have contralateral hemiparesis and contralateral reduction of the rigidity.

VII. Clinical Correlations

A. Infarction of the internal capsule
  • most frequently results from occlusion of the lenticulostriate branches of the middle cerebral artery and results in:
    1. **Contralateral tactile hypesthesia**
    2. **Contralateral anesthesia**
    3. **Contralateral hemiparesis (with the Babinski sign)**
    4. **Contralateral lower facial weakness**
    5. **Contralateral homonymous hemianopia**
B. Thalamic syndrome (Dejerine and Roussy)
  • is usually caused by occlusion of a posterior thalamoperforating artery.
  • has classic signs: contralateral hemiparesis; contralateral hemianesthesia; elevated pain threshold; spontaneous, agonizing, burning pain (hyperpathia); and athetotic posturing of the hand (thalamic hand).

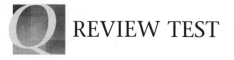

1. Which of the following thalamic nuclei has a motor function?

(A) Lateral dorsal nucleus
(B) Mediodorsal nucleus
(C) Ventral lateral nucleus
(D) Ventral posterior nucleus
(E) Lateral posterior nucleus

2. Spinothalamic fibers project to which of the following thalamic nuclei?

(A) VPM nucleus
(B) Pulvinar
(C) Ventral anterior nucleus
(D) VPL nucleus
(E) Anterior nucleus

3. Cerebellar fibers project to which of the following thalamic nuclei?

(A) VPM nucleus
(B) Lateral dorsal nucleus
(C) Lateral posterior nucleus
(D) Ventral lateral nucleus
(E) Anterior nucleus

4. The globus pallidus projects to which set of thalamic nuclei?

(A) Centromedian, ventral anterior, and ventral lateral nuclei
(B) Ventral anterior, ventral lateral, and anterior nuclei
(C) Ventral lateral, lateral dorsal, and lateral posterior nuclei
(D) Mediodorsal, VPL, and VPM nuclei
(E) Centromedian, lateral dorsal, and lateral ventral nuclei

5. Tritiated leucine [(3H)-leucine] is injected into the medial mamillary nucleus for anterograde transport; radioactive label would be found in the

(A) arcuate nucleus hypothalami
(B) anterior nucleus thalami
(C) ventral anterior nucleus thalami
(D) dorsomedial nucleus thalami
(E) supraoptic nucleus

6. Infarction of what structure could give rise to left hypesthesia, left homonymous hemianopia, left facial weakness, tongue deviation to the left side, and plantar extensor on the left side?

(A) Left internal capsule
(B) Right internal capsule
(C) Left pulvinar
(D) Right pulvinar
(E) MGB

7. A capsular stroke is most commonly caused by occlusion of which of the following arteries?

(A) Anterior cerebral artery
(B) Recurrent artery of Heubner
(C) Lateral striate arteries
(D) Posterior communicating artery
(E) Direct branches of the internal carotid artery

Questions 8 to 13

The response options for items 8 to 13 are the same. Select one answer for each item in the set.

(A) Anterior nucleus
(B) Centromedian nucleus
(C) Lateral geniculate nucleus
(D) Mediodorsal nucleus
(E) Pulvinar
(F) Ventral anterior nucleus
(G) Ventral lateral nucleus
(H) VPL nucleus
(I) VPM nucleus

Match each of the following descriptions with the appropriate thalamic nucleus.

8. Receives input from the ipsilateral central tegmental tract

9. Has reciprocal connections with the inferior parietal lobule

10. Receives input from the contralateral lateral spinothalamic tract

11. Projects to the putamen

12. Receives the dentatothalamic tract

13. Plays a role in the expression of affect, emotion, and behavior (limbic function)

Questions 14 to 18

The response options for items 14 to 18 are the same. Select one answer for each item in the set.

(A) Anterior nucleus
(B) Ventral lateral nucleus
(C) Medial geniculate (nucleus) body
(D) VPM nucleus
(E) VPI nucleus

Match each pathway with the appropriate nucleus to which it gives input.

14. Brachium of the inferior colliculus

15. Thalamic fasciculus (H_1)

16. Mamillothalamic tract

17. Dentatothalamic tract

18. Gustatory (taste) pathway

ANSWERS AND EXPLANATIONS

1–C. The ventral lateral nucleus receives motor input from the extrapyramidal (striatal) motor system (globus pallidus and substantia nigra) and from the cerebellum (dentate nucleus).

2–D. Spinothalamic fibers project to the VPL nucleus, which receives the medial lemniscus.

3–D. Cerebellar fibers (dentatocerebellar) project to the ventral lateral and VPL nuclei, which project to the motor cortex (area 4).

4–A. The globus pallidus, a nucleus of the extrapyramidal (striatal) motor system, projects to three thalamic nuclei: the centromedian, the ventral anterior, and the ventral lateral nuclei of the thalamus.

5–B. Radioactive label is found in the anterior nucleus of the thalamus, which receives input from the mammillary nucleus via the mamillothalamic tract. The arcuate nucleus of the hypothalamus projects to the portal vessels of the infundibulum via the tuberohypophysial (tuberoinfundibular) pathway; the ventral anterior nucleus of the thalamus receives input from the globus pallidus and the substantia nigra; the dorsomedial nucleus of the thalamus receives input from the amygdala, temporal neocortex and substantia nigra; and the supraoptic nucleus of the hypothalamus synthesizes vasopressin and oxytocin and projects to the pituitary.

6–B. Infarction of the internal capsule gives rise to contralateral symptoms. Thus, infarction to the right internal capsule would result in left-sided symptoms, including tactile hypesthesia, contralateral anesthesia, contralateral hemiparesis (with the Babinski sign), contralateral lower facial weakness, and contralateral homonymous hemianopia.

7–C. A capsular stroke is most commonly caused by occlusion of the lateral striate branches of the middle cerebral artery.

8–I. The VPM nucleus receives taste input via the ipsilateral central tegmental tract. The VPM nucleus receives sensory input from the head and oral cavity.

9–E. The pulvinar, the largest thalamic nucleus, has reciprocal connections with the inferior parietal lobule.

10–H. The VPL nucleus receives input from the contralateral lateral spinothalamic tract.

11–B. The centromedian nucleus projects to the putamen; this thalamic nucleus also has reciprocal connections with the motor cortex.

12–G. The ventral lateral nucleus receives contralateral cerebellar input via the dentatothalamic tract.

13–D. The mediodorsal nucleus plays a role in the expression of affect, emotion, and behavior (limbic function). It receives input from the amygdala and has reciprocal connections with the prefrontal cortex. Lesions of the mediodorsal nucleus are found in patients with the Korsakoff amnestic state.

14–C. The medial geniculate body receives auditory input via the brachium of the inferior colliculus.

15–B. The ventral lateral nucleus receives input from the globus pallidus via the thalamic fasciculus (H_1).

16–A. The anterior nucleus receives input from the mamillary nuclei via the mamillothalamic tract. This is a major link in the Papez circuit.

17–B. The ventral lateral nucleus receives cerebellar input from the dentate nucleus via the dentatothalamic tract.

18–D. The VPM nucleus receives SVA (taste) fibers from the central tegmental tract.

Visual System

I.　Introduction: The Visual System

- is served by the **optic nerve**, **CN II**, which is a special somatic afferent (**SSA**) nerve.

II.　The Retina

- is the innermost layer of the eye.
- is derived from the optic vesicle of the diencephalon.
- contains efferent fibers that give rise to the optic nerve, which is actually a fiber tract of the diencephalon.
- is sensitive to wavelengths from 400 nm to 700 nm.

A.　Structures of the ocular fundus

1. **Optic disk (optic papilla)**
   - is located 3.5 mm nasal to the fovea centralis.
   - contains unmyelinated axons from the ganglion cell layer of the retina.
   - is the blind spot (contains no rods or cones).
   - contains a central cup, a peripheral disk margin, and retinal vessels.
2. **Macula lutea**
   - is a yellow-pigmented area that surrounds the fovea centralis.
3. **Fovea centralis**
   - is located within the macula lutea, 2.5 disk diameters temporal to the optic disk.
   - contains only cones and is the site of highest visual acuity.
   - is avascular and receives nutrients by diffusion via the choriocapillaris.
   - subserves color or day (photopic) vision.
4. **Retinal blood supply**
   - is supplied by the **choriocapillaris** of the choroid layer and the **central retinal artery**, a branch of the ophthalmic artery.
   - Occlusion of the central retinal artery results in blindness.

B.　Cells of the retina (Figure 17-1)

- constitute a chain of three neurons that project visual impulses via the optic nerve and the lateral geniculate body (LGB) to the visual cortex.
1. **Rods and cones**
   - are first-order receptor cells that respond directly to light stimulation.
   - generate only graded potentials.
   - utilize glutamate as a neurotransmitter.

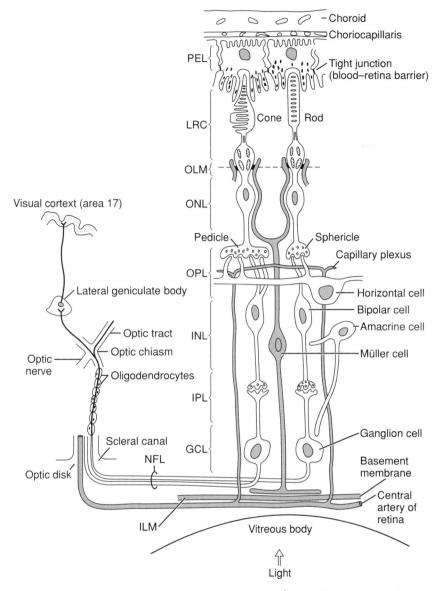

Figure 17-1.   Histology of the retina. The retina has 10 layers: (*1*) pigment epithelium layer (PEL), (*2*) layer of rods and cones (LRC), (*3*) outer limiting membrane (OLM), (*4*) outer nuclear layer (ONL), (*5*) outer plexiform layer (OPL), (*6*) inner nuclear layer (INL), (*7*) inner plexiform layer (IPL), (*8*) ganglion cell layer (GCL), (*9*) nerve fiber layer (NFL), and (*10*) inner limiting membrane (ILM). The tight junctions binding the pigment epithelial cells make up the blood–retina barrier. Retinal detachment usually occurs between the pigment layer and the layer of rods and cones. The central artery of the retina perfuses the retina to the outer plexiform layer, and the choriocapillaris supplies the outer five layers of the retina. The Müller cells are radial glial cells that have support function. Myelin of the CNS is produced by oligodendrocytes, which are not normally found in the retina. (Adapted with permission from Dudek RW: *High-Yield Histology*. Baltimore, Williams & Wilkins, 1997, p 64.)

     a. **Rods (100 million)**
- contain **rhodopsin** (visual purple).
- are sensitive to low-intensity light.
- subserve night (scotopic) vision.

     b. **Cones (7 million)**
- contain the photopigment **iodopsin**.
- operate only at high illumination levels.
- are concentrated in the fovea centralis.
- are responsible for day (photopic) vision, color vision, and high visual acuity.

2. **Bipolar neurons**
- are second-order neurons that relay stimuli from the rods and cones to the ganglion cells.
- generate only graded potentials.
- utilize glutamate as a neurotransmitter.

3. **Ganglion cells**
- are third-order neurons that form the optic nerve (CN II).
- are retinal cells with voltage-gated sodium channels that generate action potentials.
- project directly to the hypothalamus, superior colliculus, pretectal nucleus, and LGB.
- utilize glutamate as a neurotransmitter.

4. **Interneurons**

     a. **Horizontal cells**
- interconnect photoreceptors and bipolar cells.
- inhibit neighboring photoreceptors (lateral inhibition).
- generate only graded potentials.
- utilize gamma-aminobutyric acid (GABA) as a neurotransmitter.
- play a role in the differentiation of colors.

     b. **Amacrine cells**
- are small cells that have no axons and few dendrites.
- receive input from bipolar cells and project inhibitory signals to ganglion cells.
- mediate lateral interactions at the bipolar–ganglion cell synapse.
- utilize GABA, glycine, dopamine, and acetylcholine (ACh) as neurotransmitters.

5. **Müller cells**
- are radial glial cells that have a support function similar to that of astrocytes.
- extend from the inner limiting layer to the outer limiting layer.

C. **Meridional divisions of the retina**
1. The visual field illustrated in Figure 17-2 is the environment seen by one eye (**monocular field**) or by both eyes (**binocular field**).
2. The vertical meridian divides the retina into **nasal and temporal hemiretinae**; the horizontal meridian divides the retina into upper and lower hemiretinae (**upper and lower quadrants**).

     a. **Temporal hemiretina**
- receives image input from the nasal visual field.
- has ganglion cells that project to the ipsilateral LGB, layers 2, 3, and 5.

     b. **Nasal hemiretina**
- receives image input from the temporal visual field.
- has ganglion cells that project to the contralateral LGB, layers 1, 4, and 6.

     c. **Upper retinal quadrants**
- receive image input from the lower visual fields.
- have ganglion cells that project via the LGB to the upper banks of the calcarine fissure.

     d. **Lower retinal quadrants**
- receive image input from the upper visual fields.
- have ganglion cells that project via the LGB to the lower banks of the calcarine fissure.

D. **Concentric divisions of the retina and retinotopy**
1. **Macular area**
- is a small area surrounding the fovea centralis that serves central vision (high visual acuity).
- contains cones.
- predominantly projects to the posterior part of the visual cortex.

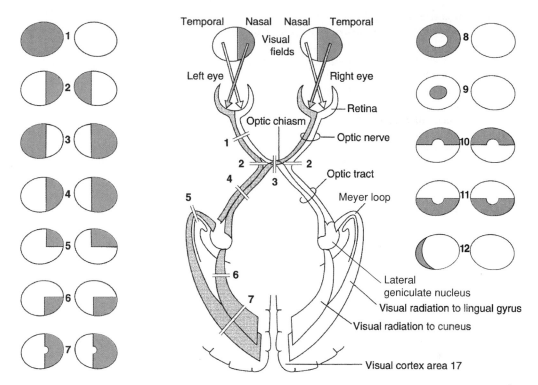

Figure 17-2.   Visual pathway from the retina to the visual cortex showing visual field defects. (**1**) Ipsilateral blindness. (**2**) Binasal hemianopia. (**3**) Bitemporal hemianopia. (**4**) Right hemianopia. (**5**) Right upper quadrantanopia. (**6**) Right lower quadrantanopia. (**7**) Right hemianopia with macular sparing. (**8**) Left constricted field as a result of end-stage glaucoma; bilateral constricted fields may be seen in hysteria. (**9**) Left central scotoma as seen in optic (retrobulbar) neuritis in multiple sclerosis. (**10**) Upper altitudinal hemianopia as a result of bilateral destruction of the lingual gyri. (**11**) Lower altitudinal hemianopia as a result of bilateral destruction of the cunei. (**12**) Left temporal crescent defect due to a lesion of the right visual cortex (area 17). (Reprinted with permission from Fix JD: *High-Yield Neuroanatomy,* 3rd ed. Philadelphia, Lippincott Williams & Wilkins, 2005, p 119.)

   2. **Paramacular area**
- is a large area surrounding the macular area that contains predominantly rods.
- projects to the visual cortex anterior to the macular representation.

   3. **Monocular area**
- represents the peripheral monocular field.
- projects to the visual cortex anterior to the paramacular representation.
- Lesions result in a contralateral crescentic defect.

III.   Visual Pathway (see Figures 1-2 and 17-2)

- transmits visual impulses from the retina to the LGB and from the LGB to the primary visual cortex (area 17) of the occipital lobe.
- consists of the following structures:

A. Ganglion cells
- constitute the ganglion cell layer of the retina, with axons that form the optic nerve, CN II.
- project from the nasal hemiretina to the contralateral LGB.
- project from the temporal hemiretina to the ipsilateral LGB.

B. **Optic nerve (CN II)**
- is a myelinated tract of the central nervous system (CNS; diencephalon) and is **not a true nerve**.
- is invested by the pia–arachnoid and dura mater.
- receives its blood supply from the central retinal artery, pial arteries, posterior ciliary arteries, and the arterial circle of Willis.
- is surrounded by the subarachnoid space.
- is **incapable of regeneration**.
- Compression results in **optic atrophy**.
- Transection at the chiasma results in **ipsilateral blindness** and a contralateral upper temporal scotoma (**junction scotoma**); inferior nasal fibers loop into the contralateral optic nerve (see Figure 17-1).

C. **Optic chiasm**
- is part of the diencephalon.
- lies dorsal to the hypophysis and diaphragma sellae.
- contains decussating fibers from the two nasal hemiretinae.
- contains noncrossing fibers from the two temporal hemiretinae.
- receives its blood supply from the anterior cerebral and internal carotid arteries.
- Midsagittal transection or pressure results in **bitemporal hemianopia** (pituitary tumor).
- Bilateral lateral compression results in **binasal hemianopia** (calcified internal carotid arteries).

D. **Optic tract**
- contains fibers from the ipsilateral temporal hemiretina and the contralateral nasal hemiretina.
- contains **pupillary reflex fibers**.
- projects to the LGB and via the brachium of the superior colliculus to the pretectal nuclei and superior colliculus.
- receives its blood supply from the posterior communicating artery and the anterior choroidal artery.
- Transection results in **contralateral homonymous hemianopia** and in **transsynaptic degeneration of the ipsilateral LGB**.

E. **Lateral geniculate body (LGB)**
- is a thalamic relay nucleus subserving vision.
- receives fibers from the ipsilateral temporal hemiretina, which terminate in layers 2, 3, and 5.
- receives fibers from the contralateral nasal hemiretina, which terminate in layers 1, 4, and 6.
- projects, via the geniculocalcarine tract, the visual radiation to the primary visual cortex (area 17). The stripe of Gennari marks the calcarine cortex.
- is irrigated by branches of the posterior cerebral artery and the anterior choroidal artery.
- Destruction results in a **contralateral homonymous hemianopia**.

F. **Geniculocalcarine tract (visual radiation)** (Figure 17-3)
- extends from the LGB to the banks of the calcarine sulcus, the visual cortex (area 17).
- is irrigated by branches of the middle cerebral artery, anterior choroidal artery, and calcarine artery (a branch of the posterior cerebral artery).
- Transection results in **contralateral homonymous hemianopia**.
- has two divisions (see Figure 17-3):
  1. **Upper division**
     - projects to the upper bank of the calcarine sulcus, the **cuneus**.
     - contains input from the superior retinal quadrants, representing inferior visual field quadrants.
     - Transection results in **contralateral lower homonymous quadrantanopia**.
  2. **Lower division**
     - loops from the LGB anteriorly (Meyer loop), then posteriorly to terminate in the lower bank of the calcarine sulcus, the **lingual gyrus**.

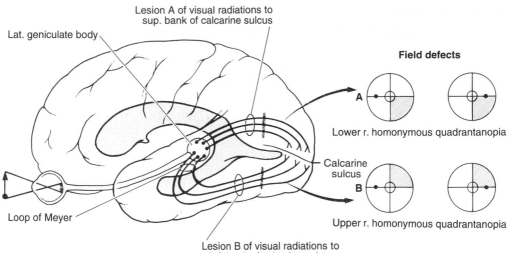

Lesion A of visual radiations to
sup. bank of calcarine sulcus

Lat. geniculate body

Field defects

A

Lower r. homonymous quadrantanopia

Calcarine
sulcus

B

Loop of Meyer

Upper r. homonymous quadrantanopia

Lesion B of visual radiations to
inf. bank of calcarine sulcus

Figure 17-3. Relationships of the left upper and left lower divisions of the geniculocalcarine tract to the lateral ventricle and the calcarine sulcus. Transection of the upper division (**A**) results in right lower homonymous quadrantanopia; transection of the lower division (**B**) results in right upper homonymous quadrantanopia.

- contains input from the inferior retinal quadrants, representing superior visual field quadrants.
- Transection of Meyer loop results in a **contralateral upper homonymous quadrantanopia**.

G. Visual (striate) cortex (area 17)
- is located on the banks of the calcarine sulcus.
- receives retinal input via the ipsilateral LGB.
- receives its blood supply from the calcarine artery, a branch of the posterior cerebral artery; anastomosis with the middle cerebral artery may be substantial (**macular sparing**).
- Lesions result in a **contralateral homonymous hemianopia** with macular sparing. Bilateral destruction of both cunei results in a **lower altitudinal hemianopia**, and bilateral destruction of the lingual gyri results in an **upper altitudinal hemianopia**.
- **Retinotopic organization** of the visual cortex includes:
  1. **Posterior third of the visual cortex**
     - receives macular input (central vision).
  2. **Intermediate area of the visual cortex**
     - receives paramacular input (peripheral input).
  3. **Anterior area of the visual cortex**
     - receives monocular input.

IV. Pupillary Light Reflexes and Pathway (Figure 17-4)

A. Pupillary light reflexes
- result when light shined into one eye causes both pupils to constrict.
  1. **Direct pupillary light reflex**
     - is the response in the stimulated eye.
  2. **Consensual pupillary light reflex**
     - is the response in the unstimulated eye.

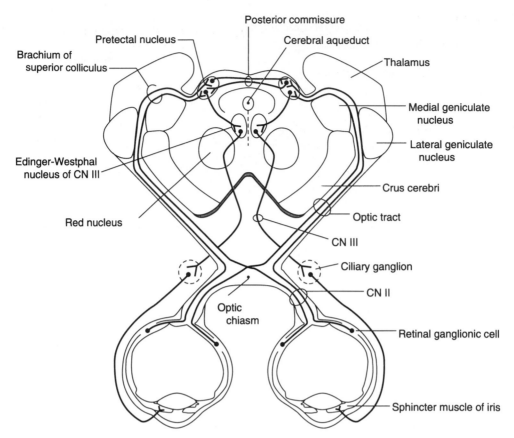

Figure 17-4. Diagram of the pupillary light pathway. Light shining into one eye causes both pupils to constrict. The response in the stimulated eye is called the direct pupillary light reflex; the response in the opposite eye is called the consensual pupillary light reflex. (Reprinted with permission from Fix JD: *High-Yield Neuroanatomy,* 3rd ed. Philadelphia, Lippincott Williams & Wilkins, 2005, p 123.)

B. Pupillary light reflex pathway
- comprises an afferent limb, **CN II,** and an efferent limb, **CN III.**
- consists of the following structures:
  1. **Ganglion cells of the retina**
     - project bilaterally to the pretectal nuclei.
  2. **Pretectal nucleus of the midbrain**
     - projects crossed (in the posterior commissure) and uncrossed fibers to the rostral Edinger-Westphal nucleus.
  3. **Edinger-Westphal nucleus of the midbrain**
     - gives rise to preganglionic parasympathetic fibers, which exit the midbrain with the oculomotor nerve and synapse with postganglionic parasympathetic neurons of the ciliary ganglion.
  4. **Ciliary ganglion of the orbit**
     - gives rise to postganglionic parasympathetic fibers, which innervate the sphincter muscle of the iris.

V.   Pupillary Dilation Pathway

- is mediated by the sympathetic division of the autonomic nervous system (ANS).
- Interruption at any level results in **Horner syndrome.**
- consists of the following structures:

A. **Hypothalamus**
   - has neurons that project directly to the ciliospinal center (T1–T2) of the intermediolateral cell column (Figure 17-5).

B. **Ciliospinal center of the spinal cord**
   - projects preganglionic sympathetic fibers via the sympathetic trunk to the superior cervical ganglion.

C. **Superior cervical ganglion**
   - projects postganglionic sympathetic fibers via the perivascular plexus of the carotid system to the dilator muscle of the iris and to the palpebral muscles of Müller. Postganglionic sympathetic fibers pass through the cavernous sinus and enter the orbit via the superior orbital fissure.

VI. The Convergence-Accommodation Reaction (see Figure 17-5)

- is essential for visual fixation and acuity at close range.
- is initiated by conscious visual fixation on a near object or by a blurred retinal image.

A. **Reflex changes**
   - with accommodative effort, three reflex changes are evoked:
     1. **Convergence**
        - occurs as the eyes focus on a near point.
        - is mediated by medial recti innervation via the oculomotor nerve (CN III).

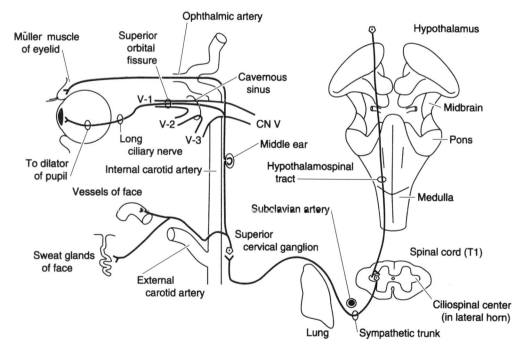

Figure 17-5. Pupillary dilation pathway (oculosympathetic pathway). Hypothalamic fibers project to the ipsilateral and ciliospinal center of the intermediolateral cell column at T1. The ciliospinal center projects preganglionic sympathetic fibers to the superior cervical ganglion. The superior cervical ganglion projects perivascular postganglionic sympathetic fibers via the tympanic cavity, cavernous sinus, and superior orbital fissure to the dilator muscle of the iris. Interruption of this pathway at any level results in Horner syndrome. (Reprinted with permission from Fix JD: *High-Yield Neuroanatomy,* 3rd ed. Philadelphia, Lippincott Williams & Wilkins, 2005, p 67.)

2. **Accommodation**
   - is adjustment of the eyes for various distances.
   - occurs as contraction of the ciliary muscle results in a thickening of the lens and an increase in refractive power.
   - is mediated by the caudal Edinger-Westphal nucleus via CN III.
3. **Pupillary constriction**
   - results in an increase in depth of field and depth of focus.
   - is mediated by the rostral Edinger-Westphal nucleus via CN III.

B. **The convergence-accommodation pathway** (see Figure 17-5)
   1. **Visual cortex (area 17)**
      - projects to the visual association cortex (area 19).
   2. **Visual association cortex (area 19)**
      - projects via the corticotectal tract to the pretectal area of the midbrain.
   3. **Pretectal area**
      - projects to Perlia nucleus.
   4. **Perlia nucleus of the oculomotor complex, CN III**
      - projects to the rostral and caudal Edinger-Westphal nuclei and the medial rectus subnuclei of CN III.

VII. Centers for Ocular Motility

A. **Frontal eye field**
   - is located in the caudal part of the middle frontal gyrus (area 8).
   - is a cortical center for voluntary eye movements, which are fast, saccadic, searching movements.
   - Stimulation (irritative lesion) results in **contralateral conjugate deviation of the eyes**.
   - Destruction (destructive lesion) results in **transient ipsilateral conjugate deviation of the eyes.**

B. **Occipital eye fields (area 18 and 19)**
   - are the cortical centers for involuntary pursuit or tracing movements.
   - Stimulation results in **contralateral conjugate deviation of the eyes**.
   - Lesions result in difficulty following a slow-moving object.

C. **Subcortical center for vertical conjugate gaze**
   - is located at the level of the posterior commissure.
   - includes the **rostral interstitial nucleus of the medial longitudinal fasciculus (MLF)**, which projects to the oculomotor and trochlear nuclei.
   - is involved in **Parinaud syndrome** (see Chapter 14 IV A).

D. **Subcortical center for lateral conjugate gaze** (Figure 17-6)
   - is located in the abducent nucleus of CN VI. Some authorities place the subcortical center in the parapontine reticular formation (PPRF); others place it in the nucleus prepositus.
   - receives input from the contralateral frontal eye field.
   - projects via the contralateral MLF to the medial rectus subnucleus of the oculomotor complex.
   - projects via abducent fibers to the ipsilateral lateral rectus muscle.
   - Damage to the MLF between the abducent and oculomotor nuclei results in **medial rectus palsy** (see VIII B).

VIII. Clinical Correlations

A. **Anisocoria (unequal pupils)**
   - is a condition in which the two pupils are not equal.
   - is present in 10% of the population.
   - is seen in **Horner syndrome** and **third nerve palsies.**

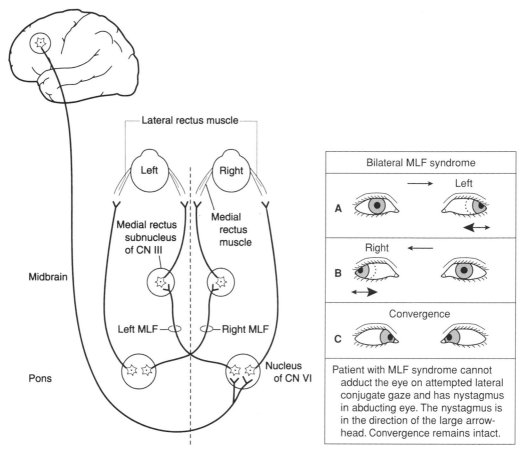

Figure 17-6. Connections of the pontine center for lateral conjugate gaze. Lesions of the medial longitudinal fasciculus (MLF) between the abducent and oculomotor nuclei result in a medial rectus palsy on attempted lateral conjugate gaze and horizontal nystagmus in the abducting eye. Convergence remains intact (*inset*). A unilateral MLF lesion would affect the ipsilateral medial rectus only. (Reprinted with permission from Fix JD: *High-Yield Neuroanatomy,* 3rd ed. Philadelphia, Lippincott Williams & Wilkins, 2005, p 125.)

B. **MLF syndrome (internuclear ophthalmoplegia [INO])** (Figure 17-7; see Figure 17-6)
  - is a condition in which there is damage (demyelination) to the MLF between the abducent and oculomotor nuclei.
  - results in **medial rectus palsy** on attempted lateral conjugate gaze and **monocular horizontal nystagmus** in the abducting eye (convergence is normal).

C. **One-and-a-half syndrome**
  - consists of a bilateral MLF lesion and a unilateral lesion of the abducent nucleus.
  - On attempted lateral conjugate gaze, the only muscle that functions is the intact lateral rectus.

D. **Argyll Robertson pupil (pupillary light-near dissociation)** (see Figure 17-7)
  - is the absence of a miotic reaction to light, both direct and consensual, with preservation of miotic reaction to near stimulus (accommodation-convergence).
  - may be present in tertiary **syphilis, diabetes mellitus**, and **lupus erythematosus**.

E. **Afferent pupil (Marcus Gunn pupil)** (see Figure 17-7)
  - results from a **lesion in the afferent limb of the pupillary light reflex** (e.g., **retrobulbar neuritis** of the optic nerve seen in **multiple sclerosis**).

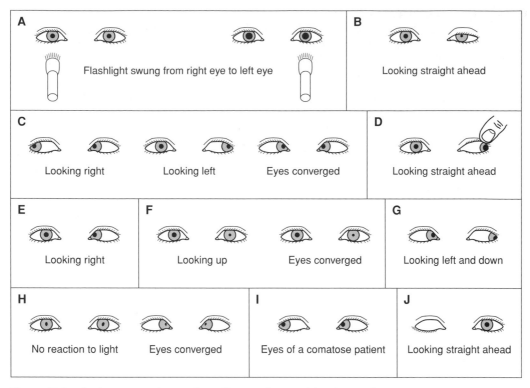

Figure 17-7. Ocular motor palsies and pupillary syndromes. **(A)** Relative afferent (Marcus Gunn) pupil, left eye. **(B)** Horner syndrome, left eye. **(C)** Internuclear ophthalmoplegia, right eye. **(D)** Third nerve palsy, left eye. **(E)** Sixth nerve palsy, right eye. **(F)** Paralysis of upward gaze and convergence (Parinaud syndrome). **(G)** Fourth nerve palsy, right eye. **(H)** Argyll Robertson pupil. **(I)** Destructive lesion of the right frontal eye field. **(J)** Third nerve palsy with ptosis, right eye. (Reprinted with permission from Fix JD: *High-Yield Neuroanatomy,* 3rd ed. Philadelphia, Lippincott Williams & Wilkins, 2005, p 124.)

- can be diagnosed by the **swinging flashlight test**.
    1. Light shined into the normal eye results in brisk **pupillary constriction** in both the normal eye and in the affected eye (consensual reaction).
    2. Light is then immediately shined into the affected eye with the afferent lesion, which results in **dilation of the afferent pupil**. The consensual stimulation of the constrictor pupillae muscle is much greater than the direct stimulation through a defective optic nerve.

F. **Transtentorial herniation (uncal herniation)** (see Figure 17-7)
   - occurs as the result of **increased supratentorial pressure**, commonly due to a brain tumor or a hematoma (subdural or epidural).
     1. The pressure cone forces the parahippocampal uncus through the tentorial incisure.
     2. The impacted parahippocampal uncus forces the contralateral crus cerebri against the tentorial edge (Kernohan notch) and brings pressure to bear on the ipsilateral CN III and the posterior cerebral artery, resulting in the following neurologic deficits:
        a. **Ipsilateral hemiparesis** due to pressure on the corticospinal tract in the crus cerebri
        b. **A fixed and dilated pupil, ptosis, and a down-and-out eye** due to pressure on the ipsilateral oculomotor nerve
        c. **Contralateral homonymous hemianopia** due to compression of the ipsilateral posterior cerebral artery, which irrigates the visual cortex

G. Papilledema (choked disk)
- is a noninflammatory congestion of the optic disk caused by increased intracranial pressure.
- is most commonly caused by **brain tumors, subdural hematoma,** and **hydrocephalus.**
- usually does not alter visual acuity or result in visual field defects.
- is usually asymmetric and is greater on the side of the supratentorial lesion.

H. Adie pupil (Holmes-Adie pupil)
- is a large tonic pupil that reacts slowly to light but does not react to near (light-near dissociation).
- is commonly seen in females with absent knee or ankle jerks.

I. Ptosis (see Figure 17-7)
- is a drooping eyelid seen in many syndromes.
  1. Oculomotor ptosis
  - is due to paralysis of the levator palpebrae (e.g., transtentorial herniation).
  2. Oculosympathetic ptosis
  - is due to paralysis of the Müller muscle as seen in Horner syndrome. This is a very slight ptosis, or pseudoptosis (e.g., Pancoast tumor).
  3. Myasthenic ptosis
  - is seen in myasthenia gravis.
  - usually increases with increasing fatigue.
  - immediately improves after an injection of a cholinesterase inhibitor (edrophonium).
  - is usually bilateral and asymmetric.

REVIEW TEST

1. Interruption of the MLF at pontine levels

(A) results in miosis and ptosis
(B) results in paralysis of upward gaze on command
(C) results in paralysis of lateral gaze on command
(D) abolishes convergence
(E) abolishes accommodation

2. A 75-year-old coal miner complains of progressive loss of vision. Visual field examination shows visual loss in the upper right quadrant in both visual fields. The lesion would most likely be in the

(A) right angular gyrus
(B) left cuneus
(C) left temporal lobe
(D) right occipital pole
(E) right lingual gyrus

Questions 3 to 10

The response options for items 3 to 10 are the same. Select one answer for each item in the set.

(A) Bitemporal hemianopia
(B) Binasal hemianopia
(C) Left upper homonymous quadrantanopia
(D) Right lower homonymous quadrantanopia
(E) Left homonymous hemianopia

Match each defect below with the condition it causes.

3. Transection of the right optic tract

4. Transection of the right Meyer loop

5. Midsagittal section of the optic chiasm

6. Tumor of the right LGB

7. Pituitary tumor

8. Tumor of the left cuneus

9. Trauma to the right lingual gyrus

10. Bilateral lateral constriction of the optic chiasm

Questions 11 to 17

The response options for items 11 to 17 are the same. Select one answer for each item in the set.

(A) Anisocoria
(B) Argyll Robertson pupil
(C) Fixed, dilated pupil
(D) Horner syndrome
(E) Marcus Gunn pupil

Match each description below with the syndrome or defect most closely associated with it.

11. Results from interruption of the cervical sympathetic trunk

12. Is present in 10% of the population

13. Is characterized by uncal herniation

14. Is characterized by the absence of the miotic reaction to light but with the presence of the miotic reaction to near stimulus

15. The pupil dilates when light is shined from the normal pupil into the afferent pupil

16. Is frequently seen in multiple sclerosis

17. Is associated with syphilis

Questions 18 to 23

The response options for items 18 to 23 are the same. Select one answer for each item in the set.

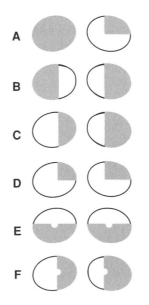

Match the description of the lesion sites in items 18 to 23 with the appropriate visual field defect shown in the figure.

18. Occlusion of the left posterior cerebral artery

19. Transection of the left optic nerve at the chiasm

20. Craniopharyngioma

21. Left temporal lobotomy

22. Bilateral trauma to the cuneate gyri

23. Transection of the left optic tract

Questions 24 to 32

The response options for items 24 to 32 are the same. Select one answer for each item in the set.

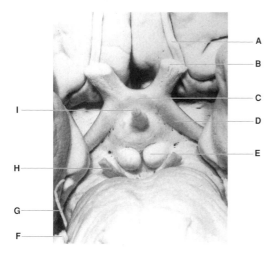

Match the description of the lesion sites in items 24 to 32 with the appropriate deficit or pathologic finding shown in the photograph of the base of the brain.

24. Transection results in polyuria and polydipsia

25. Transection results in ipsilateral ptosis

26. Transection results in homolateral extortion of the globe

27. Destruction results in an absent corneal reflex on the side of testing

28. Pathology is seen in Wernicke encephalopathy

29. Transection results in a contralateral hemianopia

30. Midsagittal section results in a bitemporal hemianopia

31. Transection results in total blindness in the left eye

32. Compression is seen in Foster Kennedy syndrome

ANSWERS AND EXPLANATIONS

1–C. Interruption of the pontine MLF results in a medial rectus palsy on attempted conjugate lateral gaze. Convergence remains intact. This syndrome, called INO or MLF syndrome, is commonly seen in multiple sclerosis.

2–C. Ablation of the anterior temporal lobe destroys the visual radiations that project to the lower bank of the calcarine sulcus. The field deficit is an upper right homonymous quadrantanopia, which is also called Meyer loop quadrantanopia.

3–E. Transection of the right optic tract results in a left homonymous hemianopia.

4–C. Transection of the Meyer loop on the right side results in a left upper quadrantanopia ("pie in the sky"). The Meyer loop is the inferior geniculocalcarine pathway, which conveys information from the inferior retinal quadrants to the inferior bank of the calcarine sulcus, the lingual gyrus.

5–A. A midsagittal section of the optic chiasm interrupts the decussating fibers from the nasal hemiretinae and results in a bitemporal hemianopia.

6–E. A lesion of the right LGB produces a left homonymous hemianopia. A lesion of the optic tract, the LGB, or the visual pathway all produce the same field deficit, a contralateral homonymous hemianopia.

7–A. A pituitary tumor most commonly produces a bitemporal hemianopia. The pituitary (hypophysis) gland lies ventral to the optic chiasm.

8–D. Destruction of the left cuneus produces a right lower homonymous quadrantanopia. Upper retinal quadrants project to the upper banks of the calcarine sulcus.

9–C. Destruction of the right lingual gyrus produces a left upper homonymous quadrantanopia. Lower retinal quadrants project to the lower banks of the calcarine sulcus.

10–B. Bilateral constriction of the optic chiasm damages the nondecussating fibers from the temporal hemiretinae and produces a binasal hemianopia.

11–D. Horner syndrome results from interruption of the cervical sympathetic trunk.

12–A. Anisocoria, unequal pupils, is present in 10% of the population.

13–C. In transtentorial herniation, the hippocampal uncus is forced by increased pressure (brain tumor) through the tentorial incisure. Pressure on the oculomotor nerve (CN III) results in a fixed, dilated pupil and an eye that looks down and out. Pressure on the basis pedunculi, affecting the corticospinal tracts, results in a contralateral hemiparesis.

14–B. The Argyll Robertson pupil is characterized by absence of the miotic reaction to light but with presence of the miotic reaction to near stimulus.

15–E. The Marcus Gunn pupil is an afferent pupil, with a lesion in the afferent limb of the pupillary light pathway.

16–E. The Marcus Gunn pupil is commonly seen in multiple sclerosis.

17–B. The Argyll Robertson pupil is associated with neurosyphilis.

238

18–F. Occlusion of the left posterior cerebral artery results in a right homonymous hemianopia with macular sparing; macular sparing is due to a dual blood supply to the visual cortex.

19–A. Transection of the left optic nerve at the chiasm results in total blindness on the left side and a scotoma in the right upper temporal quadrant. Fibers from the lower nasal quadrant loop into the contralateral optic nerve before decussating in the optic chiasma. The field defect is called a junction scotoma.

20–B. Craniopharyngiomas and pituitary tumors put pressure on the decussating fibers of the optic chiasma, causing a bitemporal hemianopia.

21–D. A left temporal lobotomy transects Meyer loop, which projects to the inferior bank of the calcarine fissure, resulting in a right upper quadrantanopia.

22–E. Bilateral trauma to the cuneate gyri results in a lower altitudinal hemianopia.

23–C. Transection of the left optic tract results in a right hemianopia with macular sparing.

24–I. Transection of the infundibulum interrupts the supraopticohypophyseal tract. This results in diabetes insipidus with polydipsia and polyuria (e.g., craniopharyngioma).

25–H. Destruction of the oculomotor nerve results in paralysis of the levator palpebrae muscle with a severe ipsilateral ptosis.

26–G. The trochlear nerve intorts, elevates, and abducts the globe. In fourth nerve palsy, the ipsilateral eye is extorted. The patent's chin points to the side of the lesion. Remember, head tilt is associated with fourth nerve palsy.

27–F. The ophthalmic division of the trigeminal nerve mediates the afferent limb of the corneal reflex.

28–E. In Wernicke encephalopathy, petechial hemorrhages in the mamillary bodies are commonly found, along with capillary hyperplasia, and astrocytic gliosis. Wernicke encephalopathy is due to a thiamine (vitamin B_1) deficiency.

29–D. Severance of the optic tract results in contralateral hemianopia.

30–C. A midsagittal section through the optic chiasm results in bitemporal hemianopia.

31–B. Transection of the optic nerve (fasciculus) results in total blindness of the ipsilateral eye.

32–A. Foster Kennedy syndrome involves the olfactory tract and the optic nerve. This disorder may be due to a tumor (olfactory groove meningioma). The signs are ipsilateral anosmia, ipsilateral optic atrophy, and contralateral papilledema.

Autonomic Nervous System

I. Overview: The Autonomic Nervous System (ANS)

- is a general visceral efferent (**GVE**) motor system that controls and regulates smooth muscle, cardiac muscle, and glands.
- has three divisions: the **sympathetic**, the **parasympathetic**, and the **enteric**.
- consists of two types of projection neurons: **preganglionic neurons** and **postganglionic neurons** (sympathetic ganglia have interneurons).
- forms output that is influenced by the hypothalamus.

II. Divisions of the Autonomic Nervous System

A. Sympathetic division (Figure 18-1; Table 18-1)
- is also called the **thoracolumbar**, or **adrenergic, system**.
- stimulates activities that are mobilized during emergency stress situations, the fight, fright, and flight responses, which include increased heart rate and force of contraction and increased blood pressure.
  1. **Preganglionic neurons** (see Figures 6-2 and 6-3)
     - are located in the intermediolateral cell column (T1–L3).
     - project via ventral roots and white communicating rami to the sympathetic trunk or via splanchnic nerves to prevertebral (collateral) ganglia. They synapse at both locations with postganglionic neurons.
  2. **Postganglionic neurons** (see Figures 6-2 and 6-3)
     - are located in the sympathetic trunk (paravertebral ganglia) and in prevertebral (collateral) ganglia.
     - in the sympathetic trunk, project via gray communicating rami to spinal nerves and innervate blood vessels, arrector pili muscles, and sweat glands.
     - in prevertebral ganglia, project to abdominal and pelvic viscera.
  3. **Interneurons**
     - are called **small intensely fluorescent (SIF) cells**.
     - are located in sympathetic ganglia.
     - are dopaminergic and inhibitory.
  4. **Neurotransmitters**
     a. **Acetylcholine** (ACh)
        - is the neurotransmitter of **preganglionic neurons**.
     b. **Norepinephrine**
        - is the neurotransmitter of **postganglionic sympathetic neurons**, with the exception of sweat glands and some blood vessels that receive cholinergic sympathetic innervation.

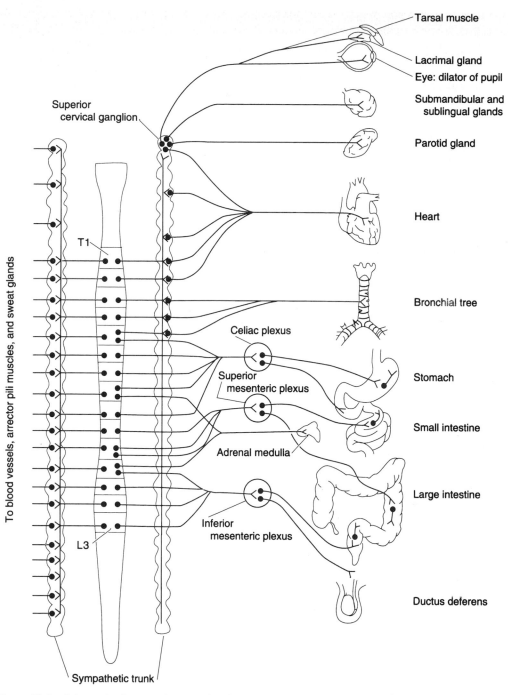

Figure 18-1. Schematic diagram showing the sympathetic (thoracolumbar) innervation of the ANS. The entire sympathetic innervation of the head is via the superior cervical ganglion. Gray communicating rami are found at all spinal cord levels, white communicating rami are found only in spinal segments T1 to L3. (Reprinted with permission from Fix JD: *High-Yield Neuroanatomy,* 3rd ed. Philadelphia, Lippincott Williams & Wilkins, 2005, p 128.)

TABLE 18–1	*Sympathetic and Parasympathetic Activity on Organ Systems*	
Structure	**Sympathetic Function**	**Parasympathetic Function**
Eye		
Radial muscle of iris	Dilates pupil (mydriasis)	
Circular muscle of iris		Constricts pupil (miosis)
Ciliary muscle		Contracts for near vision
Lacrimal gland		Stimulates secretion
Salivary glands	Viscous secretion	Watery secretion
Sweat glands		
Thermoregulatory	Increases	
Apocrine (stress)	Increases	
Heart		
Sinoatrial node	Accelerates	Decelerates (vagal arrest)
Atrioventricular node	Increases conduction velocity	Decreases conduction velocity
Contractility	Increases	Decreases (atria)
Vascular smooth muscle		
Skin, splanchnic vessels	Contracts	
Skeletal muscle vessels	Relaxes	
Bronchiolar smooth muscle	Relaxes	Contracts
Gastrointestinal tract		
Smooth muscle		
Walls	Relaxes	Contracts
Sphincters	Contracts	Relaxes
Secretion and motility	Decreases	Increases
Genitourinary tract		
Smooth muscle		
Bladder wall	Little or no effect	Contracts
Sphincter	Contracts	Relaxes
Penis, seminal vesicles	Ejaculation	Erection
Adrenal medulla	Secretes epinephrine and norepinephrine	
Metabolic functions		
Liver	Gluconeogenesis and glycogenolysis	
Fat cells	Lipolysis	
Kidney	Renin release	

    c. **Epinephrine**
- is produced by the chromaffin cells of the adrenal medulla.
- exists in a 4:1 ratio to norepinephrine.

    d. **Dopamine**
- is the neurotransmitter of the **SIF cells**.

    e. **Vasoactive intestinal polypeptide (VIP)**
- is co-localized with ACh in some postganglionic parasympathetic fibers.
- is a vasodilator.

B. Parasympathetic division (Figure 18-2; see Table 18-1)
- is called the **craniosacral**, or **cholinergic**, **system**.
- stimulates activities that conserve energy and restore body resources, including reduction of heart rate and increases in digestion and absorption of food.

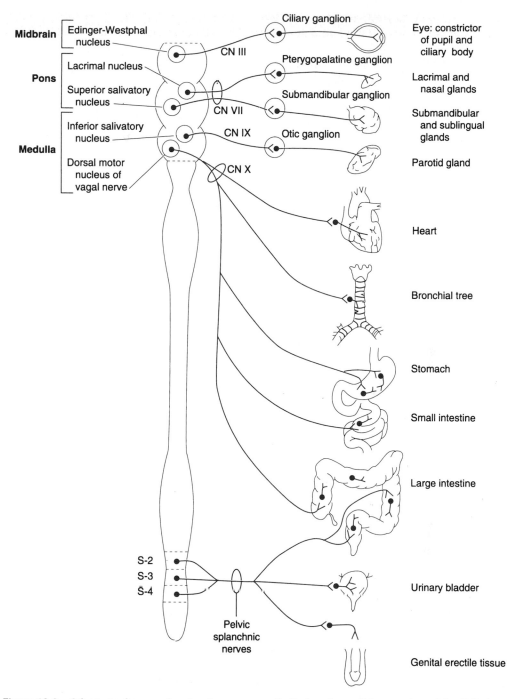

Figure 18-2. Schematic diagram showing the parasympathetic (craniosacral) innervation of the ANS. Sacral outflow includes segments S2 to S4. Cranial outflow is mediated via four cranial nerves: CN III, CN VII, CN IX, and CN X. (Reprinted with permission from Fix JD: *High-Yield Neuroanatomy,* 3rd ed. Philadelphia, Lippincott Williams & Wilkins, 2005, p 129.)

- **uses ACh** as the neurotransmitter for both preganglionic and postganglionic synapses.
    1. **Cranial division**
        - is associated with four cranial nerves.
            a. **Oculomotor nerve (CN III)** (see IV A 2; Figure 17-4)
            b. **Facial nerve (CN VII)** (see Figure 13-6)

(1) **Superior salivatory nucleus**
  • projects preganglionic fibers to the pterygopalatine and submandibular ganglia.
(2) **Pterygopalatine ganglion**
  • projects postganglionic fibers to the lacrimal gland and to the mucosa of the nose and palate.
(3) **Submandibular ganglion**
  • projects postganglionic fibers to the submandibular and sublingual glands.

c. **Glossopharyngeal nerve (CN IX)** (see Figure 9-5)
(1) **Inferior salivatory nucleus**
  • projects preganglionic fibers to the otic ganglion.
(2) **Otic ganglion**
  • projects postganglionic fibers to the parotid gland.

d. **Vagal nerve (CN X)** (see Figures 9-3 and 9-4)
(1) **Dorsal motor nucleus**
  • projects preganglionic fibers to intramural (terminal) ganglia within or adjacent to visceral organs.
(2) **Intramural (terminal) ganglia**
  • innervate, via short postganglionic fibers, viscera of the thorax and abdomen as far as the left colic flexure.
(3) **Nucleus ambiguus**
  • projects preganglionic fibers to the intramural ganglia of the heart (sinoatrial and atrioventricular nodes).

2. **Sacral division**
  • originates from the sacral parasympathetic nucleus of sacral segments S2 to S4.
  • postganglionic neurons lie on, near, or in the wall of the innervated viscus (intramural ganglia).
  • innervates via pelvic nerves the lower abdomen and pelvic viscera, including the colon distal to the left colic flexure, urinary bladder (detrusor muscle), and genital viscera.
  • is involved with **micturition**, **defecation**, and **sexual function**.

3. **Neurotransmitters**
  a. **ACh**
  b. **VIP**
    • is co-localized with ACh.
    • stimulates secretomotor neurons and vasodilator neurons.
  c. **Nitric oxide**
    • is a newly discovered neurotransmitter responsible for relaxation of smooth muscle.
    • is responsible for penile erection (see Chapter 22 IX).

C. **Enteric division**
  • consists of intramural (enteric) ganglia and plexuses of the gastrointestinal tract, including the submucosal (Meissner) plexus and the myenteric (Auerbach) plexus.
  • is influenced by postganglionic adrenergic sympathetic input.
  • is influenced by preganglionic cholinergic parasympathetic input.
  • functions independently when deprived of central nervous system (CNS) innervation.
  • plays a major role in the control of **gastrointestinal motility**.

III.   Visceral Afferent Fibers and Pain

• All sympathetic and parasympathetic nerves contain both general visceral afferent (**GVA**) and **GVE** fibers.

A. **GVA fibers and innervated structures**
  • Most visceral reflexes and organic sensations are mediated by parasympathetic afferent fibers.

1. **GVA cell bodies**
   - are found in dorsal root ganglia, inferior ganglia of the glossopharyngeal nerve (CN IX), the vagal nerve (CN X), and the geniculate ganglion of the facial nerve (CN VII).
2. **GVA pain fibers**
   - are found in the white communicating rami.
   - accompany sympathetic nerves exclusively.
   - have their cell bodies in the dorsal root ganglia of the thoracolumbar region (T1–L3).
3. **GVA reflex fibers**
   - accompany both sympathetic and parasympathetic nerves.
   - terminate centrally in the solitary nucleus and mediate the gag reflex.
4. **Carotid sinus**
   - is a slight dilation of the common carotid artery at the bifurcation. It contains baroreceptors that when stimulated cause bradycardia and a decrease in blood pressure.
   - is innervated by GVA fibers from CN IX.
5. **Carotid body (glomus caroticum)**
   - is a small structure just above the bifurcation of the common carotid artery; it contains chemoreceptors that respond to carbon dioxide, oxygen, and pH levels.
   - is innervated by GVA fibers from CN IX and CN X.

B. **Visceral pain**
   - results from the following conditions:
     1. **Distention of any viscus**
     2. **Spasms or strong contractions**, especially when accompanied by ischemia
     3. **Mechanical stimulation**, especially when the organ is hyperemic
     4. **Myocardial ischemia** with the release of kinins

C. **Referred visceral pain**
   - is the false reference or localization of a painful visceral stimulus to a somatic dermatome of the same spinal cord segment.
   - can be explained by the **convergence-projection mechanism**:
     1. For example, in angina pectoris, painful impulses from the myocardium are projected to sensory dorsal horn relay neurons of thoracic segments T1 to T4. These same relay neurons also receive cutaneous input from their corresponding dermatomes.
     2. Painful impulses are projected to the somesthetic cortex via the spinothalamic and thalamocortical tracts. These impulses are misperceived as coming from nociceptors of the left chest (T2–T4) and radiating down the left arm (T1 and T2).

IV. Autonomic Innervation of Selected Organs (see Table 18-1)

A. **Eye**
   1. **Sympathetic input**
      a. **Hypothalamic neurons** project directly to the intermediolateral cell column at T1 and T2, the ciliospinal center of Budge.
      b. The **intermediolateral cell column** (T1–T2) projects preganglionic fibers via the sympathetic trunk to the superior cervical ganglion.
      c. The **superior cervical ganglion** projects postganglionic fibers via the internal carotid artery to the cavernous sinus.
      d. Pupillodilator fibers reach the dilator pupillae muscle of the iris via the superior orbital fissure and via the nasociliary and long ciliary nerves (CN V). Some pupillodilator fibers accompany the caroticotympanic nerves prior to entering the orbit; this explains Horner syndrome (ptosis, enophthalmos, miosis, flushing, and hemihidrosis) with otitis media.
      e. Fibers to the tarsal muscles of **Müller** reach the eyelids via the **ophthalmic artery** (in the optic canal).
      f. Interruption of sympathetic input to the eye at any level results in **Horner syndrome**.

2. **Preganglionic versus postganglionic Horner syndrome**
   a. Instill 1% hydroxyamphetamine into the conjunctional sac.
   b. A dilated iris indicates preganglionic (central) Horner syndrome, and an undilated iris indicates postganglionic Horner syndrome.
   c. This test is used to rule out other causes of miosis (e.g., anisocoria).

3. **Parasympathetic input** (see Figure 17-4)
   a. The **Edinger-Westphal nucleus** projects preganglionic fibers via the oculomotor nerve (CN III) to the ciliary ganglion.
   b. The **ciliary ganglion** projects postganglionic fibers via the short ciliary nerves to the sphincter pupillae (which acts to contract the pupil) and ciliary muscle (which affects lens shape in accommodation).
   c. **Postganglionic fibers** mediate the efferent limb of the pupillary light reflex.
   d. Interruption of the parasympathetic input results in **internal ophthalmoplegia** (a fixed [unresponsive] and dilated pupil) and cycloplegia (paralysis of accommodation).

B. **Blood vessels**
   • receive their innervation from the **sympathetic** division of the ANS.
   1. **Arteries and arterioles**
      a. Constriction of cutaneous and splanchnic blood vessels results from sympathetic stimulation of α-receptors.
      b. Dilation of skeletal muscle arteries results from sympathetic stimulation of β-receptors.
      c. Blood vessels are not affected by parasympathetic stimulation.
   2. **Large veins and venules**
      • are moderately innervated.
   3. **Capillaries**
      • seem to have no innervation.
   4. **Cerebral blood vessels**
      • respond to circulating metabolites (carbon dioxide and oxygen).

C. **Heart**
   1. **Sympathetic input**
      a. The **intermediolateral cell column** (T1–T5) projects preganglionic fibers to the upper thoracic ganglia and to the three cervical ganglia of the sympathetic trunk.
      b. The **rostral sympathetic trunk** projects postganglionic fibers via cardiac nerves to the ventricular and atrial walls and the pacemaker tissue.
      c. **Stimulation of cardiac nerves** results in an increase in heart rate and in the force of cardiac contractility (via β_1-adrenergic receptors).
   2. **Parasympathetic input**
      a. The **nucleus ambiguus** of CN X projects preganglionic fibers via the vagal nerve to the intramural ganglia of the atria and the sinoatrial node.
      b. **Postganglionic fibers** from the intramural ganglia innervate the heart.
      c. **Vagal stimulation** lowers the strength and rate of cardiac contraction.

D. **Bladder (control of micturition)**
   • Control is predominantly parasympathetic.
   1. **Sympathetic input**
      • is from T12 to L3 via the inferior mesenteric plexus and via the inferior hypogastric plexus to the detrusor muscle and the internal sphincter.
      • Damage to sympathetic fibers has no effect on bladder function.
   2. **Parasympathetic input**
      • is from S2–S3 via the pelvic splanchnic nerves to the detrusor muscle and the internal sphincter.
      • Stimulation results in emptying the bladder.
      • Paralysis produces an atonic bladder, with no reflex or voluntary control.

3. **Somatomotor input**
   - is from S2 to S4 via the pudendal nerves to the external sphincter muscle.
4. **Sensory input to spinal cord**
   - is via hypogastric, pelvic, and pudendal nerves.
   - Damage results in an atonic bladder with overflow incontinence (dribbling).
5. **Ascending pathway for bladder sensation**
   - controls the urge to void.
   - is found with sacral fibers of the lateral spinothalamic tract.
   - Transection results in loss of the urge to void and overflow incontinence.
6. **Upper motor neuron (UMN) input**
   - controls volitional micturition.
   - is from the paracentral lobule via the corticosacral tract (between the denticulate ligament and the lateral horn).
   - Bilateral transection results in an uninhibited neurogenic bladder. Sensation is normal, but the patient has no control over voiding; the bladder fills and suddenly empties without cortical control.

V.   Clinical Correlations

A. **Megacolon (Hirschsprung disease)**
   - is also called **congenital aganglionic megacolon**.
   - is characterized by extreme dilation and hypertrophy of the colon with fecal retention and by the absence of ganglion cells in the myenteric plexus.
   - results from the **failure of neural crest cells to migrate into the colon**.

B. **Familial dysautonomia (Riley-Day syndrome)**
   - affects Jewish children predominantly.
   - is an **autosomal recessive trait** characterized by abnormal sweating, blood pressure instability (orthostatic hypotension), difficulty in feeding due to inadequate muscle tone in the gastrointestinal tract, and progressive sensory loss.
   - results from a **loss of neurons in autonomic and sensory ganglia**.

C. **Raynaud disease**
   - is a painful disorder of the terminal arteries of the extremities.
   - is characterized by idiopathic paroxysmal bilateral cyanosis of the digits, due to arterial and arteriolar contraction caused by cold or emotion.
   - may be treated by **preganglionic sympathectomy**.

D. **Peptic ulcer**
   - results from **excessive production of hydrochloric acid** because of increased parasympathetic (tone) stimulation.

E. **Botulism**
   - occurs when *Clostridium botulinum* toxin blocks the release of ACh from presynaptic vesicles in motor end plates and in synapses of autonomic ganglia.
   - leads to paralysis of striated muscles, the striking deficit.
   - Dry eyes and mouth and gastrointestinal ileus are the autonomic deficits.
   - is characterized by the absence of sensory impairment.

REVIEW TEST

1. Postganglionic sympathetic cholinergic fibers innervate the

(A) sweat glands
(B) lacrimal gland
(C) ductus deferens
(D) trigone of the urinary bladder
(E) detrusor muscle

2. Which of the following ganglia does not contain postganglionic parasympathetic neurons?

(A) Otic
(B) Celiac
(C) Pterygopalatine
(D) Submandibular
(E) Ciliary

3. Destruction of the ciliary ganglion results in which of the following deficits?

(A) Severe ptosis
(B) Loss of corneal reflex
(C) Loss of lacrimation
(D) Loss of direct pupillary reflex
(E) Miosis

Questions 4 to 8

The response options for items 4 to 8 are the same. Select one answer for each item in the set.

(A) Hirschsprung disease
(B) Horner syndrome
(C) Peptic ulcer disease
(D) Riley-Day syndrome
(E) Raynaud disease

Match each of the characteristics below with the condition it best describes.

4. Results from increased parasympathetic stimulation

5. Is a painful vasospastic disorder affecting the digits

6. Is an autosomal recessive trait characterized by abnormal sweating and blood pressure instability

7. Results from congenital absence of ganglion cells in the myenteric plexus

8. Consists of anisocoria and lack of sweating

Questions 9 to 14

The response options for items 9 to 14 are the same. Select one answer for each item in the set.

(A) ACh
(B) Dopamine
(C) Nitric oxide
(D) Norepinephrine
(E) VIP

Match the characteristics below with the appropriate neurotransmitter.

9. Is a vasodilator

10. Is the neurotransmitter of the SIF cells

11. Innervates apocrine sweat glands

12. Innervates eccrine (merocrine) sweat glands

13. Is the transmitter responsible for penile erection

14. Is the neurotransmitter of the arrector pili muscle

ANSWERS AND EXPLANATIONS

1–A. Postganglionic sympathetic cholinergic fibers innervate the eccrine (merocrine) sweat glands and some blood vessels; blood vessels, however, are predominantly innervated by postganglionic sympathetic adrenergic fibers. Apocrine sweat glands of the axilla are innervated by adrenergic fibers; these glands secrete in response to mental stress.

2–B. The celiac ganglion is a sympathetic prevertebral (collateral) ganglion that contains postganglionic neurons.

3–D. Destruction of the ciliary ganglion interrupts postganglionic parasympathetic fibers, which innervate the sphincter muscle of the iris and the ciliary muscle; this results in loss of the direct pupillary reflex, mydriasis, and paralysis of accommodation. In addition, postganglionic sympathetic vasomotor fibers are interrupted, resulting in a hyperemic globe. Postganglionic sympathetic pupillodilator fibers reach the iris via the nasociliary and long ciliary nerve. Severe ptosis results from an oculomotor paralysis involving the fibers that innervate the levator palpebrae muscle. Mild ptosis results from a lesion of the oculosympathetic fibers, which innervate the smooth tarsal muscle (Horner syndrome).

4–C. Peptic ulcer disease results from increased parasympathetic tone.

5–E. Raynaud disease is a benign symmetric disease characterized by painful vasospasms affecting the digits.

6–D. Riley-Day syndrome, familial dysautonomia, is an autosomal recessive trait characterized by abnormal sweating and blood pressure instability.

7–A. Congenital aganglionic megacolon, or Hirschsprung disease, results from failure of the neural crest cells to migrate into the wall of the distal colon (sigmoid colon and rectum) and form the myenteric plexus. It is characterized by extreme dilation and hypertrophy of the colon, with fecal retention.

8–B. Anisocoria (unequal pupils) and hemianhidrosis (lack of sweating on half of the face) are consistent with Horner syndrome, which also involves ptosis, miosis, and hemianhidrosis.

9–E. VIP is a vasodilator found in postganglionic parasympathetic fibers, co-localized with ACh.

10–B. Dopamine is the neurotransmitter of the SIF cells.

11–D. Norepinephrine innervates apocrine sweat glands; these glands of the axilla and anal region respond to emotional stress.

12–A. ACh innervates eccrine (merocrine) sweat glands, which respond to heat stress.

13–C. Nitric oxide is the transmitter responsible for penile erection.

14–D. Norepinephrine is the neurotransmitter of the arrector pili muscles.

Hypothalamus

I. Overview: The Hypothalamus

- is a division of the diencephalon.
- lies within the floor and ventral part of the walls of the third ventricle.
- functions primarily in the **maintenance of homeostasis**.
- subserves three systems: the **autonomic nervous system** (ANS), the **endocrine system**, and the **limbic system**.

II. Surface Anatomy of the Hypothalamus (see Figures 1-2 and 1-5)

- is visible only from the ventral aspect of the brain.
- lies between the optic chiasm and the interpeduncular fossa (posterior perforated substance).
- lies below the hypothalamic sulcus.
- includes the following **ventral surface structures**:

A. Infundibulum
   - is the stalk of the hypophysis.
   - contains the hypophyseal portal vessels.
   - contains the supraopticohypophyseal and tuberohypophyseal tracts.

B. Tuber cinereum
   - is the prominence between the infundibulum and the mamillary bodies.
   - includes the **median eminence**, which contains the **arcuate nucleus** (infundibular nucleus).

C. Mamillary bodies
   - contain the **mamillary nuclei**.

D. Optic chiasm
   - is the floor of the optic recess of the third ventricle.

E. Arterial circle of Willis
   - surrounds the ventral surface of the hypothalamus and provides its blood supply.

III. Hypothalamic Regions and Nuclei

- The hypothalamus is divided into a lateral area and a medial area, which are separated by the fornix and the mamillothalamic tract.

A. **Lateral hypothalamic area**
   • is traversed by the **medial forebrain bundle**.
   • includes two major nuclei:
      1. **Lateral preoptic nucleus**
         • is the anterior telencephalic portion.
      2. **Lateral hypothalamic nucleus** (Figure 19-1)
         • when stimulated, induces eating.
         • Lesions cause anorexia and starvation.

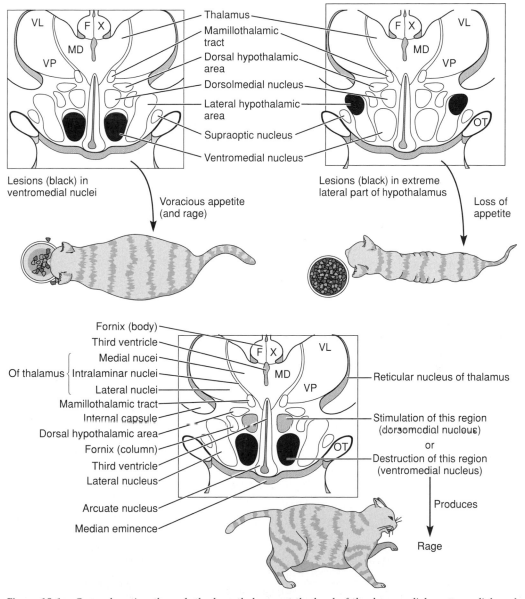

Figure 19-1. Coronal section through the hypothalamus at the level of the dorsomedial ventromedial, and lateral hypothalamus nuclei. Lesions or stimulation of these nuclei result in obesity, cachexia, and rage. The column of the fornix separates the medial from the lateral hypothalamic zones. A lesion of the optic tract results in a contralateral hemianopia. FX = fornix; MD = medial dorsal nucleus of thalamus; OT = optic tract; VL = ventral lateral nucleus of thalamus; VP = ventral posterior nucleus of thalamus.

B. Medial hypothalamic area (Figure 19-2)
- includes the periventricular area that borders the third ventricle.
- is divided into four regions, from anterior to posterior:
    1. **Preoptic region**
        - is the anterior telencephalic portion.
        - contains the **medial preoptic nucleus**, which regulates the release of gonadotropic hormones from the adenohypophysis. The medial preoptic nucleus contains the sexually dimorphic nucleus, whose development is dependent on testosterone levels.
    2. **Supraoptic region**
        - lies dorsal to the optic chiasm.
        a. **Suprachiasmatic nucleus**
            - receives direct input from the retina.
            - plays a role in the **control of circadian rhythms**.
        b. **Anterior nucleus**
            - plays a role in **temperature regulation**.
            - stimulates the parasympathetic nervous system.
            - Destruction results in **hyperthermia**.
        c. **Paraventricular nucleus**
            - Neurosecretory cells synthesize and release antidiuretic hormone (**ADH**), **oxytocin**, and corticotropin-releasing hormone (**CRH**).
            - regulates water balance (conservation of water).
            - gives rise to the supraopticohypophyseal tract, which projects to the neurohypophysis.
            - Destruction results in **diabetes insipidus**.
        d. **Supraoptic nucleus**
            - synthesizes **ADH** and **oxytocin**.
            - projects to the neurohypophysis via the supraopticohypophyseal tract.

Paraventricular and supraoptic nuclei
- regulate water balance
- produce ADH and oxytocin
- destruction causes diabetes insipidus
- paraventricular nucleus projects to autonomic nuclei of brainstem and spinal cord

Anterior nucleus
- thermal regulation (dissipation of heat)
- stimulates parasympathetic NS
- destruction results in hyperthermia

Preoptic area
- contains sexual dimorphic nucleus
- regulates release of gonadotropic hormones

Suprachiasmatic nucleus
- receives input from retina
- controls circadian rhythms

Dorsomedial nucleus
- stimulation results in obesity and savage behavior

Posterior nucleus
- thermal regulation (conservation of heat)
- destruction results in inability to thermoregulate
- stimulates the sympathetic NS

Lateral nucleus
- stimulation induces eating
- destruction results in starvation

Mamillary body
- receives input from hippocampal formation via fornix
- projects to anterior nucleus of thalamus
- contains hemorrhagic lesions in Wernicke's encephalopathy

Ventromedial nucleus
- satiety center
- destruction results in obesity and savage behavior

Midbrain

CN III

Pons

Arcuate nucleus
- produces hypothalamic releasing factors
- contains DOPA-ergic neurons that inhibit prolactin release

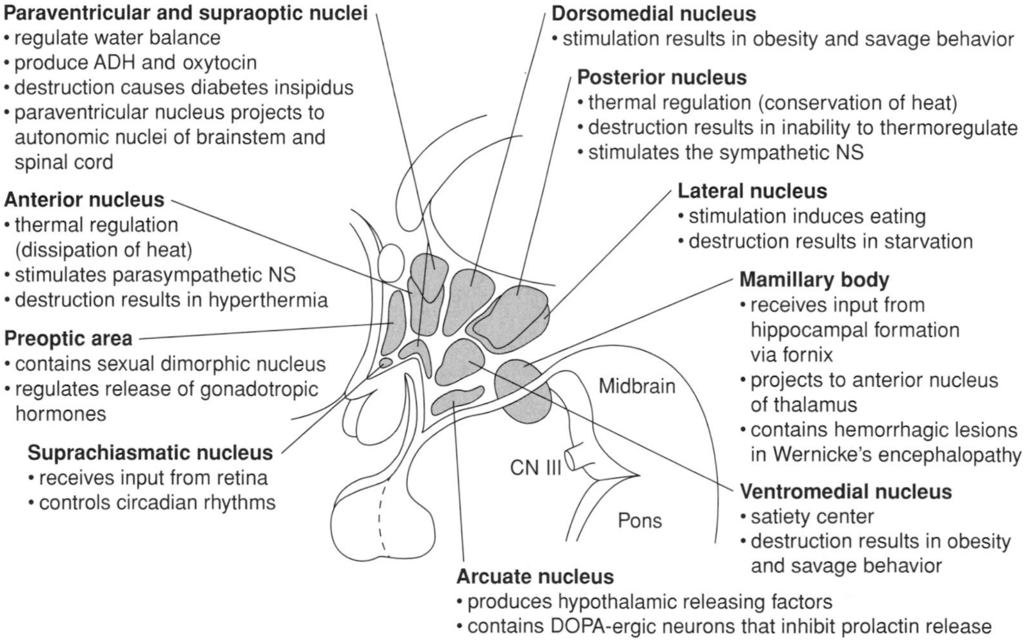

Figure 19-2. Major hypothalamic nuclei and their functions. NS = nervous system. (Modified with permission from Fix JD: *High-Yield Neuroanatomy,* 3rd ed. Philadelphia, Lippincott Williams & Wilkins, 2005, p 132.)

3. **Tuberal region**
   - lies dorsal to the tuber cinereum.
   a. **Dorsomedial nucleus** (see Figure 19-1)
      - when stimulated in animals, results in savage behavior.
   b. **Ventromedial nucleus** (see Figure 19-1)
      - is considered a **satiety center**.
      - when stimulated, inhibits the urge to eat.
      - Bilateral destruction results in hyperphagia, obesity, and savage behavior.
   c. **Arcuate (infundibular) nucleus**
      - is located in the tuber cinereum.
      - is a periventricular nucleus.
      - contains neurons that produce **hypothalamic-releasing factors** and gives rise to the tuberohypophyseal tract, which terminates in the hypophyseal portal system of the infundibulum.
      - effects, via hypothalamic-releasing factors, the release or nonrelease of adenohypophyseal hormones into the systemic circulation.
      - contains dopaminergic neurons; **dopamine** is the **prolactin-inhibiting factor (PIF)**.
4. **Mamillary region**
   - lies dorsal to the mamillary bodies.
   a. **Mamillary nuclei**
      - receive input from the **hippocampal formation** (specifically the subiculum) via the **fornix**.
      - receive input from the dorsal and ventral tegmental nuclei and the raphe nuclei via the mamillary peduncle.
      - project to the anterior nucleus of the thalamus via the mamillothalamic tract.
      - contain hemorrhagic lesions in Wernicke encephalopathy.
   b. **Posterior nucleus**
      - plays a role in **thermal regulation** (i.e., conservation and increased production of heat).
      - Lesions result in **poikilothermia**, the inability to thermoregulate.

IV.   Major Hypothalamic Connections (Figures 19-3 and 19-4)

A. **Afferent connections to the hypothalamus**
   - **derive** from the following structures:
   1. **Septal area and nuclei and orbitofrontal cortex**
      - via the medial forebrain bundle
   2. **Hippocampal formation**
      - primarily from the subiculum via the fornix
   3. **Amygdaloid complex**
      - via the stria terminalis and ventral amygdalofugal pathway
   4. **Primary olfactory cortex (area 34)**
      - via the medial forebrain bundle
   5. **Mediodorsal nucleus of the thalamus**
      - via the inferior thalamic peduncle
   6. **Brainstem nuclei**
      a. **Tegmental nuclei (dorsal and ventral)**
         - project via the mamillary peduncle.
      b. **Raphe nuclei (dorsal and superior central)**
         - project serotonergic fibers via the medial forebrain bundle and the mamillary peduncle (see Figure 22-4).
      c. **Locus ceruleus**
         - projects noradrenergic fibers via the medial forebrain bundle (see Figure 22-4).

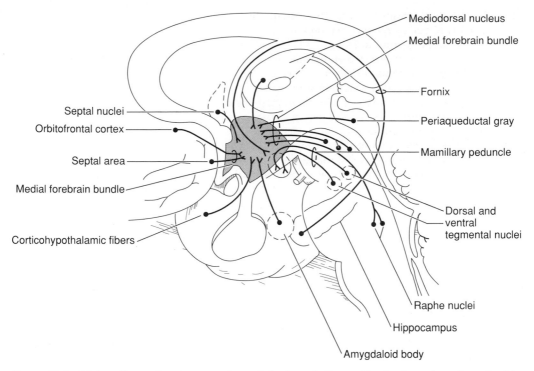

Figure 19-3. Major afferent (input) connections of the hypothalamus. The fornix projects from the hippocampal formation to the mamillary bodies. The medial forebrain bundle conducts afferent and efferent fibers.

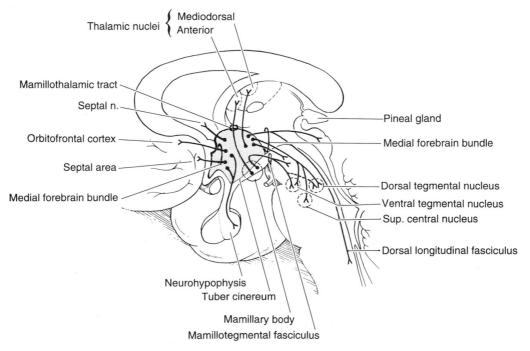

Figure 19-4. Major efferent (output) connections of the hypothalamus. The medial forebrain bundle conducts afferent and efferent fibers. The hypothalamus projects directly to the autonomic visceral nuclei of the brainstem and spinal cord.

B. **Efferent connections from the hypothalamus**
- **project** to the following structures:
  1. **Septal area and nuclei**
     - via the medial forebrain bundle
  2. **Anterior nucleus of the thalamus**
     - via the mamillothalamic tract
  3. **Mediodorsal nucleus of the thalamus**
     - via the inferior thalamic peduncle
  4. **Amygdaloid complex**
     - via the stria terminalis and the ventral amygdalopetal pathway
  5. **Brainstem nuclei and spinal cord**
     - via the dorsal longitudinal fasciculus and the medial forebrain bundle
  6. **Adenohypophysis**
     - via the tuberohypophyseal tract and hypophyseal portal system
  7. **Neurohypophysis**
     - via the supraopticohypophyseal tract

V. Major Fiber Systems

A. **Fornix** (see Figures 1-4, 1-5, 19-2, 20-3, and 20-6)
- has five parts: the **alveus**, **fimbria**, **crus**, **body**, and **column**.
- projects from the hippocampal formation to the mamillary nucleus, anterior nucleus of the thalamus, and septal area.
- is the largest projection to the hypothalamus.
- Bilateral transection results in an acute amnestic syndrome.

B. **Medial forebrain bundle** (see Figures 19-3 and 19-4)
- traverses the entire lateral hypothalamic area.
- interconnects the septal area and nuclei, the hypothalamus, and the midbrain tegmentum.

C. **Mamillothalamic tract** (see Figure 20-3)
- projects from the mamillary nuclei to the anterior nucleus of the thalamus.

D. **Mamillary peduncle** (see Figure 19-3)
- conducts fibers from the dorsal and ventral tegmental nuclei and the raphe nuclei to the mamillary body.

E. **Mamillotegmental tract** (see Figure 19-4)
- conducts fibers from the mamillary nuclei to the dorsal and ventral tegmental nuclei.

F. **Stria terminalis** (see Figure 20-3)
- is the most prominent pathway from the amygdaloid complex.
- interconnects the septal area, the hypothalamus, and the amygdaloid complex.
- lies in the sulcus terminalis between the caudate nucleus and the thalamus.

G. **Ventral amygdalofugal pathway** (see Figure 20-3)
- interconnects the amygdaloid complex and the hypothalamus.

H. **Supraopticohypophyseal tract** (Figure 19-5)
- conducts fibers from the supraoptic and paraventricular nuclei to the **neurohypophysis** (the release site for ADH and oxytocin).

I. **Tuberohypophyseal (tuberoinfundibular) tract** (see Figure 19-5)
- conducts fibers from the arcuate nucleus to the hypophyseal portal system of the infundibulum.

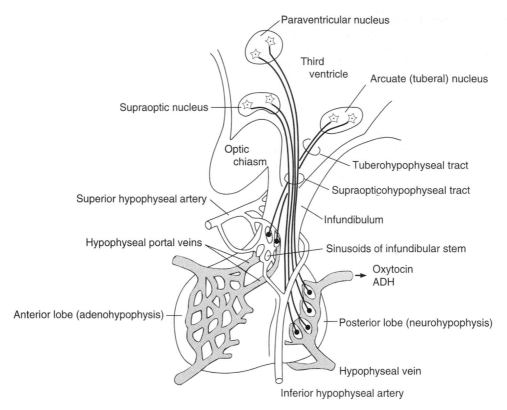

Figure 19-5. Hypophyseal portal system. The paraventricular and supraoptic nuclei produce ADH and oxytocin and transport the substances via the supraopticohypophyseal tract to the capillary bed of the neurohypophysis. The arcuate nucleus of the infundibulum transports releasing hormones via the tuberohypophyseal tract to the sinusoids of the infundibular stem, which drain into the secondary capillary plexus in the adenohypophysis. (Modified with permission from Fix JD: *High-Yield Neuroanatomy,* 3rd ed. Philadelphia, Lippincott Williams & Wilkins, 2005, p 133.)

J. **Dorsal longitudinal fasciculus** (see Figure 19-4)
- extends from the hypothalamus to the caudal medulla.
- projects to the parasympathetic nuclei of the brainstem.

K. **Hypothalamospinal tract**
- contains direct descending autonomic fibers that influence preganglionic sympathetic neurons of the intermediolateral cell column and preganglionic neurons of the sacral parasympathetic nucleus.
- interruption above T1 results in Horner syndrome.

VI.   Functional Considerations

A. **Autonomic function**
- The ANS is regulated by hypothalamic nuclei.
  1. **Anterior hypothalamus**
     - has an excitatory effect on the parasympathetic nervous system.
  2. **Posterior hypothalamus**
     - has an excitatory effect on the sympathetic nervous system.

B. **Temperature regulation**
   1. **Anterior hypothalamus**
      - helps **regulate and maintain body temperature**.
      - Destruction causes **hyperthermia**.
   2. **Posterior hypothalamus**
      - helps **produce and conserve heat**.
      - Destruction causes the **inability to thermoregulate**.

C. **Water balance regulation**
   - ADH controls water excretion by the kidneys.

D. **Food intake regulation**
   - two hypothalamic nuclei play roles in the control of appetite:
   1. **Ventromedial nucleus** (see III B 3 b)
   2. **Lateral hypothalamic nucleus**
      - is called the **hunger** or **feeding center**.
      - Destruction causes **starvation** and **emaciation**.

E. **Hypothalamic-releasing and release-inhibiting factors**
   - are produced in the **arcuate nucleus** of the median eminence.
   - are transported via the tuberohypophyseal tract to the hypophyseal portal system.
   - effect the release or nonrelease of adenohypophyseal hormones.
   - are, with the exception of dopamine, **peptides** (hypophysiotropins), which include:
   1. Thyrotropin-releasing hormone (**TRH**)
   2. Gonadotropin-releasing hormone (**GnRH**)
   3. **Somatostatin** (growth hormone–inhibiting hormone)
   4. Growth hormone–releasing hormone (**GHRH**)
   5. **CRH**
   6. **PIF** and prolactin-releasing factor (**PRF**) (**PIF** is dopamine.)

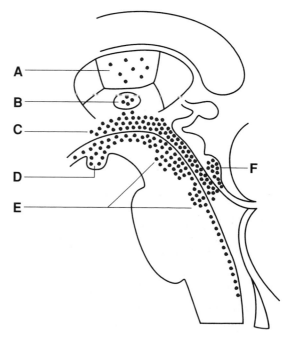

Figure 19-6. Midsagittal section through the brainstem and diencephalon showing the distribution of lesions in Wernicke encephalopathy. (A) Mediodorsal nucleus of the thalamus. (B) Massa intermedia. (C) Perventricular area. (D) Mamillary nuclei. (E) Midbrain and pontine tegmentum. (F) Inferior colliculus. Lesions in the mamillary nuclei are associated with Wernicke encephalopathy and thiamine (vitamin B_1) deficiency. (Modified with permission from Fix JD: *High-Yield Neuroanatomy,* 3rd ed. Philadelphia, Lippincott Williams & Wilkins, 2005, p 140.)

VII. Clinical Correlations

A. **Craniopharyngioma**
- is a congenital epidermoid tumor thought to originate from remnants of the Rathke pouch.
- is usually calcified.
- is the most common **supratentorial tumor** found in children.
- Pressure on the chiasm results in a **bitemporal hemianopia**. Pressure on the hypothalamus causes **hypothalamic syndrome**, with adiposity, diabetes insipidus, disturbance of temperature regulation, and somnolence.

B. **Pituitary adenoma**
- constitutes 15% of cases of clinically symptomatic **intracranial tumors**.
- is rarely seen in children.
- when endocrine active, produces endocrine abnormalities (e.g., amenorrhea and galactorrhea from a prolactin-secreting adenoma, the most common type).
- Pressure on the chiasm results in a **bitemporal hemianopia** (most cases show asymmetry of field defects). Pressure on the hypothalamus may cause **hypothalamic syndrome**.

C. **Wernicke encephalopathy** (Figure 19-6)
- is due to a thiamine (vitamin B_1) deficiency.
- is characterized by the triad: **ocular palsies, ataxic gait**, and **mental confusion**.
- Lesions are found in the hypothalamus (primarily in the mamillary bodies) and in the periaqueductal gray of the midbrain.

REVIEW TEST

1. The sexually dimorphic nucleus is located in the

(A) anterior nucleus
(B) arcuate nucleus
(C) medial preoptic nucleus
(D) posterior nucleus
(E) ventromedial nucleus

2. A 40-year-old woman who has taken birth control pills has a 4-month history of amenorrhea and a bitemporal hemianopia that began as a bitemporal quadrantanopia. What is the most likely cause of these deficits?

(A) Sella turcica meningioma
(B) Cavernous sinus meningioma
(C) Pituitary adenoma
(D) Optic glioma
(E) Aneurysm of the anterior communicating artery

3. Which of the following statements concerning the hypothalamus is correct?

(A) It is a division of the subthalamus.
(B) It contains the tuberculum cinereum.
(C) Its suprachiasmatic nucleus receives input from retina.
(D) It is not related to the limbic system
(E) Its dorsomedial and the ventromedial nuclei are separated by the striae medullares.

4. Which of the following is a hypothalamic structure?

(A) alveus
(B) arcuate
(C) fimbria
(D) crus
(E) column

Questions 5 to 11

The response options for items 5 to 11 are the same. Select one answer for each item in the set.

(A) Fornix
(B) Medial forebrain bundle
(C) Stria terminalis
(D) Mamillary peduncle
(E) Dorsal longitudinal fasciculus

Match each description below with the structure it best describes.

5. Extends from the posterior hypothalamic nucleus to the caudal medulla

6. Interconnects the hypothalamus and the amygdaloid complex

7. Is the largest projection to the hypothalamus

8. Connects the septal area to the midbrain tegmentum

9. Conducts fibers from the hippocampal formation to the mamillary nucleus

10. Lies between the caudate nucleus and the thalamus

11. Separates the medial hypothalamus from the lateral hypothalamus

Questions 12 to 20

The response options for items 12 to 20 are the same. Select one answer for each item in the set.

(A) Anorexia
(B) Craniopharyngioma
(C) Diabetes insipidus
(D) Hyperthermia
(E) Inability to thermoregulate
(F) Obesity and savage behavior
(G) Pituitary adenoma
(H) Wernicke encephalopathy

Match each description below with the appropriate clinical condition.

12. Amenorrhea and galactorrhea

13. Hemorrhagic lesions in the mamillary bodies

14. Associated with the Rathke pouch

15. Destruction of the anterior hypothalamic nuclei

16. Stimulation of the ventromedial nuclei

17. Bilateral lesions of the ventromedial hypothalamic nuclei

18. Bilateral lesions of the posterior hypothalamic nuclei

19. Destruction of the supraoptic and paraventricular nuclei

20. Is due to a thiamine (vitamin B$_1$) deficiency

ANSWERS AND EXPLANATIONS

1–C. The sexually dimorphic nucleus is located in the medial preoptic nucleus of the preoptic region.

2–C. A pituitary adenoma is characterized by amenorrhea and visual field defects, specifically a bitemporal hemianopia. The amenorrhea-galactorrhea syndrome includes visual abnormalities, amenorrhea, galactorrhea, and elevated serum prolactin.

3–C. The suprachiasmatic nucleus of the hypothalamus receives direct input from the retina and plays a role in the control of circadian rhythms. The tuberculum cinereum overlies the spinal trigonal nucleus. The limbic system has reciprocal connections with the hypothalamus. The striae medullares separate the dorsal aspect of the pons from the dorsal aspect of the medulla oblongata.

4–B. The arcuate nucleus is a periventricular nucleus in the tuber cinereum. It contains neurons that produce hypothalamic-releasing factors and gives rise to the tuberohypophysial tract. The alveus, fimbria, crus, and column are components of the fornix.

5–E. The dorsal longitudinal fasciculus extends from the posterior hypothalamic nucleus to the caudal medulla and projects to autonomic centers of the brainstem. It contains both ascending and descending fibers.

6–C. The amygdaloid complex is interconnected with the hypothalamus via the stria terminalis and the ventral amygdalofugal pathway.

7–A. The fornix contains 2.7 million fibers and is the largest projection to the hypothalamus.

8–B. The medial forebrain bundle interconnects the septal area, the hypothalamus, and the midbrain tegmentum.

9–A. The fornix projects from the subiculum of the hippocampal formation to the mamillary nucleus of the hypothalamus. The fornix projects to the anterior nucleus of the thalamus, septal nuclei, lateral preoptic region, and the nucleus of the diagonal band of Broca.

10–C. The stria terminalis lies in the sulcus terminalis with the vena terminalis, separates the head of the caudate nucleus from the thalamus, and interconnects the amygdaloid nuclear complex with the hypothalamus.

11–A. The column of the fornix lies between the medial and lateral hypothalamus.

12–G. Amenorrhea and galactorrhea result from a prolactin-secreting pituitary adenoma, the most common type of pituitary adenoma.

13–H. Hemorrhagic lesions in the mamillary bodies and in the periaqueductal gray of the midbrain are seen in Wernicke encephalopathy.

14–B. Craniopharyngiomas, congenital epidermoid tumors, are derived from the Rathke pouch; they are the most common supratentorial tumors found in children.

15–D. Destruction of the anterior hypothalamic nuclei results in hyperthermia.

16–A. Stimulation of the ventromedial nuclei inhibits the urge to eat, resulting in emaciation (cachexia or anorexia). Destruction of these nuclei results in hyperphagia and savage behavior.

17–F. Bilateral lesions of the ventromedial hypothalamic nuclei result in hyperphagia and savage behavior.

18–E. Bilateral lesions of the posterior hypothalamic nuclei result in the inability to thermoregulate (poikilothermia). Bilateral destruction of only the posterior aspect of the lateral hypothalamic nucleus results in anorexia and emaciation.

19–C. Destruction of the supraoptic and paraventricular nuclei or the supraopticohypophyseal tract results in diabetes insipidus with polydipsia and polyuria.

20–H. Wernicke encephalopathy is due to a thiamine (vitamin B_1) deficiency.

Olfactory, Gustatory, and Limbic Systems

I.   Olfactory System

- mediates the special visceral afferent (SVA) modality of **smell** via the olfactory nerve (**CN I**).
- is the only sensory system that has no precortical relay in the thalamus.
- projects to the thalamus, hypothalamus, amygdala, and hippocampal formation.

A. **Olfactory pathway** (Figure 20-1; see Figure 1-2)
   1. **Olfactory receptor cells**
      - are chemoreceptors.
      - number 25 million on each side.
      - are replaced throughout life (they may regenerate).
      - are found in the nasal mucosa.
      - are **first-order neurons** in the olfactory pathway.
      - are unmyelinated bipolar neurons whose central processes are CN I.
      - have axons that enter the olfactory bulb and synapse in the olfactory glomeruli with **mitral and tufted cells**.
   2. **Olfactory bulb**
      - lies on the cribriform plate of the ethmoid bone and receives the olfactory nerve.
      - contains **mitral and tufted cells** (second-order neurons) that project via the olfactory tract and the lateral olfactory stria to the primary olfactory cortex and the amygdaloid nucleus.
   3. **Olfactory tract**
      - contains the **anterior olfactory nucleus**.
      - gives rise to the **medial and lateral olfactory striae**.
      - projects to the contralateral olfactory tract via the anterior commissure.
   4. **Lateral olfactory stria**
      - projects to the primary olfactory cortex and the amygdaloid nucleus.
   5. **Primary olfactory cortex**
      - overlies the **uncus** of the parahippocampal gyrus (area 34).
      - receives input from the lateral olfactory stria.
      - consists of **prepiriform** and **periamygdaloid cortices**.
      - projects to the mediodorsal nucleus of the thalamus via the amygdaloid nucleus to the hypothalamus and via the entorhinal cortex (area 28) to the hippocampal formation.
   6. **Mediodorsal nucleus of the thalamus**
      - projects to the **orbitofrontal cortex**, where the **conscious perception of smell** takes place.

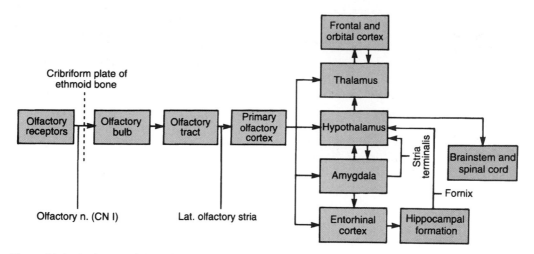

Figure 20-1. Pathways of the olfactory system. The olfactory nerve enters the olfactory bulb via the cribriform plate. Mitral and tufted cells of the olfactory bulb project via the lateral olfactory stria to the primary olfactory cortex (prepiriform and periamygdaloid cortices). The primary olfactory cortex projects to the hypothalamus, thalamus, amygdaloid nucleus, and entorhinal area. The olfactory system is the only sensory system that projects directly to the cortex of the telencephalon without a precortical relay in the thalamus.

B. **Clinical correlations**
1. **Anosmia**, the loss of smell, may occur as a result of a lesion of the olfactory nerve; anosmia is ipsilateral.
2. Olfactory nerves may be damaged by **fractures of the cribriform plate**; by **meningitis, meningiomas, or gliomas**; or by **abscesses of the frontal lobes**.
3. **Olfactory hallucinations** may be a consequence of lesions of the parahippocampal uncus.
4. **Foster Kennedy syndrome**
   - results from a **meningioma of the olfactory groove**, which compresses the olfactory tract and the optic nerve.
   - results in ipsilateral anosmia, optic atrophy, and contralateral papilledema.
5. **Fracture of the cribriform plate of the ethmoid bone** may result in anosmia and cerebrospinal rhinorrhea.

II.   Gustatory System

- mediates the SVA modality of **taste**.
- mediates gustation, which, like smell, is a chemical sense. In the colloquial sense, taste may be an olfactory sensation.

A. **Gustatory pathway** (Figure 20-2)
1. **Taste receptor cells**
   - are chemoreceptors.
   - are modified epithelial cells, not neurons.
   - are continuously being regenerated.
   - are located in the taste buds of the tongue, epiglottis, and palate.
   - are innervated by SVA fibers of the facial nerve (CN VII), the glossopharyngeal nerve (CN IX), and the vagal nerve (CN X).
2. **First-order neurons**
   - are **pseudounipolar ganglion cells** in the geniculate ganglion of CN VII, in the petrosal ganglion of CN IX, and in the nodose ganglion of CN X.
   - project centrally, via the solitary tract, to the solitary nucleus.

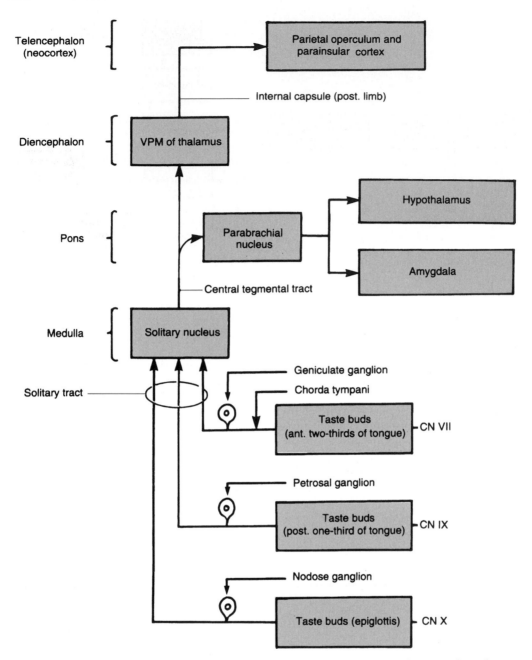

Figure 20-2. Gustatory pathway. CN VII, CN IX, and CN X transmit taste (SVA) information from the anterior two-thirds of the tongue, the posterior third of the tongue, and the epiglottis to the solitary tract and nucleus; from the solitary nucleus via the central tegmental tract to the medial parabrachial nucleus; and to the VPM nucleus of the thalamus, hypothalamus, and amygdaloid complex. The gustatory cortex is located in the parietal operculum and in the parainsular cortex.

3. **Solitary nucleus**
   - receives taste input from the tongue and epiglottis.
   - projects ipsilaterally via the **central tegmental tract** to the ventral posteromedial (VPM) nucleus of the thalamus.
4. **Parabrachial nucleus of the pons**
   - receives taste input from the solitary nucleus.
   - projects taste input to the hypothalamus and amygdala.

5. **Ventral posteromedial nucleus**
   - projects to the gustatory cortex of the parietal operculum (area 43) and parainsular cortex.
6. **Gustatory cortex of the insular area** (area 43)
   - projects via the entorhinal cortex (area 28) to the hippocampal formation.

B. **Taste perception**
   1. **Taste testing**
      - should involve the anterior two-thirds of the tongue. Do not stimulate the posterior third of the tongue for reasons of inconvenience.
   2. **Taste buds** on the tongue detect:
      a. **Sweetness** at the apex of the tongue
      b. **Saltiness** posterolateral to the apex of the tongue
      c. **Bitterness** on the circumvallate papillae
      d. **Sourness** on the anterior two-thirds of the dorsal surface of the tongue

C. **Clinical correlation: Ageusia** (gustatory anesthesia, or lack of sense of taste)
   - is most commonly caused by heavy smoking.
   - is most frequently associated with peripheral lesions of CN VII (Bell palsy and disease of the middle ear [chorda tympani]) and CN IX.

III. Limbic System

- is considered to be the anatomic substrate underlying behavioral and emotional expression.
- plays a role in feeling, feeding, fighting, fleeing, and undertaking mating activity.
- expresses itself through the hypothalamus via the autonomic nervous system (ANS).

A. **Major components and connections** (Figure 20-3)
   - include structures of the telencephalon, diencephalon, and midbrain.
   1. **Orbitofrontal cortex** (see Figure 1-2)
      - mediates the conscious perception of **smell**.
      - has reciprocal connections with the mediodorsal nucleus of the thalamus.
      - is interconnected via the medial forebrain bundle with the septal area and hypothalamic nuclei.
   2. **Mediodorsal nucleus of the thalamus**
      - has reciprocal connections with the orbitofrontal and prefrontal cortices and the hypothalamus.
      - receives input from the amygdaloid nucleus.
      - plays a role in **affective behavior and memory**.
   3. **Anterior nucleus of the thalamus**
      - receives input from the mamillary nucleus via the mamillothalamic tract and fornix.
      - projects to the cingulate gyrus.
      - is a major link in the limbic **circuit of Papez**.
   4. **Septal area** (see Figures 1-4 and 23-1B)
      - is a telencephalic structure.
      - consists of a cortical septal area, which includes the paraterminal gyrus and the subcallosal area.
      - consists of a subcortical septal area (the septal nuclei), which lies between the septum pellucidum and the anterior commissure.
   - has reciprocal connections with the hippocampal formation via the fornix.
   - has reciprocal connections with the hypothalamus via the medial forebrain bundle.
   - projects via the **stria medullaris** (thalami) to the **habenular nucleus**.
   5. **Limbic lobe** (see Figure 23-1B)
      - includes the **subcallosal area**, the **paraterminal gyrus**, the **cingulate gyrus and isthmus**, and the **parahippocampal gyrus**, which includes the **uncus** (see Figure 1-4).
      - contains, buried in the parahippocampal gyrus, the **hippocampal formation** and the **amygdaloid nuclear complex**.

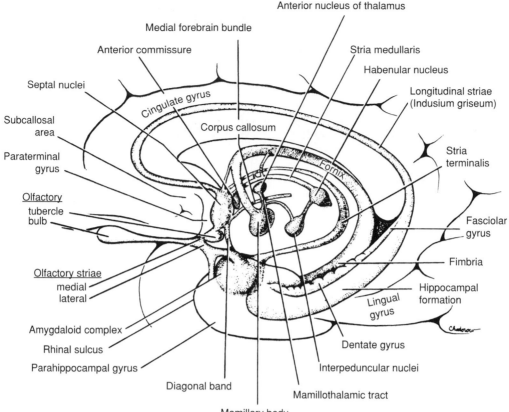

Figure 20-3. Major subcortical structures of the limbic system. The fornix projects from the hippocampal formation to the septal nuclei (precommissural fornix) and to the mamillary body (postcommissural fornix). The major pathway from the amygdaloid nucleus is the stria terminalis, which terminates in the septal nuclei and in the hypothalamus. The stria medullaris of the thalamus connects the septal nuclei to the habenular nucleus. (Reprinted with permission from Carpenter MB, Sutlin J: *Human Neuroanatomy.* Baltimore, Williams & Wilkins, 1983, p 618.)

6. **Hippocampal formation** (Figure 20-4)
  - functions in learning, memory, and recognition of novelty.
  - receives major input via the entorhinal cortex.
  - projects major output via the fornix.
  a. **Major structures of the hippocampal formation**
    - project output via the fornix to the septal area and the mamillary nuclei.
    - receive input via the fornix from the septal area.
    - receive input via the entorhinal cortex (area 28) as the alvolear pathway to the hippocampus and the perforant pathway to the dentate gyrus.
    (1) **Dentate gyrus** (see Figure 1-4)
      - has a three-layered archicortex.
      - contains **granule cells** that receive hippocampal input and project it to the pyramidal cells of the hippocampus and subiculum.
    (2) **Hippocampus (cornu ammonis)**
      - has a three-layered archicortex.
      - contains **pyramidal cells** that project via the fornix to the septal area and the hypothalamus.
      - is divided into four cytoarchitectural areas (CA1–CA4); CA1 (Sommer sector) is especially vulnerable to hypoxia (Figure 20-5).

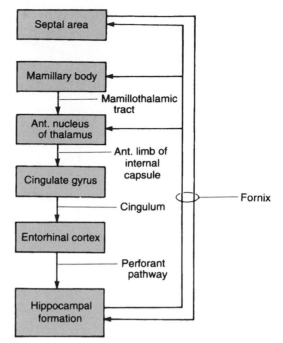

Figure 20-4. Limbic connections. Major afferent and efferent connections of the hippocampal formation. The circuit of Papez is hippocampal formation → mamillary nucleus → anterior thalamic nucleus → cingulate gyrus → hippocampal formation. The hippocampal formation consists of three components: the hippocampus per se (cornu ammonis), the subiculum, and the dentate gyrus. The hippocampus projects to the septal area, the subiculum projects to the mamillary nuclei, and the dentate gyrus does not project beyond the hippocampal formation.

    (3) **Subiculum**
- receives input via the hippocampal pyramidal cells.
- projects via the fornix to the mamillary nuclei and the anterior nucleus of the thalamus.

  b. **Major afferent connections to the hippocampal formation** (see Figures 20-4 and 20-5)
    (1) **Cerebral association cortices** (areas 19, 22, and 7)
    (2) **Septal area**
    (3) **Anterior nucleus of the thalamus,** via the cingulate gyrus, cingulum, and entorhinal cortex

  c. **Major efferent connections from the hippocampal formation** (see Figures 20-4 and 20-5)
    (1) **Mamillary nucleus of the hypothalamus**
    (2) **Septal area**
    (3) **Anterior nucleus of the thalamus**

7. **Amygdaloid complex (amygdala)** (Figure 20-6)
- is a basal ganglion underlying the parahippocampal uncus.
- produces activities associated with feeding and nutrition when stimulated.
- may cause rage and aggressive behavior when stimulated.
- is divided into a corticomedial group and a basolateral group. The corticomedial group receives olfactory input, and the basolateral receives prodigious cortical input.

  a. **Major afferent connections to the amygdaloid complex** (see Figure 20-6)
- **from** the following structures:
    (1) **Olfactory bulb and olfactory cortex**
    (2) **Cerebral cortex** (limbic and sensory association cortices)
    (3) **Hypothalamus**

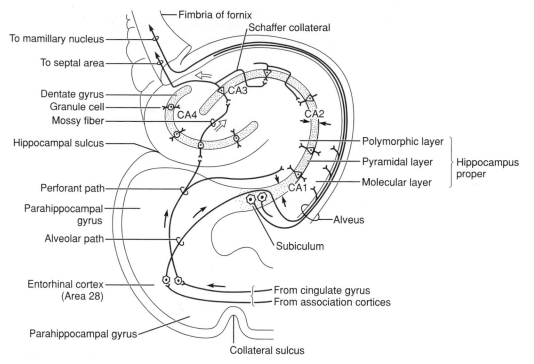

Figure 20-5.   Major connections of the hippocampal formation. The hippocampal formation (HF) consists of three parts: hippocampus, dentate gyrus, and subiculum. The two major hypothalamic output pathways are (*1*) granule cell via mossy fiber to pyramidal cell via precommissural fornix to septal nuclei and (*2*) subicular neuron via postcommissural fornix to the medial mamillary nucleus. The HF plays an important role in learning and memory, and lesions of the HF result in short-term memory defects. In Alzheimer disease, loss of cells in the HF and entorhinal cortex leads to loss of memory and cognitive function. CA = cornu ammonis. The sector CA1 is very sensitive to hypoxia (cardiac arrest or stroke).

  b. Major efferent connections from the amygdaloid complex (see Figure 20-6)
   • **to** the following structures:
    (1) Cerebral cortex (limbic and sensory association cortices)
    (2) Hypothalamus
    (3) Brainstem and spinal cord
 8. Hypothalamus
  • is a major part of the limbic system that projects to the brainstem and spinal cord (see Chapter 19).
 9. Limbic midbrain nuclei
  a. Ventral tegmental area (see Figure 22-2)
   • projects ascending dopaminergic fibers to all limbic structures.
  b. Raphe nuclei of the midbrain (see Figure 22-4)
   • project ascending serotonergic fibers to all limbic structures.
  c. Locus ceruleus (see Figure 22-3)
   • projects ascending noradrenergic fibers to all limbic structures.

B. Major limbic fiber systems (see Figures 20-3, 20-4, and 20-6)
 1. Fornix (see Figures 1-4, 1-5, and 20-3)
  • projects from the hippocampal formation to the hypothalamus (mamillary nucleus), the anterior nucleus of the thalamus, and the septal area.
  • projects from the septal area to the hippocampal formation.

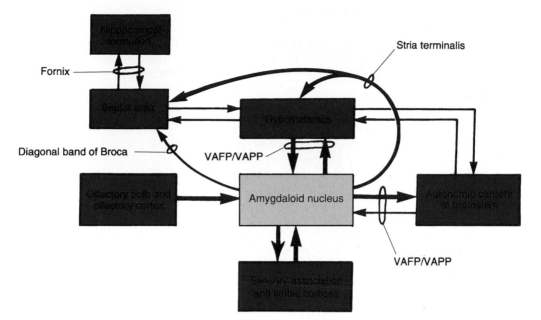

Figure 20-6.   Major connections of the amygdaloid nucleus. The amygdaloid nucleus receives input from three major sources: the olfactory system, the sensory association and limbic cortices, and the hypothalamus. The major output from the amygdaloid nucleus is via two channels: the stria terminalis projects to the hypothalamus and the septal area, and the ventral amygdalofugal pathway (VAFP) projects to the hypothalamus, brainstem, and spinal cord. A smaller efferent bundle, the diagonal band of Broca, projects to the septal area. Afferent fibers from the hypothalamus and brainstem enter the amygdaloid nucleus via the ventral amygdalopetal pathway (VAPP).

2. **Stria terminalis**
   - lies between the thalamus and the caudate nucleus.
   - projects from the amygdala to the hypothalamus and the septal area.
3. **Ventral amygdalofugal pathway**
   - projects from the amygdala to the hypothalamus, thalamus, brainstem, and spinal cord.
4. **Stria medullaris (thalami)**
   - projects from the septal area to the habenular nucleus.
5. **Diagonal band of Broca**
   - forms the medial border of the anterior perforated substance.
   - interconnects the amygdaloid nucleus and the septal area.
6. **Tractus retroflexus (habenulointerpeduncular tract)**
   - projects from the habenular nucleus (epithalamus) to the interpeduncular nucleus (midbrain).

C. **Papez circuit** (see Figure 20-4)
   - is a circular pathway that interconnects the major limbic structures.
   - contains the following stations:
   1. **Hippocampal formation**
      - projects via the **fornix** to the mamillary nucleus.
   2. **Mamillary body**
      - projects via the **mamillothalamic tract** to the anterior nucleus of the thalamus.
   3. **Anterior nucleus of the thalamus**
      - projects to the **cingulate gyrus**.
      - receives the mamillothalamic tract.
   4. **Cingulate gyrus**
      - projects via the entorhinal cortex to the hippocampal formation (see Figure 20-5).

D. **Functional and clinical considerations**
  1. **Hippocampus**
     - has a low threshold for seizure activity.
     - is involved in learning and memory.
     - Bilateral ablation results in the **inability to form long-term memories**.
  2. **Cingulate gyrus**
     - Lesions result in **akinesia, mutism, apathy**, and **indifference to pain**.
  3. **Amygdaloid nucleus**
     - modulates hypothalamic and endocrine activities.
     - has the highest concentration of opiate receptors in the brain.
     - has a high concentration of estradiol receptors.
     - Bilateral lesions result in **placidity**, with **loss of fear, rage, and aggression**.
  4. **Klüver-Bucy syndrome**
     - results from ablation of the temporal poles, including the amygdaloid nuclei, the hippocampal formations, and the anterior temporal neocortex.
     - may result from temporal lobe surgery for epilepsy, viral encephalitis (e.g., herpes simplex virus affects primarily the temporal lobes), and temporal lobe contusions due to head trauma.
     - is characterized by placidity, hypersexuality, hyperphagia, and psychic blindness (visual agnosia).
  5. **Mamillary bodies and the mediodorsal nucleus of the thalamus**
     - are damaged by chronic alcoholism and thiamine (vitamin B_1) deficiency, which results in **Korsakoff syndrome** (amnestic–confabulatory syndrome). This syndrome is considered to be a late chronic stage of Wernicke encephalopathy (see Figure 19-6). Clinical signs include memory disturbances (amnesia), confabulation, and temporospatial disorientation.

REVIEW TEST

1. Rhinorrhea would most likely result from a fracture of which bone?

(A) Ethmoid
(B) Frontal
(C) Lacrimal
(D) Nasal
(E) Palatine

2. A patient presents with visual agnosia and is referred to a psychiatric unit. Psychic blindness would most likely result from bilateral lesions of the

(A) accumbens septi nucleus
(B) amygdala
(C) hippocampus
(D) superior colliculus
(E) subiculum

3. Who wrote the classic paper *A Proposed Mechanism of Emotion*, which describes a major pathway of the limbic system?

(A) Klüver and Bucy
(B) Wernicke and Korsakoff
(C) Papez
(D) Liepmann
(E) Brodmann

4. A 40-year-old female was referred to a psychiatric unit with signs of nymphomania that were first manifest after a car accident. The responsible lesion would most likely be in the

(A) dentate gyrus
(B) cornu ammonis
(C) subiculum
(D) amygdala
(E) alveus

5. A 40-year-old man was admitted to the hospital and was examined by a staff neurologist. Examination revealed the following: alcohol abuse, paralysis of conjugate gaze, nystagmus, confusion, and memory loss. These symptoms are likely due to a deficiency in

(A) vitamin A
(B) vitamin B_1
(C) vitamin B_6
(D) vitamin B_{12}
(E) niacin

6. Bilateral ablation of what structure results in the inability to form long-term memories?

(A) hippocampus
(B) amygdala
(C) cingulate gyrus

(D) hypothalamus
(E) ventral tegmental area

7. A 50-year-old female presents with ipsilateral anosmia, optic atrophy, and contralateral papilledema. The syndrome is

(A) Foster Kennedy
(B) Edinger-Westphal
(C) Brown-Séquard
(D) Klüver-Bucy
(E) Wernicke-Korsakoff

Questions 8 to 12

The response options for items 8 to 12 are the same. Select one answer for each item in the set.
(A) Stria terminalis
(B) Stria medullaris
(C) Medial forebrain bundle
(D) Tractus retroflexus
(E) Diagonal band of Broca

Match the characteristic with the structure it best describes.

8. Consists of septohabenular fibers

9. Forms the medial border of the anterior perforated substance

10. Lies between the thalamus and the caudate nucleus

11. Projects from the epithalamus to the midbrain tegmentum

12. Is a major efferent pathway from the amygdala

Questions 13 to 16

The response options for items 13 to 16 are the same. Select one answer for each item in the set.
(A) Amygdala
(B) Hippocampal formation
(C) Both A and B
(D) Neither A nor B

Match each characteristic with the structure it most appropriately describes.

13. Is located in the temporal lobe

14. Is destroyed in Klüver-Bucy syndrome

15. Projects via the stria terminalis

16. Receives direct olfactory input

ANSWERS AND EXPLANATIONS

1–A. Rhinorrhea would most likely result from a fracture of the cribriform plate of the ethmoid bone, which could tear the arachnoid membrane and result in a leakage of cerebrospinal fluid into the nasal cavity.

2–B. Bilateral lesions of the amygdalae result in psychic blindness, the inability to recognize objects visually. Subjects can see objects but do not understand what they see. Bilateral lesions of the hippocampus result in memory loss (e.g., viral encephalitis). Lesions of the superior colliculus result in paralysis of upward and downward gaze.

3–C. Papez wrote *A Proposed Mechanism of Emotion*; the circuit is hippocampal formation → mamillary body → anterior thalamic nucleus → cingulate gyrus → entorhinal cortex → hippocampal formation (see Figure 20-4). Klüver-Bucy syndrome is characterized by placidity, hypersexuality, hyperphagia, and psychic blindness (visual agnosia). Wernicke Korsakoff syndrome is characterized by alcohol abuse resulting in thiamine deficiency, conjugate gaze palsies, ataxia, confusion, and memory loss. Liepmann is known for his classic book on ataxias. Brodmann is known for his brain maps, called the Brodmann areas.

4–D. Bilateral ablation of the inferior temporal cortex results in damage to the amygdala resulting in hypersexuality, hyperphagia, docility, and psychic blindness (Klüver-Bucy syndrome).

5–B. The lack of thiamine B₁ results in Wernicke-Korsakoff syndrome; the classic clinical triad of Wernicke encephalopathy is confusion, gait ataxia, and ophthalmoplegia. Korsakoff syndrome is profound memory impairment and confabulation. Vitamin A deficiency results in impaired night vision; when ingested in excess, vitamin A may cause pseudotumor cerebri. Pyridoxine (vitamin B₆) is used to prevent isoniazid neuropathy. Vitamin B₁₂ deficiency results in anemia and subacute combined degeneration. Niacin (nicotinic acid) is used to prevent pellagra.

6–A. Bilateral ablation of the hippocampus results in the inability to form long-term memories. The hippocampus plays a major role in learning and memory.

7–A. Foster Kennedy syndrome includes ipsilateral anosmia, optic atrophy, and contralateral papilledema; pressure on the olfactory tract causes ipsilateral anosmia, pressure on the optic nerve causes ipsilateral optic atrophy and a central scotoma and contralateral papilledema. Edinger and Westphal described this parasympathetic nucleus of the rostral midbrain (p. 283). Brown-Séquard is associated with a spinal cord lesion, spinal cord hemisection. Klüver and Bucy described the limbic lobe syndrome (p. 439). Wernicke-Korsakoff syndrome consists of Wernicke encephalopathy and Korsakoff psychosis.

8–B. The stria medullaris (thalami) contains septohabenular fibers (i.e., fibers that project from the septal nuclei to the habenular nuclei). The stria medullaris (singular) should not be confused with the striae medullares (plural). The striae medullares (rhombencephali) arise from the arcuate nuclei of the medulla and are seen on the floor of the rhomboid fossa.

9–E. The diagonal band of Broca is the medial border of the anterior perforated substance. This fiber bundle contains amygdaloseptal and septoamygdalar fibers. The nucleus of the diagonal band projects via the fornix to the hippocampal formation.

10–A. The stria terminalis and the vena terminalis lie in the sulcus terminalis between the thalamus and the caudate nucleus.

11–D. The tractus retroflexus contains habenulointerpeduncular fibers that project from the habenular nuclei of the epithalamus to the interpeduncular nucleus of the midbrain tegmentum.

12–A. The stria terminalis is a major efferent pathway from the amygdala. It projects to the septal area and to the bed nucleus of the stria terminalis.

13–C. Both the hippocampal formation and the amygdala are found in the parahippocampal gyrus of the temporal (limbic) lobe.

14–C. The hippocampal formation and the amygdala are both involved in Klüver-Bucy syndrome.

15–A. The amygdala projects via the stria terminalis and via the ventral amygdalofugal pathway. The stria terminalis is the most prominent projection from the amygdaloid complex.

16–A. The amygdala receives both direct and indirect olfactory input.

Basal Ganglia and the Striatal Motor System

I. Basal Ganglia (Figure 21-1)

- consists of subcortical nuclei (gray matter) within the cerebral hemispheres.

A. Components
1. **Caudate nucleus**
2. **Putamen**
3. **Globus pallidus**
4. **Amygdala (amygdaloid nuclear complex)** (See Chapter 20 III A 7)
5. **Claustrum**
   - is located between the putamen and the insular cortex and between the external capsule and the extreme capsule.

B. Groupings of the basal ganglia
1. **Striatum (neostriatum)**
   - consists of the **caudate nucleus** and the **putamen**, which are similar in structure and connections and have a common embryologic origin.
2. **Lentiform nucleus**
   - consists of the **putamen** and the **globus pallidus**.
3. **Corpus striatum**
   - consists of the **lentiform nucleus** and the **caudate nucleus**.

II. Striatal Motor System (see Figure 21-1)

- is also called the **extrapyramidal motor system**.
- plays a role in the initiation and execution of somatic motor activity, especially willed movement.
- is involved in automatic stereotyped motor activity of a postural and reflex nature.
- exerts its influences on motor activities via the thalamus, motor cortex, and corticobulbar and corticospinal systems.

A. Components of the striatal system
- consist of the following nuclei:
1. **Striatum (caudatoputamen or neostriatum)**
   a. **Caudate nucleus (caudatum)**
   b. **Putamen**

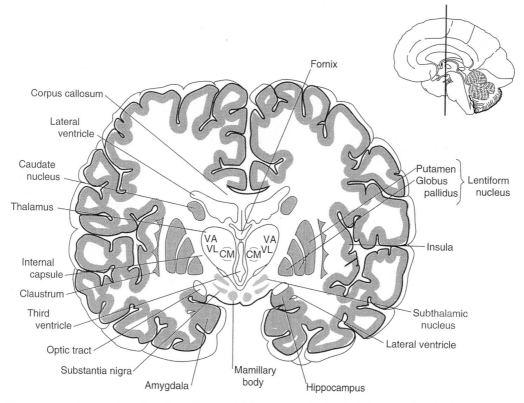

Figure 21-1. A coronal section through the mid thalamus at the level of the mamillary bodies. The basal ganglia are all prominent at this level and include the striatum and the lentiform nucleus. The subthalamic nucleus and substantia nigra are important components of the striatal motor system. (Modified with permission from Fix JD: *High-Yield Neuroanatomy*, 3rd ed. Philadelphia, Lippincott Williams & Wilkins, 2005, p. 142.)

  2. Globus pallidus (pallidum or paleostriatum)
    a. Medial (internal) segment
      • is adjacent to the internal capsule.
    b. Lateral (external) segment
      • is adjacent to the putamen.
  3. Subthalamic nucleus
    • lies between the internal capsule and the thalamus and between the internal capsule and the lenticular fasciculus.
  4. Thalamus
    a. Ventral anterior nucleus
    b. Ventral lateral nucleus
    c. Centromedian nucleus
  5. Substantia nigra
    a. Pars compacta
      • contains dopaminergic neurons, which contain the pigment melanin.
    b. Pars reticularis
      • contains gamma-aminobutyric acid (GABA) –ergic neurons.
  6. Pedunculopontine nucleus
    • lies in the lateral tegmentum of the caudal midbrain.

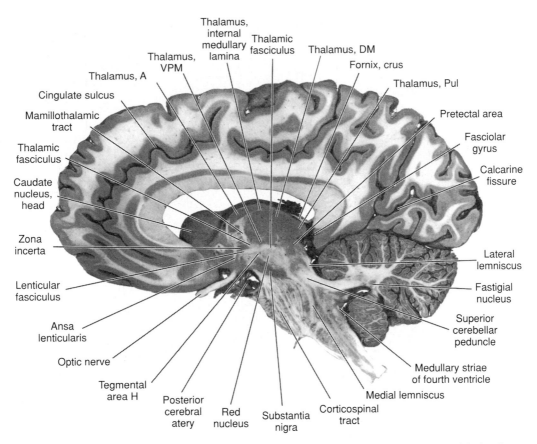

Figure 21-2. A parasagittal section through the caudate nucleus and the substantia nigra. (Modified with permission from Woolsey TA, Hanaway J, Gado MH: *The Brain Atlas: A Visual Guide to the Human Central Nervous System*, 2nd ed. Hoboken, John Wiley & Sons, 2003, p. 128.)

B. **Major connections of the striatal system** (Figure 21-2)
  1. **Striatum (caudate nucleus and putamen)**
     - receives its largest input from the **neocortex**, from virtually all neocortical areas.
     - receives input from the **thalamus** (centromedian nucleus) and from the **substantia nigra**.
     - projects fibers to two major nuclei: the **globus pallidus** and the **substantia nigra** (pars reticularis).
  2. **Globus pallidus** (Figure 21-3)
     - receives input from two major nuclei: the **striatum** and the **subthalamic nucleus**.
     - projects fibers to three major nuclei: the **subthalamic nucleus**, the **thalamus** (ventral anterior, ventral lateral, and centromedian nuclei), and the **pedunculopontine nucleus**.
  3. **Subthalamic nucleus**
     - receives input from the **globus pallidus** and from the **motor cortex**.
     - projects fibers to the globus pallidus.
  4. **Thalamus** (see Figure 16-1)
     a. **Input to the thalamus**
        (1) **Globus pallidus**
           - projects to the **ventral anterior**, **ventral lateral**, and **centromedian nuclei**.

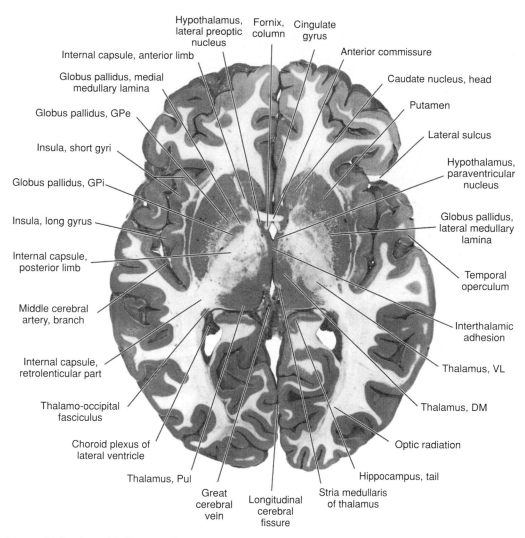

Figure 21-3. An axial (horizontal) section through the anterior commissure and the massa intermedia. (Modified with permission from Woolsey TA, Hanaway J, Gado MH: *The Brain Atlas: A Visual Guide to the Human Central Nervous System,* 2nd ed. Hoboken, John Wiley & Sons, 2003, p. 100.)

      (2) Substantia nigra
- projects from the pars reticularis to the **ventral anterior, ventral lateral,** and the **mediodorsal nuclei** of the thalamus.

    b. Projections from the thalamus
      (1) Motor cortex (area 4)
- from the **ventral lateral** and **centromedian nuclei**

      (2) Premotor cortex (area 6)
- from the **ventral anterior** and **ventral lateral nuclei**

      (3) Supplementary motor cortex (area 6)
- from the **ventral lateral** and **ventral anterior nuclei**

      (4) Striatum
- from the **centromedian nucleus**

  5. Substantia nigra
- receives major input from the **striatum.**
- projects fibers to the **striatum** and the **thalamus** (ventral anterior, ventral lateral, and mediodorsal nuclei).

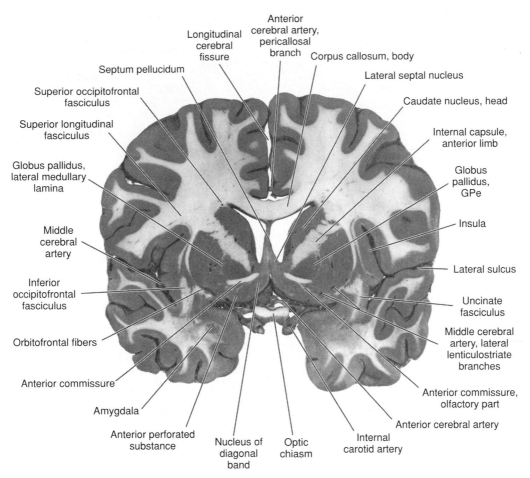

Figure 21-4. A coronal section through the lentiform nucleus and the amygdaloid nucleus; the lentiform nucleus consists of the putamen and the globus pallidus. The amygdaloid nucleus appears as a circular profile below the uncus. (Modified with permission from Woolsey TA, Hanaway J, Gado MH: *The Brain Atlas: A Visual Guide to the Human Central Nervous System*, 2nd ed. Hoboken, John Wiley & Sons, 2003, p. 60.)

6. **Pedunculopontine nucleus**
   - receives GABA-ergic input from the **globus pallidus**.
   - projects glutaminergic fibers to the **globus pallidus** and to the **substantia nigra**.

C. **Major neurotransmitters of the neurons of the striatal system** (Figure 21-4)
   1. **Glutamate-containing neurons** (see Figure 22-10)
      - project from the cerebral cortex to the striatum.
      - project from the subthalamic nucleus to the globus pallidus.
      - excite **striatal GABA-ergic** and **cholinergic neurons**.
   2. **GABA-containing neurons** (see Figure 22-9)
      - are the predominant neurons of the striatal system.
      - are found in the striatum, globus pallidus, and substantia nigra (pars reticularis).
      - give rise to the following **GABA-ergic projections**: striatopallidal, striatonigral, pallidothalamic, and nigrothalamic projections.
      - degenerate in Huntington disease.
   3. **Dopamine-containing neurons** (see Figure 22-2)
      - are found in the pars compacta of the substantia nigra.
      - give rise to the dopaminergic nigrostriatal projection.

- are thought to regulate the production of striatal peptides and peptide mRNA.
- degenerate in Parkinson disease.

4. Neurons containing acetylcholine (ACh) (see Figure 22-1)
- are local circuit neurons found in the striatum.

5. Neuropeptide-containing neurons (see Figures 22-6 through 22-8)
- include **enkephalin, dynorphin, substance P, somatostatin, neurotensin, neuropeptide Y,** and **cholecystokinin.**
- are also found in the basal ganglia.
- coexist with the major neurotransmitters (e.g., GABA and/or enkephalin and GABA and/or substance P).

D. Ventral striatopallidal complex and its connections
- play a role in initiating movements in response to motivational and emotional activity (e.g., limbic functions).

  1. Ventral striatum
  - consists of the **nucleus accumbens** and the olfactory tubercle.
  - receives input from the olfactory, prefrontal, and hippocampal cortices.
  - projects to the ventral pallidum.

  2. Ventral pallidum
  - consists of the **substantia innominata.**
  - receives input from the ventral striatum.
  - projects to the medial dorsal nucleus of the thalamus.

E. Clinical correlations
  1. Parkinson disease
  - is a common condition that is associated with degeneration and depigmentation of neurons in the substantia nigra.
  - results in the **depletion of dopamine** in the caudate nucleus and putamen.
  - includes clinical manifestations of **bradykinesia** and **hypokinesia** (difficulty in initiating and performing volitional movements); **rigidity** (cog-wheel and lead-pipe rigidity); and **resting tremor** (pill-rolling tremor).

  2. MPTP-induced parkinsonism
  - is caused by 1-methyl-4-phenyl-1,2,3,6-tetrahydropyridine (MPTP), a **meperidine analog** found in illicit recreational drugs.
  - results in the destruction of dopaminergic neurons, which are located in the substantia nigra.

  3. Progressive supranuclear palsy
  - is associated with **Parkinson disease.** Progressive supranuclear palsy together with Parkinson disease is called the Parkinson-plus syndrome.
  - is characterized by supranuclear ophthalmoplegia, primarily downgaze paresis, which is followed by paresis of other eye movements. As the disease progresses, the remainder of the motor cranial nerves become involved, resulting in the clinical picture of pseudobulbar palsy. (See Glossary.)
  - is characterized by neuronal cell loss in the globus pallidus, red nucleus, substantia nigra, periaqueductal gray, and dentate nucleus.
  - spares the cerebral and the cerebellar cortices.
  - results in neurofibrillary tangles in the surviving neurons.

  4. Huntington disease (chorea major)
  - is an inherited **autosomal dominant movement disorder** associated with severe degeneration of the cholinergic and GABA-ergic neurons, which are located in the caudate nucleus and putamen.
  - is usually accompanied by **gyral atrophy** in the frontal and temporal lobes.
  - can be traced to a single gene defect on chromosome 4.
  - is characterized by impaired initiation and slowness of saccadic eye movements; patients cannot make a volitional saccade without moving the head.
  - results in clinical manifestations of **choreiform movements** and **progressive dementia.**

- results in **hydrocephalus ex vacuo** due to the loss of neurons located in the head of the caudate nucleus, and to a lesser extent in the putamen.
- Prenatal and postnatal diagnosis using DNA techniques is available.

5. **Other choreiform dyskinesias**

   a. **Sydenham chorea (St. Vitus dance)**
      - is the most common cause of chorea overall.
      - occurs mainly in girls as a sequela to rheumatic fever.

   b. **Chorea gravidarum**
      - occurs usually during the second trimester of pregnancy.
      - in many cases, a history of Sydenham chorea can be obtained.

6. **Ballism and hemiballism**
   - are extrapyramidal motor disorders most often resulting from a vascular lesion (infarct) of the subthalamic nucleus.
   - are characterized by **violent flinging** (ballistic) **movements of one or both extremities;** symptoms appear on the contralateral side.
   - may be treated with dopamine-blocking drugs or with GABA-mimetic agents.
   - may be treated surgically by **ventrolateral thalamotomy**.

7. **Hepatolenticular degeneration (Wilson disease)**
   - is an autosomal recessive disorder due to a **defect in the metabolism of copper** (ceruloplasmin).
   - has its gene locus on chromosome 13.
   - results in clinical manifestations of **tremor, rigidity**, and **choreiform or athetotic movements**. Tremor is the most common neurologic sign.
   - has psychiatric symptoms, including psychosis, personality disorders, and dementia.
   - results in a **corneal Kayser-Fleischer ring**, which is pathognomonic.
   - is marked by lesions in the liver (cirrhosis) and in the lentiform nuclei (necrosis and cavitation of the putamen).
   - is diagnosed by low serum ceruloplasmin, elevated urinary excretion of copper, and increased copper concentration in liver biopsy.
   - is treated with the copper-chelating agent D-penicillamine and pyridoxine for anemia.

8. **Tardive dyskinesia**
   - is a syndrome of repetitive choreic movements affecting the face, limbs, and trunk.
   - results from treatment with antipsychotic drugs (e.g., phenothiazines, butyrophenones, or metoclopramide).

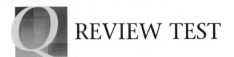

REVIEW TEST

1. A six-year old girl has brief, irregular contractions in her feet; symptoms are suspected to be a result of an untreated strep infection. What is the diagnosis?

(A) chorea major
(B) Sydenham chorea
(C) chorea gravidarum
(D) ballism
(E) hemiballism

2. Which thalamic nucleus projects to the striatum?

(A) Centromedian nucleus
(B) Mediodorsal nucleus
(C) Ventral lateral nucleus
(D) Ventral anterior nucleus
(E) Ventral posterolateral nucleus

3. The globus pallidus projects to the thalamus via the

(A) fasciculus retroflexus
(B) stria medullaris
(C) ansa lenticularis
(D) ansa peduncularis
(E) stria terminalis

4. The predominant neurons of the striatal system contain

(A) GABA
(B) glutamate
(C) serotonin
(D) acetylcholine
(E) dopamine

5. An ophthalmologist sees a Kayser-Fleischer ring while examining Descemet's membrane with a slit lamp; what trace metal is found in the membrane?

(A) aluminum
(B) copper
(C) iron
(D) mercury
(E) magnesium

6. A 50-year-old woman has resting tremor, cogwheel rigidity, bradykinesia, and shuffling gait. The incidence of this disease in patients over 50 years of age is:

(A) 1%
(B) 2%
(C) 3%
(D) 4%
(E) 5%

Questions 7 to 15

The response options for items 7 to 15 are the same. Select one answer for each item in the set.

(A) Chorea gravidarum
(B) Hepatolenticular degeneration
(C) Hemiballism
(D) Huntington disease
(E) Parkinson disease
(F) Sydenham chorea
(G) Tardive dyskinesia

Match each of the characteristics with the appropriate lettered movement disorder.

7. Is the overall most common cause of chorea

8. Results from a loss of dopaminergic neurons in the pars compacta of the substantia nigra

9. A corneal Kayser-Fleischer ring is pathognomonic for this dyskinesia

10. Results from a lesion of the subthalamic nucleus

11. Is characterized by repetitive choreic movements affecting the face, limbs, and trunk, which results from treatment with antipsychotic drugs

12. Can be traced to a single gene defect on chromosome 4

13. Has its gene locus on chromosome 13

14. Is characterized by cortical atrophy and loss of neurons in the head of the caudate nucleus

15. Central nervous system lesions are characterized by necrosis and cavitation of the putamen

ANSWERS AND EXPLANATIONS

1–B. Sydenham chorea (St. Vitus dance) is the most common chorea. It occurs mainly in girls as a sequela to rheumatic fever, which may develop after a strep infection. Chorea major (Huntington disease) is an inherited disorder that manifests as choreiform movements and progressive dementia; chorea gravidarum occurs during the second trimester of pregnancy; and ballism and hemiballism are violent flinging movement of one or both extremities as a result of an infarct of the subthalamic nucleus.

2–A. The striatum (caudate nucleus and putamen) receives thalamic input from the centromedian nucleus, the largest of the intralaminar nuclei.

3–C. The globus pallidus projects to the thalamus via the lenticular and thalamic fasciculi and via the ansa lenticularis. The ansa peduncularis (part of the inferior thalamic peduncle) interconnects the amygdaloid nucleus and the hypothalamus. It also interconnects the orbitofrontal cortex and the thalamus (mediodorsal nucleus). The fasciculus retroflexus (habenulointerpeduncular tract) interconnects the habenular nucleus and the interpeduncular nucleus. The stria medullaris (thalami) interconnects the septal area (nuclei) and the habenular nuclei. The stria terminalis projects from the amygdaloid complex to the septal area and the hypothalamus.

4–A. GABA-containing neurons are the predominant neurons of the striatal system. They are found in the striatum, globus pallidus, and substantia nigra (pars reticularis).

5–B. Wilson disease is an autosomal recessive disorder that results from a defect in the metabolism of copper. Wilson disease is diagnosed by low serum ceruloplasmin, elevated urinary excretion of copper, and increased copper concentration in liver biopsy. Tremor is the most common symptom and is known as the wing-beating tremor.

6–A. The incidence of Parkinson disease is 1% of the population of 50 years of age.

7–F. Sydenham chorea (St. Vitus dance) is the most common cause of chorea overall. Magnetic resonance imaging (MRI) studies show an increased signal in the head of the caudate nucleus with T_2-weighted images. Quantitative MRI reveals an increase in the size of the caudate nucleus, putamen, and globus pallidus. In Huntington disease, there is massive loss of neurons in the caudatoputamen.

8–E. Parkinson disease results from a loss of dopaminergic neurons in the pars compacta of the substantia nigra.

9–B. Hepatolenticular degeneration, Wilson disease, is an autosomal recessive disorder due to a defect in the metabolism of copper. The Kayser-Fleisher ring is a green band of pigmentation found around the limbus in Descemet membrane; it is a pathognomonic of Wilson disease.

10–C. Hemiballism results from a contralateral lesion (usually vascular) of the subthalamic nucleus. It is characterized by violent flinging (ballistic) movements of one or both extremities.

11–G. Tardive dyskinesia is a syndrome characterized by repetitive choreic movements affecting the face and trunk, which results from treatment with antipsychotic drugs (e.g., phenothiazines, butyrophenones, or metoclopramide).

12–D. Huntington disease has its gene locus on chromosome 4 (gene location 4p16.3)

13–B. In Wilson disease the abnormal gene has been assigned to the esterase D locus on chromosome 13.

14–D. Huntington disease is characterized by cortical atrophy and loss of neurons in the head of the caudate nucleus, which results in hydrocephalus ex vacuo.

15–B. Wilson disease is characterized by necrosis and cavitation of the putamen.

Neurotransmitters and Pathways

I. Introduction

A. Neurotransmitters (chemical messengers)
- are substances released on excitation from presynaptic neurons. They produce the effects of nerve stimulation in postsynaptic neurons or in receptor cells.

B. Neurochemical pathways and loci
- can be classified according to the chemical composition of their neurotransmitters.
  1. **Monoaminergic pathways**
     - make use of **monoamines** as neurotransmitters; they contain one amine group. Monoamines include **dopamine, norepinephrine, epinephrine**, and **serotonin**.
       a. **Catecholaminergic pathways**
          - make use of a monoamine that contains a catechol nucleus. Catecholamines include **dopamine, norepinephrine**, and **epinephrine**.
          - include dopaminergic, noradrenergic (norepinephrinergic), and adrenergic (epinephrinergic) pathways.
       b. **Indolaminergic pathways**
          - make use of a monoamine that contains an indole nucleus. **Serotonin** is an indolamine.
          - include serotonergic pathways.
  2. **Cholinergic pathways**
     - make use of **acetylcholine** (ACh) as a neurotransmitter.
  3. **Peptidergic pathways**
     - make use of **peptides** as neurotransmitters.
  4. **Gamma-aminobutyric acid (GABA) –ergic pathways**
     - make use of **GABA** as a neurotransmitter.
  5. **Glutamatergic pathways**
     - make use of **glutamate** as a neurotransmitter.
  6. **Glycinergic pathways**
     - make use of **glycine** as a neurotransmitter.
  7. **L-Arginine–nitric oxide pathway**
     - makes use of the gaseous neurotransmitter **nitric oxide**. (Figure 22-1)

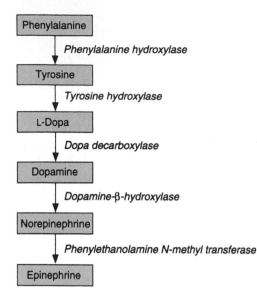

Figure 22-1. Synthesis of catecholamines from phenylalanine. Epinephrine, which is derived from norepinephrine, is found primarily in the adrenal medulla.

II. Acetylcholine

A. Characteristics of ACh
- can be identified indirectly by the marker choline acetyltransferase.
- is the major transmitter of the peripheral nervous system (PNS), neuromuscular junction, parasympathetic nervous system, preganglionic sympathetic fibers, and postganglionic sympathetic fibers to the sweat glands.
- is found in neurons of the somatic and visceral motor nuclei in the brainstem and spinal cord.

B. Major cholinergic pathways (Figure 22-2)
1. Septal nuclei
- project via the fornix to the hippocampal formation.

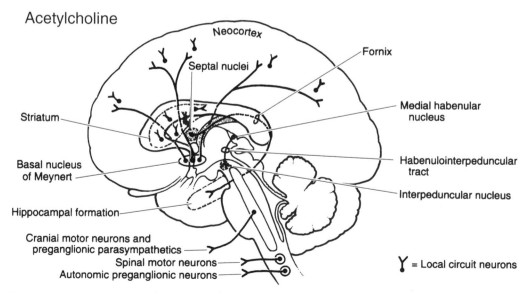

Figure 22-2. Distribution of ACh-containing neurons and their axonal projections. The basal nucleus of Meynert projects to the entire cortex; this nucleus degenerates in Alzheimer disease. Striatal ACh–local circuit neurons degenerate in Huntington chorea.

2. **Basal nucleus of Meynert**
   - is located in the substantia innominata of the basal forebrain, between the globus pallidus and the anterior perforated substance.
   - projects to the entire neocortex.
   - receives input from the locus ceruleus, raphe nuclei, substantia nigra, amygdaloid nucleus, and orbitofrontal and temporal cortices.
   - degenerates in **Alzheimer disease**.
3. **Striatum (caudate nucleus and putamen)**
   - contains ACh in its local circuit neurons.
   - has cholinergic neurons that degenerate in **Huntington disease** and **Alzheimer disease**.
4. **Neocortex**
   - contains ACh in its local circuit neurons.

III. Dopamine

A. **Characteristics of dopamine**
   - is a **catecholamine**.
   - can be identified by the marker tyrosine hydroxylase.
   - plays a role in cognitive, motor, and neuroendocrine functions.
   - is **depleted in Parkinson disease**.
   - has **increased production in schizophrenics** (dopamine hypothesis of schizophrenia).

B. **Major dopaminergic pathways** (Figure 22-3)
   1. **Nigrostriatal pathway**
      - The substantia nigra projects to the striatum.
      - Destruction of dopaminergic nigral neurons results in **parkinsonism**.

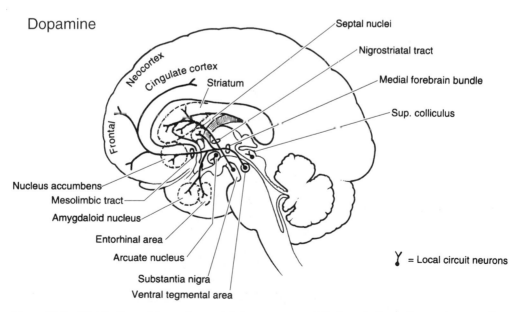

Figure 22-3. Distribution of dopamine-containing neurons and their projections. Two major ascending dopamine pathways arise in the midbrain: the nigrostriatal tract from the substantia nigra and the mesolimbic tract from the ventral tegmental area. In Parkinson disease, loss of dopaminergic neurons occurs in the substantia nigra and in the ventral tegmental area.

2. **Mesolimbic pathway**
   - The ventral tegmental area projects to all cortical and subcortical structures of the limbic system.
   - is linked to behavior and schizophrenia.
3. **Tuberohypophyseal (tuberoinfundibular) pathway**
   - The arcuate nucleus of the hypothalamus projects to the portal vessels of the infundibulum.
   - Released dopamine inhibits the release of **prolactin** from the adenohypophysis.

IV. Norepinephrine (Noradrenalin)

A. **Characteristics of norepinephrine**
   - is a **catecholamine**.
   - can be localized by the marker dopamine β-hydroxylase.
   - is the transmitter of the postganglionic sympathetic neurons.
   - may play a role in the genesis and maintenance of **mood**. The catecholamine hypothesis of mood disorders states that reduced norepinephrine activity is related to **depression** and that increased norepinephrine activity is related to **mania**.

B. **Noradrenergic pathways** (Figure 22-4)
   1. **Locus ceruleus**
      - contains the largest concentration of noradrenergic neurons in the central nervous system (CNS).
      - is located in the pons and midbrain.
      - projects to all parts of the CNS.
      - receives input from the cortex, limbic system, reticular formation, raphe nuclei, cerebellum, and spinal cord.
      - shows a significant loss of neurons in Alzheimer disease and Parkinson disease.
      - is hypothesized to play a role in **anxiety** and **panic disorders**.

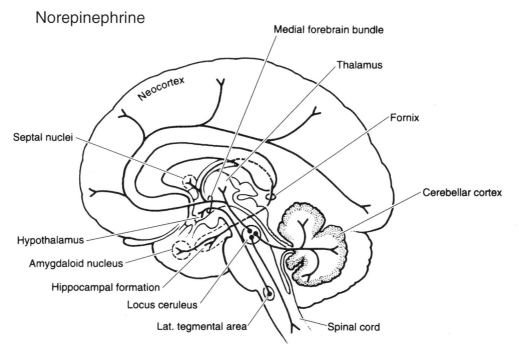

Figure 22-4. Distribution of norepinephrine-containing neurons and their projections. The locus ceruleus, located in the pons and midbrain, is the chief source of noradrenergic fibers. The locus ceruleus projects to all parts of the CNS.

2. **Lateral tegmental area**
   - is located in the medulla and pons.
   - projects via the central tegmental tract and the medial forebrain bundle to the hypothalamus and thalamus.

V.   Serotonin (5-Hydroxytryptamine [5-HT])

A. **Characteristics of 5-HT**
   - can be identified by the marker tryptophan hydroxylase.
   - plays an important role in influencing arousal, sensory perception, emotion, and higher cognitive functions.
   - The **permissive serotonin hypothesis** states that reduced 5-HT activity permits reduced levels of catecholamines to cause depression and elevated levels to cause mania.
   - **Severe depression** and **insomnia** are associated with low 5-HT levels, and **mania** is associated with high 5-HT activity. Dysfunction of 5-HT is believed to underlie obsessive-compulsive disorder.
   - Tricyclic antidepressants and fluoxetine increase 5-HT availability by reduction of its reuptake.

B. **Major serotonergic pathways** (Figure 22-5)
   - 5-HT neurons are found only in the **raphe nuclei** of the brainstem. Raphe nuclei project diffusely to the entire CNS (see Figure 22-4).
   1. **Raphe nuclei of the medulla**
      - project to the dorsal horns of the spinal cord.
   2. **Raphe nuclei of the pons**
      - project to the spinal cord and cerebellum.
   3. **Raphe nuclei of the midbrain**
      - project to widespread areas of the diencephalon and the telencephalon, including the striatum.

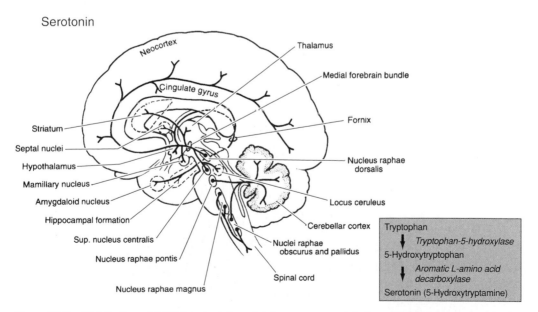

Figure 22-5.   Distribution of 5-HT (serotonin)-containing neurons and their projections. Serotonin-containing neurons are found in nuclei of the raphe. They project widely to the forebrain, cerebellum, and spinal cord. The *inset* shows the synthetic pathway of serotonin.

C. **Pineal gland (epiphysis cerebri)**
   - contains the highest concentration of 5-HT in the body.
   - contains pinealocytes, which convert 5-HT to melatonin.

VI. Opioid Peptides

A. **Endorphins** (Figure 22-6)
   - are derived from **pro-opiomelanocortin** (POMC), the precursor of adrenocorticotropic hormone (ACTH).
   - include β-endorphin, the major endorphin found in the brain.
   - appear to play a major role in **endocrine function**.
   - Endorphinergic neurons are found almost exclusively in the **hypothalamus** (arcuate and premamillary nuclei). These neurons project to the hypothalamus, amygdala, nucleus accumbens, septal area, thalamus, and locus ceruleus (midbrain and pons).

B. **Enkephalins** (Figure 22-7)
   - are derived from **proenkephalin**.
   - are the most widely distributed and abundant opioid peptides.
   - are found in the highest concentrations in the **globus pallidus**.
   - are synthesized in striatal neurons, which project to the globus pallidus.
   - are located mainly in local circuits of the limbic and striatal systems.
   - coexist with dopamine, norepinephrine, ACh, and GABA.
   - play a role in **pain suppression** in the dorsal horn of the spinal cord.

C. **Dynorphins**
   - are derived from **prodynorphin**.
   - follow, in general, the distribution map for enkephalin.
   - have high concentrations in the **hypothalamus** and **amygdala**.

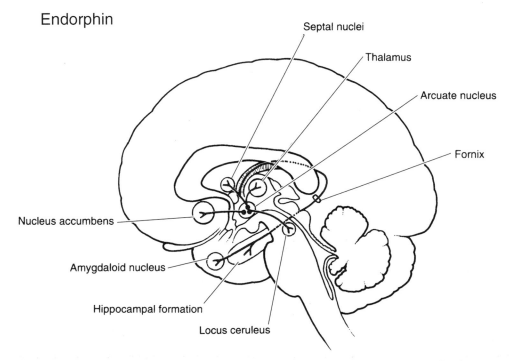

Figure 22-6. Distribution of endorphin-containing neurons and their projections. Endorphinergic neurons are found almost exclusively in the hypothalamus (arcuate nucleus).

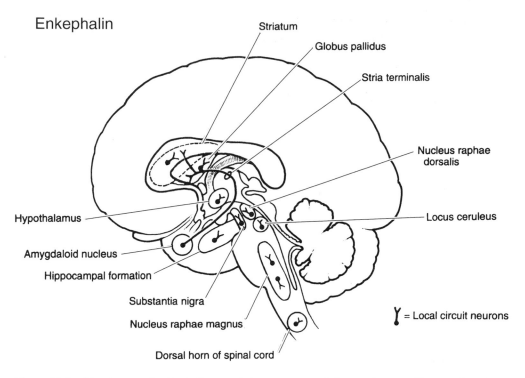

Figure 22-7. Distribution of enkephalin-containing neurons and their projections. They are found primarily in local circuits of the limbic and striatal systems. Enkephalinergic neurons of the brainstem and spinal cord play a role in pain suppression mechanisms.

VII. Nonopioid Neuropeptides

A. Substance P (Figure 22-8)
- is an excitatory neurotransmitter.
- is contained in dorsal root ganglion cells, which project to the substantia gelatinosa.
- plays a role in **pain transmission** (in Aδ and C fibers).
- is synthesized in striatal neurons, which project to the globus pallidus and the substantia nigra.
- is found in highest concentration in the **substantia nigra** (striatonigral and pallidonigral tracts).

B. Somatostatin (Figure 22-9)
- is also called somatotropin release–inhibiting factor.
- Somatostatinergic neurons are found in the anterior hypothalamus and in the preoptic region, striatum, amygdala, cerebral cortex, and in dorsal root ganglion cells. Somatostatinergic neurons from the anterior hypothalamus project their axons to the median eminence, where somatostatin enters the hypophyseal portal system and regulates the release of growth hormone (GH) and thyroid-stimulating hormone (TSH).
- The concentration of somatostatin in the neocortex and hippocampus is significantly reduced in **Alzheimer disease**.

VIII. Amino Acids

- are, from a quantitative standpoint, the major transmitters in the mammalian CNS.

Substance P

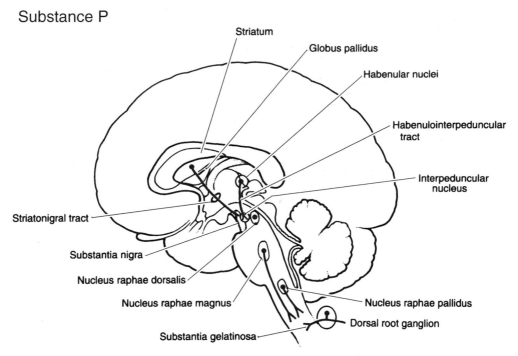

Figure 22-8. Distribution of substance P–containing neurons and their projections. Substance P is the neurotransmitter for nociceptive neurons of the dorsal root ganglia. Striatal substance P neurons project via the striatonigral tract to the substantia nigra.

Somatostatin

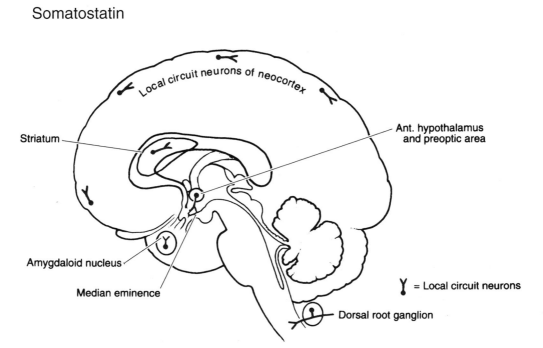

Figure 22-9. Distribution of somatostatin-containing neurons and their projections. Somatostatin is found primarily in the anterior hypothalamus and preoptic area. Somatostatinergic neurons project to the hypophyseal portal system and thus regulate the release of growth hormone.

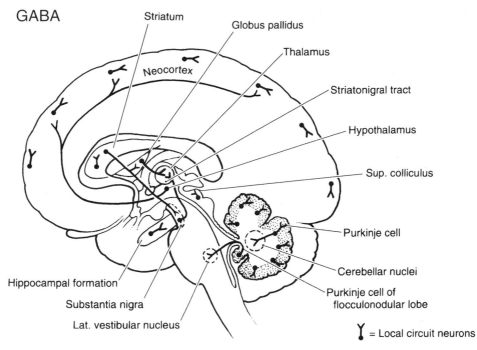

Figure 22-10. Distribution of GABA-containing neurons and their projections. GABA-ergic neurons are the major inhibitory cells of the CNS. GABA local circuit neurons are found in the neocortex, allocortex, and in the cerebellar cortex (Purkinje cells). Striatal GABA-ergic neurons project to the globus pallidus and the substantia nigra. Pallidal GABA-ergic neurons project to the thalamus and the subthalamic nucleus.

A. **Inhibitory amino acid transmitters**
- are aliphatic amino acids that have **one acidic and one amine function**.
  1. **GABA** (Figure 22-10)
     - can be localized by the marker glutamic acid decarboxylase.
     - is the major inhibitory neurotransmitter of the brain.
     - coexists with substance P and with enkephalin.
     - Purkinje, stellate, basket, and Golgi cells of the cerebellar cortex are GABA-ergic (see Figure 15-3).
     - GABA-ergic striatal neurons project to the globus pallidus and the substantia nigra.
     - GABA-ergic pallidal neurons project to the thalamus.
     - GABA-ergic nigral neurons project to the thalamus.
  2. **Glycine**
     - is the major inhibitory neurotransmitter of the spinal cord.
     - is used by the Renshaw cells of the spinal cord.
     - Its inhibitory action is blocked by strychnine.

B. **Excitatory amino acid transmitters**
- are aliphatic amino acids that have **two acidic functions and one alpha-amino group**.
  1. **Glutamate** (Figure 22-11)
     - is a major excitatory transmitter of the brain; 60% of brain synapses are glutamatergic.
     - is the neurotransmitter of the cerebellar granule cell.
     - is used by the corticobulbar and corticospinal tracts.
     - is used by dorsal root ganglion cells.
     - is believed to be involved in long-term potentiation of hippocampal neurons via *N*-methyl-D-aspartate (NMDA) receptors.

Glutamate and Aspartate

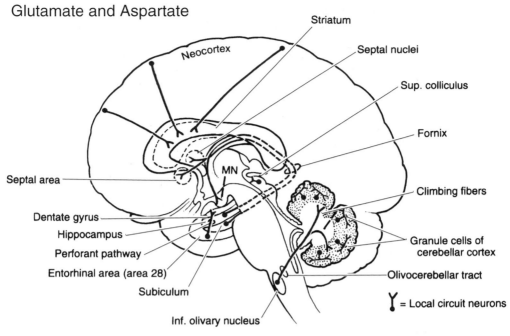

Figure 22-11. Distribution of glutamate- and aspartate-containing neurons and their projections. Glutamate is considered the major excitatory transmitter of the CNS. Cortical glutamatergic neurons project to the striatum; hippocampal and subicular glutamatergic neurons project via the fornix to the septal area and hypothalamus. Neurons of the inferior olivary nucleus project aspartatergic fibers to the cerebellum. The granule cells of the cerebellum are glutamatergic. *MN* = mamillary nucleus.

- plays a role in kindling-induced seizures.
- plays a role in **pain transmission** (in Aδ and C fibers).
- Neocortical glutamatergic neurons project to the striatum, the subthalamic nucleus, and the thalamus. The subthalamic nucleus projects glutamatergic fibers to the globus pallidus.
2. **Aspartate** (see Figure 22-11)
   - is a major excitatory transmitter of the brain.
   - is the transmitter of the climbing fibers of the cerebellum.

IX. Nitric Oxide

- is a recently discovered gaseous neurotransmitter that is produced when nitric oxide synthase converts arginine to citrulline with the formation of nitric oxide.
- is located in the olfactory system, striatum, cortex, hippocampal formation, supraoptic nucleus of the hypothalamus, and cerebellum.
- is responsible for the smooth muscle relaxation of the corpus cavernosum and thus penile erection.
- is believed to play a role in memory formation (long-term potentiation in the hippocampal formation).

X. Functional and Clinical Correlations

A. **Endogenous pain control system**
   1. **Ascending pathway**
      - Spinoreticular pain impulses project to the periaqueductal gray of the midbrain.

2. **Descending raphe–spinal pathway**
   - Excitatory neurons of the periaqueductal gray project to the nucleus raphae magnus of the pons.
   - Excitatory neurons of the nucleus raphae magnus project serotonergic fibers to enkephalinergic inhibitory neurons of the substantia gelatinosa.
   - Enkephalinergic neurons of the substantia gelatinosa inhibit afferent pain fibers (substance P) and tract neurons that give rise to the spinoreticular and spinothalamic tracts.
3. **Descending ceruleospinal pathway**
   - projects from the locus ceruleus to the spinal cord.
   - is thought to directly inhibit tract neurons that give rise to the ascending pain pathways.

B. **Parkinson disease**
   - results from **degeneration of dopaminergic neurons** found in the pars compacta of the substantia nigra.
   - results in a **reduction of dopamine** in the striatum and in the substantia nigra.
   - results in the formation of **Lewy bodies**, intraneuronal inclusions in the substantia nigra.

C. **Huntington disease (Huntington chorea)**
   - results from a **loss of ACh- and GABA-containing neurons** in the striatum (caudatoputamen).
   - results in a **loss of GABA** in the striatum and substantia nigra.

D. **Alzheimer disease**
   - results from the **degeneration of cortical neurons and cholinergic neurons** found in the basal nucleus of Meynert.
   - is associated with a **60%–90% loss of choline acetyltransferase** in the cerebral cortex.
   - is characterized histologically by the presence of neurofibrillary tangles, senile (neuritic) plaques, granulovacuolar degeneration, and Hirano bodies.
   - is twice as common in women as in men.
   - Senile plaques consist of degenerated nerve cell processes and a central core of amyloid β-protein.

E. **Myasthenia gravis**
   - is an autoimmune syndrome that occurs in the presence of antibodies to the nicotinic ACh receptor.
   - is caused by the action of antibodies that reduce the number of receptors in the neuromuscular junction, resulting in **muscle paresis**.
   - involves extraocular and eyelid muscles (e.g., in diplopia, ptosis).
   - involves bulbar muscles (e.g., in nasal speech, jaw fatigue).
   - leads to weaker limbs proximally and stronger limbs distally.
   - may be diagnosed with intravenous edrophonium.
   - may be effectively treated with thymectomy, followed by corticosteroid therapy.

F. **Lambert-Eaton myasthenic syndrome**
   - is caused by a presynaptic defect of ACh release.
   - results in weakness in the limb muscles but not in the bulbar muscles. Muscle strength improves with use, unlike in myasthenia gravis, in which muscle use results in fatigue.
   - is associated with neoplasms (e.g., lung, breast, prostate) in 50% of cases.
   - leads to autonomic dysfunction, with dry mouth, constipation, impotence, and urinary incontinence.

REVIEW TEST

Questions 1 to 19

The response options for items 1 to 19 are the same. Select one answer for each item in the set.

(A) ACh
(B) Aspartate
(C) β-Endorphin
(D) Dopamine
(E) Endorphin
(F) Enkephalin
(G) Epinephrine
(H) GABA
(I) Glutamate
(J) Glycine
(K) Nitric oxide
(L) Norepinephrine
(M) Serotonin
(N) Somatostatin
(O) Substance P

Match each of the statements with the neurotransmitter it best describes.

1. Its highest concentration is found in the pineal gland

2. Is found in pseudounipolar ganglion cells and in the substantia gelatinosa

3. Is responsible for the smooth muscle relaxation of the corpus cavernosum and thus penile erection

4. Is produced by neurons found in the locus ceruleus

5. Is the neurotransmitter of the corticostriatal pathway

6. Is produced by neurons of the raphe nuclei

7. Is the neurotransmitter of the climbing fibers of the cerebellum

8. Low levels are associated with severe depression and insomnia

9. Is produced by neurons found in the basal nucleus of Meynert

10. Is produced almost exclusively in the hypothalamus

11. A reduction of postsynaptic receptor sites for this neurotransmitter causes myasthenia gravis

12. Is the neurotransmitter of the Renshaw cells

13. Striatal levels of this neurotransmitter are reduced in Huntington disease

14. Is the neurotransmitter of the Purkinje cells

15. Is the neurotransmitter of the cerebellar granule cell

16. Is found in high concentration in the pars compacta of the substantia nigra and in the ventral tegmental area of the mesencephalon

17. Is the neurotransmitter of the mesolimbic pathway

18. Inhibits the release of prolactin from the adenohypophysis

19. Is the main neurotransmitter of the pallidothalamic and nigrothalamic tracts

Questions 20 to 24

The response options for items 20 to 24 are the same. Select one answer for each item in the set.

(A) Lambert-Eaton myasthenic syndrome
(B) Myasthenia gravis
(C) Alzheimer disease
(D) Huntington disease
(E) Parkinson disease

Match each of the cases with the disorder it best describes.

20. A 60-year-old man presents with a resting tremor in his right upper extremity that has progressively worsened over the past 3 years. He recently had a positron emission tomography scan using a radioactive marker which showed a reduction of levodopa metabolism. This reduction was likely caused by dopaminergic neuronal death. What is the diagnosis for this patient?

21. A 25-year-old woman complains of difficulty swallowing and weakness in her hands and fingers. A blood test reveals antibodies to the nicotinic acetylcholine receptor. What is the diagnosis for this patient?

22. A brain autopsy of an 85-year-old woman reveals neurofibrillary tangles and neuritic plaques. What did this patient have?

23. A 53-year-old smoker complains of weakness in his arms and legs but notes that his muscle strength seems to improve when exercising. He also complains of dry mouth and constipation. A chest radiograph reveals a mass in the left lung. What is the diagnosis?

24. A 45-year-old man complains that he has been experiencing jerky, uncontrollable movements. He reports having noticed similar symptoms for the past few years but notes that the symptoms seem to be getting worse. His family history reveals that his father had some of the same symptoms prior to his death in an automobile accident. The magnetic resonance imaging scan shows cell loss in the caudatoputamen. What is the diagnosis?

25. The major excitatory neurotransmitter in the brain is
(A) GABA
(B) ACh
(C) Glycine
(D) Aspartate
(E) Glutamate

26. The major inhibitory neurotransmitter in the brain is
(A) Somatostatin
(B) GABA
(C) Serotonin
(D) Substance P
(E) Nitric oxide

ANSWERS AND EXPLANATIONS

1–M. The highest concentration of serotonin is found in the pineal body (epiphysis cerebri). Pinealocytes convert 5-HT to melatonin.

2–O. Substance P is the neurotransmitter of pain fibers and is found in pseudounipolar ganglion cells and in the substantia gelatinosa of the spinal cord. Substance P is also found in the caudal spinal trigeminal tract.

3–K. Nitric oxide is responsible for the smooth muscle relaxation of the corpus cavernosum and thus penile erection.

4–L. The highest concentration of norepinephrinergic neurons is found in the locus ceruleus.

5–I. Glutamate is the neurotransmitter of the corticostriatal pathway.

6–M. Serotonin is produced by neurons of the raphe nuclei.

7–B. Aspartate is the neurotransmitter of the climbing fibers of the cerebellum.

8–M. Low levels of 5-HT are associated with severe depression and insomnia.

9–A. ACh is found in highest concentration in the basal nucleus of Meynert, between the anterior perforated substance and the globus pallidus, a forebrain nucleus.

10–E. Endorphin is produced almost exclusively in the hypothalamus (arcuate nucleus).

11–A. In myasthenia gravis, there is a reduced acetylcholine receptor concentration in the motor end plate due to an autoimmune reaction directed against the receptor proteins.

12–J. Glycine is the major inhibitory neurotransmitter of the spinal cord; glycine is used by Renshaw cells, inhibitory interneurons driven by axon collaterals of lower motor neurons.

13–H. Striatal levels of GABA are greatly reduced in Huntington disease. This attrition of GABA-ergic neurons in the head of the caudate nucleus results in hydrocephalus ex vacuo.

14–H. GABA is the neurotransmitter of the Purkinje cells.

15–I. Glutamate is the neurotransmitter of the cerebellar granule cells.

16–D. Dopamine is found in high concentration in the pars compacta of the substantia nigra and in the ventral tegmental area of the mesencephalon.

17–D. Dopamine is the neurotransmitter of the mesolimbic pathway. This pathway is linked to behavior and schizophrenia.

18–D. Dopamine inhibits the release of prolactin from the adenohypophysis. Dopaminergic neurons are found in the arcuate nucleus of the hypothalamus.

19–H. GABA, the most common inhibitory neurotransmitter of the brain, is the main neurotransmitter of the pallidothalamic and nigrothalamic tracts.

20–E. Parkinson disease results from degeneration of dopaminergic neurons found in the pars compacta of the substantia nigra. While Parkinson disease is typically diagnosed based on neurologic symptoms, a positron emission tomography scan with radioactive labeling can sometimes be used as a diagnostic tool.

21–B. Myasthenia gravis is an autoimmune syndrome whose symptoms usually include the presence of antibodies to the nicotinic acetylcholine receptor. Other symptoms include muscle paresis, diplopia, ptosis, jaw fatigue, and weak proximal limbs.

22–C. Alzheimer disease is characterized histologically by the presence of neurofibrillary tangles, senile (neuritic) plaques, granulovacuolar degeneration, and Hirano bodies. This disease results from the degeneration of cortical neurons and cholinergic neurons found in the basal nucleus of Meynert. It is also associated with a 60%–90% loss of choline acetyltransferase in the cerebral cortex.

23–A. Lambert-Eaton myasthenic syndrome is an autoimmune syndrome caused by a presynaptic defect of ACh release. It results in weakness in limb muscles, and muscle strength improves with use. It is associated with neoplasms (e.g., lung, breast, prostrate) in 50% of cases.

24–D. Huntington disease is a hereditary disorder that results from a loss of ACh- and GABA-containing neurons in the striatum. Some symptoms include jerky, random, uncontrollable, rapid (choreiform) movements; slowness of saccadic eye movements; and progressive dementia.

25–E. Glutamate is the major excitatory neurotransmitter; 60% of brain synapses are glutamatergic.

26–B. GABA is the major inhibitory neurotransmitter and can be localized by using glutamic acid decarboxylase as a marker.

Cerebral Cortex

I.   Overview: The Cerebral Cortex

- contains 20 billion (2×10^{10}) nerve cells.
- consists of the neocortex (90%) and the allocortex (10%).

A. Neocortex (isocortex; homogenetic cortex)
- is a six-layered cortex.

B. Allocortex (heterogenetic cortex)
- is three-layered and includes two types:
  1. **Archicortex**
     - includes the hippocampus and the dentate gyrus.
  2. **Paleocortex**
     - includes the olfactory cortex.

II.   Six Layers of the Neocortex (Figure 23-1)

- are expressed as roman numerals I through VI:

A. Molecular layer (I)
- is the superficial layer below the pia mater.

B. External granular layer (II)

C. External pyramidal layer (III)
- gives rise to association and commissural fibers.

D. Internal granular layer (IV)
- receives thalamocortical fibers from the thalamic nuclei of the ventral tier (e.g., ventral posterolateral [VPL] and ventral posteromedial [VPM] nuclei).
- in the striate cortex (area 17), receives input from the lateral geniculate body.
- myelinated fibers of this layer form the stripe of Gennari, which is visible to the naked eye.

E. Internal pyramidal layer (V)
- gives rise to corticobulbar, corticospinal, and corticostriatal fibers.
- contains the giant cells of Betz, which are found only in the motor cortex (area 4) of the precentral gyrus and the anterior paracentral lobule.

F. Multiform layer (VI)
- is the deepest layer of the cortex. It gives rise to projection, commissural, and association fibers.
- is the major source of corticothalamic fibers.

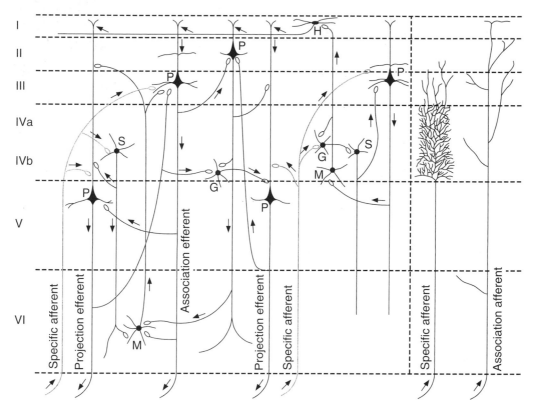

Figure 23-1.   Neurocortical circuits. G = granule cell; H = horizontal cell; M = Martinotti cell; P = pyramidal cell; S = stellate cell. Loops show synaptic junctions. (reprinted with permission from Parent A: *Carpenter's Human Neuroanatomy,* 9th ed. Baltimore, Williams & Wilkins, 1996, p. 868.)

III.   Functional Areas of the Cerebral Cortex (Figure 23-2)

- is divided into 47 cytoarchitectural areas, the **Brodmann areas**.

A. **Sensory areas**
   1. **Primary somatosensory cortex (areas 3, 1, and 2)**
      - is located in the **postcentral gyrus** and in the posterior part of the **paracentral lobule**.
      - receives input from the ventral posterior nucleus.
      - contributes to the corticospinal tract.
      - is somatotopically organized as the **sensory homunculus** (Figure 23-3A).
      - Stimulation results in contralateral numbness and tingling (paresthesia).
      - Destruction results in a contralateral loss of tactile discrimination (**hypesthesia and astereognosis**).
   2. **Secondary somatosensory cortex**
      - lies ventral to the primary somatosensory area along the superior bank of the lateral sulcus.
   3. **Somatosensory association cortex**
      a. **Superior parietal lobule (areas 5 and 7)**
         - receives input from areas 3, 1, and 2. Area 7 receives visual input from area 19.
         - Destruction results in **contralateral losses of tactile discrimination, stereognosis** (the ability to recognize form), and **statognosis** (the ability to recognize the position of body parts in space). Destruction also leads to neglect of events occurring in the contralateral portion of the external world (more commonly seen with parietal damage on the right side).

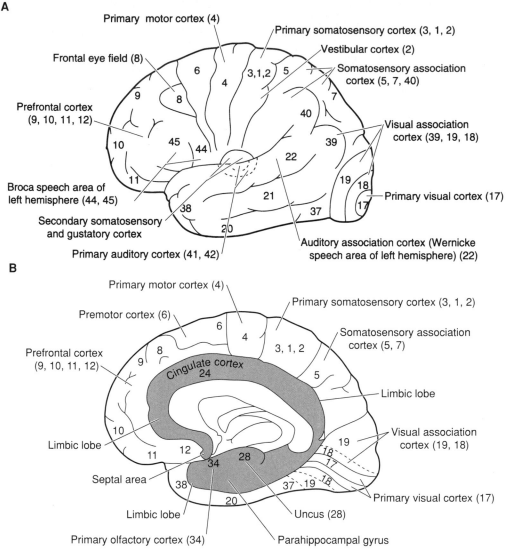

Figure 23-2. Some motor and sensory areas of the cerebral cortex. (**A**) Lateral convex surface of the hemisphere. (**B**) Medial surface of the hemisphere. The numbers refer to the Brodmann brain map, the Brodmann areas.

b. **Supramarginal gyrus (area 40)**
- interrelates somatosensory, auditory, and visual input (multimodal sensory stimuli).
- Destruction in the dominant hemisphere may result in the following deficits:
  (1) **Ideomotor or "classic" apraxia (ideokinetic apraxia)**
     - is the inability to button one's clothes or comb one's hair when asked.
     - is the inability to manipulate tools, with retention of the ability to explain their use.
  (2) **Ideational or sensory apraxia**
     - is characterized by the inability to formulate the ideational plan for executing the several components of a complex multistep act (e.g., performing the steps of lighting a cigarette when asked to do so).
     - occurs most frequently in diffuse cerebral degenerating disease, Alzheimer disease, and multi-infarct dementia.

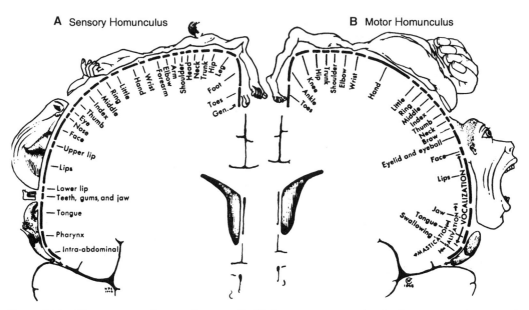

Figure 23-3. The sensory and motor homunculi. (A) Sensory representation in the postcentral gyrus. (B) Motor representation in the precentral gyrus. (Reprinted with permission from Penfield W and Rasmussen T: *The Cerebral Cortex of Man.* New York, Hafner Publishing, 1968, pp. 44 and 57.)

    (3) **Facial apraxia**
- is the inability to perform facial–oral movements on command (i.e., lick the lips).
- is the most common apraxia.

    (4) **Conduction aphasia**
- is associated with poor repetition of spoken language (results from interruption of the arcuate fasciculus; see III C 4).

4. **Primary visual cortex (area 17)**
- is located in the occipital lobe in both banks of the calcarine sulcus.
- receives input from the lateral geniculate body.
- Destruction results in **visual field deficits** (e.g., contralateral homonymous hemianopia) (see Figure 17-2).

5. **Secondary and tertiary visual cortices**
- include areas 18 and 19 of the occipital lobe.
- Lesions may result in **visual hallucinations**.

6. **Visual association cortex (angular gyrus [area 39])**
- receives input from areas 18 and 19.
- Destruction of the underlying visual radiation results in **contralateral homonymous hemianopia** or **lower quadrantanopia**.
- Destruction in the dominant hemisphere results in **Gerstmann syndrome** with the following deficits:
  - a. **Right–left confusion**
  - b. **Finger agnosia** (inability to recognize, name, or select one's own or another's fingers)
  - c. **Agraphia** (inability to express thoughts in writing with possible retention of the ability to copy written or printed words; often coexists with alexia)
  - d. **Dyscalculia** (difficulty with arithmetic)

7. **Primary auditory cortex (areas 41 and 42)**
- is located in the transverse gyri of Heschl.
- receives input from the medial geniculate body.
- unilateral destruction results in only **partial deafness** (due to bilateral cochlear representation).

8. **Auditory association cortex (area 22)**
   - is located in the posterior part of the superior temporal gyrus.
   - includes **Wernicke speech area**.
   - includes the **planum temporale** (part of Wernicke speech area), which is larger in the dominant hemisphere.
   - Lesion in the dominant hemisphere results in **Wernicke sensory aphasia**.
   - Lesion in the nondominant hemisphere results in **sensory dysprosody** (inability to perceive the pitch or rhythm of speech).

9. **Gustatory cortex (area 43)**
   - is located in the parietal operculum and parainsular cortex.
   - receives taste input from the VPM nucleus of the thalamus.

10. **Vestibular cortex (area 2)**
   - is located in the postcentral gyrus.
   - receives input from the ventral posteroinferior (VPI) and the VPL nuclei of the thalamus.

B. **Motor areas**

1. **Primary motor cortex (area 4)**
   - is located in the **precentral gyrus** and in the anterior part of the **paracentral lobule**.
   - contributes to the corticospinal tract.
   - is somatotopically organized as the **motor homunculus** (see Figure 23-3B).
   - contains the giant cells of Betz in layer V.
   - Stimulation results in contralateral movements of voluntary muscles, especially distal muscles of the limbs.
   - Ablation results in a **contralateral upper motor neuron (UMN) lesion**.
   - Bilateral lesions of the paracentral lobule (e.g., parasagittal meningiomas) result in **urinary incontinence**.

2. **Premotor cortex (area 6)**
   - is located anterior to the precentral gyrus.
   - contributes to the corticospinal tract.
   - plays a role in the **control of proximal and axial muscles**; it prepares the motor cortex for specific movements in advance of their execution.
   - Stimulation results in adversive movements of the head and trunk and flexion and extension of the extremities.
   - Lesions in the dominant hemisphere may cause **sympathetic apraxia** (motor apraxia in the left hand).

3. **Supplementary motor cortex (area 6)**
   - is located on the medial surface of the hemisphere anterior to the paracentral lobule.
   - contributes to the corticospinal tract.
   - plays a role in **programming complex motor sequences** and in **coordinating bilateral movements**; it regulates the somatosensory input into the motor cortex.
   - Stimulation results in vocalization with associated facial movements and coordinated movements of the limbs.
   - Ablation in human subjects has resulted in transient **speech deficits or aphasias**.
   - Bilateral lesions result in **hypertonus of the flexor muscles** but no paralysis.

4. **Frontal eye field (area 8)**
   - is located in the posterior part of the middle frontal gyrus.
   - projects via the corticotectobulbar tract to the contralateral lateral gaze center of the pons (abducent nucleus).
   - Stimulation (irritative lesion) results in conjugate deviation of the eyes to the opposite side.
   - Destructive lesions result in **conjugate deviation of the eyes toward the side of the lesion**.

C. **Areas of higher cortical function**

1. **Prefrontal cortex (areas 9–12)**
   a. **Characteristics of the prefrontal cortex**
      - extends from area 6 to the frontal pole (area 10).
      - has reciprocal connections with the mediodorsal nucleus of the thalamus.

b. **Frontal lobe syndrome (Phineas Gage syndrome)**
- results from **lesions of the prefrontal cortex.**
- results in the following signs:
  (1) **Inappropriate social behavior**
    - Lesions usually involve the fronto-orbital prefrontal cortex.
  (2) **Difficulty in adaptation and loss of initiative**
    - Lesions involve the dorsolateral prefrontal cortex.
  (3) **Sucking, groping, and grasping reflexes**
  (4) **Gait apraxia, incontinence, abulia** (loss of the ability to perform voluntary actions), or **akinetic mutism** (a coma-like state called coma vigil)
    - These signs result from bilateral disease.

2. **Broca speech area (areas 44 and 45)** (Figure 23-4)
   a. **Characteristics of the Broca speech area**
   - is located in the posterior part of the inferior frontal gyrus in the dominant hemisphere.
   - is connected to Wernicke speech area by the arcuate fasciculus.
   b. **Broca aphasia**
   - results from lesions in Broca speech area.
   - is also called **motor, expressive, nonfluent,** or **anterior aphasia.**
   - causes patients to speak slowly (nonfluent) and with effort; however, they have good comprehension of spoken and written language.
   - is frequently accompanied by **contralateral weakness of the lower face and arm** and a **sympathetic apraxia** of the left hand (the inability to write with the nonparalyzed hand).

3. **Wernicke speech area (area 22)** (see Figure 23-4)
   a. **Characteristics of the Wernicke speech area**
   - is located in the posterior part of the superior temporal gyrus in the dominant hemisphere.
   - is connected to Broca speech area by the arcuate fasciculus.

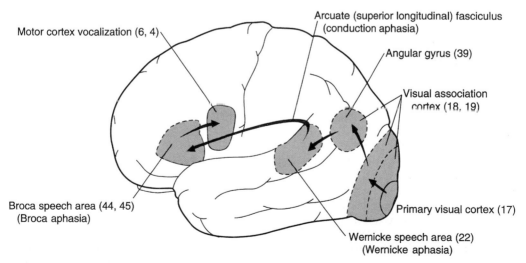

Figure 23-4. Cortical areas of the dominant hemisphere that play an important role in language production. The visual image of a word is projected from the visual cortex (17) to the visual association cortices (18 and 19) and then to the angular gyrus (39). Further processing occurs in Wernicke speech area (22), where the auditory form of the word is recalled. Via the arcuate fasciculus, this information reaches Broca speech area (44 and 45), where motor speech programs control the vocalization mechanisms of the precentral gyrus. Lesions of Broca speech area, Wernicke speech area, or the arcuate fasciculus result in dysphasias.

b. Wernicke aphasia
- results from lesions in the dominant hemisphere.
- is also called **sensory, receptive, fluent,** or **posterior aphasia**.
- Patients have poor comprehension of speech, speak faster than normal, and have difficulty in finding the right words to express themselves. They appear unaware of the deficit.

4. Arcuate fasciculus
a. Characteristics of the arcuate fasciculus
- underlies the supramarginal gyrus (area 40) and the frontoparietal operculum.
- connects the audiovisual association areas (areas 22, 39, and 40) with Broca speech area (areas 44 and 45).

b. Conduction aphasia
- results from transection of the arcuate fasciculus.
- is a **fluent aphasia** associated with poor repetition of spoken language. Speech comprehension and expression are relatively good.
- **Paraphrasic errors** (using incorrect words) are common, and **object naming is impaired** (nominal aphasia or amnestic aphasia). Patients are aware of the deficit.

5. Corpus callosum
- interconnects corresponding hemispheric areas.
- does not contain commissural fibers from the hand region of the motor or sensory strips, or from the striate cortex.
- receives its blood supply from the anterior cerebral artery and the posterior cerebral artery; the splenium is perfused by the posterior cerebral artery.
- Damage to the splenium results in left hemidyslexia.

IV. Cerebral Dominance

- is determined by the Wade test. Sodium amobarbital (Amytal) is injected into the carotid artery. If the patient becomes aphasic, the anesthetic was administered to the dominant hemisphere.

A. Dominant hemisphere
- is responsible for **propositional language** consisting of **grammar, syntax,** and **semantics**.
- is also responsible for speech and calculation.
- The left hemisphere is dominant in 95% of cases.
  1. Lesions of the dominant superior parietal lobule (Figure 23-5A)
  - result in contralateral loss of sensory discrimination (**astereognosis**) (i.e., loss of dorsal column modalities; area 5).
  - result in contralateral neglect (area 7).
  2. Lesions of the dominant inferior parietal lobule (see Figure 23-5A)
  - involve the supramarginal and angular gyri (areas 40 and 39).
  - result in the following conditions:
    a. Receptive aphasia
    b. Gerstmann syndrome
    c. Alexia with agraphia (often coexists with Gerstmann syndrome)
    d. Tactile agnosia (bimanual astereognosis)
    e. Ideomotor apraxia
    f. Ideational apraxia

B. Nondominant hemisphere
- is primarily responsible for **three-dimensional** or **spatial perception** and **nonverbal ideation** (music and poetry).
  1. Lesions of the nondominant superior parietal lobule (see Figure 23-5B)
  - result in **contralateral loss of sensory discrimination** (i.e., loss of dorsal column modalities; area 5).
  - result in **contralateral neglect** (area 7).

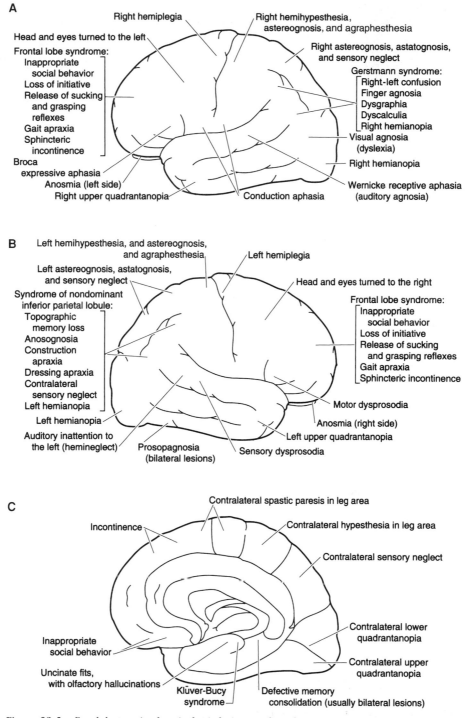

Figure 23-5. Focal destructive hemispheric lesions and resulting symptoms. (**A**) Lateral convex surface of the dominant left hemisphere. (**B**) Lateral convex surface of the nondominant right hemisphere. (**C**) Medial surface of the nondominant hemisphere. (Reprinted with permission from Fix JD: *High-Yield Neuroanatomy*, 3rd ed. Philadelphia, Lippincott Williams & Wilkins, 2005, p. 161.)

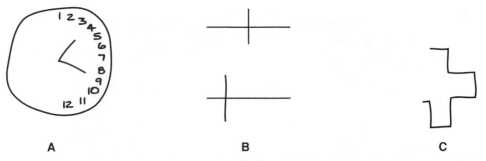

Figure 23-6. Testing for construction apraxia. (A) The patient is asked to copy the face of a clock. (B) The patient is asked to bisect a horizontal line. (C) The patient is asked to copy a cross. These drawings show contralateral neglect. The responsible lesion is found in the nondominant (right) parietal lobe. Left hemianopia by itself does not result in contralateral neglect. (Reprinted with permission from Fix JD: *High-Yield Neuroanatomy,* 3rd ed. Philadelphia, Lippincott Williams & Wilkins, 2005, p. 159.)

2. **Lesions of the nondominant inferior parietal lobule**
   - involve the supramarginal and angular gyri.
   - result in the following conditions:
     a. **Left-sided hemineglect**
        - results in a lack of awareness of the left half of space or the left half of the body.
        - results in hemi-inattention or extinction; if, with the patient's eyes closed, both hands are touched simultaneously, the left hand stimulus often is not reported.
     b. **Topographic memory loss**
        - results in the inability to negotiate familiar surroundings.
     c. **Anosognosia (denial of deficit)**
        - results in indifference to the causal disease (e.g., hemiparesis or hemianopia).
     d. **Constructional apraxia** (Figure 23-6)
        - results in the inability to draw simple designs (e.g., cross, star, or clock); the left side of the design is omitted.
        - may also occur in lesions of the dominant hemisphere.
     e. **Dressing apraxia**
        - results in the inability to dress oneself.
3. **Lesions of the nondominant inferior frontal gyrus (areas 44 and 45)**
   - correspond to Broca speech area and result in **expressive dysprosody** (the inability to articulate the pitch and rhythm of speech).
4. **Lesions of the nondominant superior temporal gyrus (area 22)**
   - correspond to Wernicke speech area and result in **receptive dysprosody** (the inability to perceive pitch and rhythm of speech).

V. Split-Brain Syndrome (Figures 23-7 and 23-8)

A. **Description of split-brain syndrome**
   - represents a **disconnection syndrome** that results from transection (commissurotomy) of the corpus callosum.

B. **Deficits**
   1. Inability of a blindfolded patient to match an object held in one hand with that held in the other hand
   2. Inability, when blindfolded, to correctly name objects placed in the left hand (**anomia**)

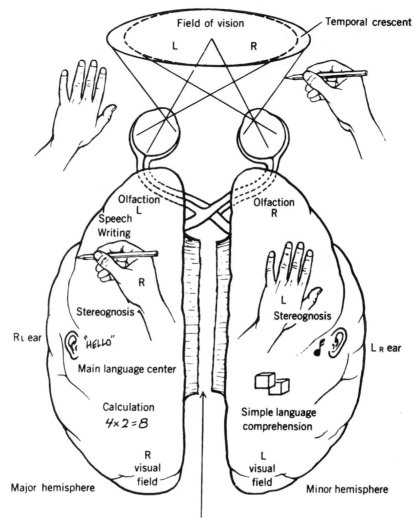

Figure 23-7. Functions of the split brain after transection of the corpus callosum. Tactile and visual perception is projected to the contralateral hemisphere; olfaction is perceived on the same side; and audition is perceived predominantly in the opposite hemisphere. The left hemisphere is dominant for language; the right hemisphere is dominant for spatial construction and nonverbal ideation. (Reprinted with permission from Noback CR and Demarest RJ: *The Human Nervous System.* Baltimore, Williams & Wilkins, 1991, p. 416.)

3. Inability to match an object seen in the right half of the visual field with one seen in the left half (the test must be performed rapidly to eliminate bilateral visual scanning)
4. **Alexia** in the left visual fields (the verbal symbols seen in the right visual cortex have no access to the language centers of the left hemisphere)

VI. Blood Supply to the Major Functional Cortical Areas

- Only **cortical branches** are discussed in this section.

A. **Anterior cerebral artery** (see Figure 3-3)
   1. **Territory of the anterior cerebral artery**
      - supplies the medial aspect of the hemisphere.

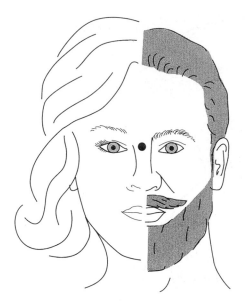

Figure 23-8. Chimeric (hybrid) figure of a face used to examine the hemispheric function of commissurotomized patients. The patient is instructed to fixate on the dot. If the patient is asked verbally to describe what he sees and he says that he sees the face of a man, then the left hemisphere predominates in vocal tasks. If asked to point to the face and he points to the woman, then the right hemisphere predominates in pointing tasks. (Reprinted with permission from Fix JD: *High-Yield Neuroanatomy,* 3rd ed. Philadelphia, Lippincott Williams & Wilkins, 2005, p. 163.)

2. **Occlusion: affected areas and deficits**
   a. **Paracentral lobule**
      - contralateral somatosensory loss in the lower extremity with paresthesia, numbness, and apallesthesia (loss of vibration sensation)
      - contralateral weakness and hyperreflexia in the lower extremity with the Babinski sign (plantar reflex is the extensor)
      - urinary incontinence with bilateral infarction
   b. **Corpus callosum: infarction**
      - dyspraxia and tactile agnosia of the left limbs

B. **Middle cerebral artery** (see Figure 3-4)
   1. **Territory of the middle cerebral artery**
      - supplies the lateral convex surface of the hemisphere.
   2. **Occlusion: affected areas and deficits**
      a. **Frontal lobe**
         (1) **Precentral gyrus**
             - contralateral facial weakness and weakness in the upper extremity
         (2) **Frontal eye field**
             - conjugate deviation of the eyes to the affected side
         (3) **Prefrontal cortex**
             - affects judgment, insight, and mood (frontal lobe syndrome).
         (4) **Inferior frontal gyrus of the dominant side**
             - Broca expressive aphasia and contralateral weakness of the lower face and arm
             - sympathetic apraxia of the left hand
      b. **Temporal lobe**
         (1) **Transverse temporal gyri of Heschl**
             - deafness with bilateral destruction
         (2) **Superior temporal gyrus of the dominant side**
             - Wernicke receptive aphasia
         (3) **Superior and middle temporal gyri (superolateral parts)**
             - auditory illusions and hallucinations
      c. **Parietal lobe**
         (1) **Postcentral gyrus and superior parietal lobule**
             - loss of sensory discrimination and stereognosis
             - hemineglect (may occur with either left or right parietal lesions)

(2) **Inferior parietal lobule of the dominant hemisphere**
- ideomotor and ideational apraxia
- Gerstmann syndrome

(3) **Inferior parietal lobule of the nondominant hemisphere**
- hemineglect syndrome
- topographic memory loss, anosognosia, and constructional and dressing apraxia

C. **Posterior cerebral artery** (see Figure 3-5)
  1. **Territory of the posterior cerebral artery**
     - supplies the occipital lobe, the inferior aspect of the temporal lobe (excluding the temporal pole), and the splenium of the corpus callosum.
  2. **Occlusion: affected areas and deficits**
     a. **Occipital lobe: visual cortex (striate and extrastriate)**
        - if bilateral, cortical blindness (pupils are reactive to light)
        - contralateral homonymous hemianopia with macular sparing
     b. **Temporal lobe (inferomedial aspect): hippocampal formation and amygdala**
        - also perfused by the anterior choroidal artery
        - if bilateral or in the dominant hemisphere, memory deficit (amnesia)
        - incapacity to create and store new long-term memories; the patient retains and may recall long-term memories.
     c. **Occipitotemporal region (ventromesial aspect)**
        - Bilateral lesions may result in **prosopagnosia** (the inability to identify a familiar face) and **achromatopsia** (acquired color blindness).

D. **Left posterior cerebral artery**
  1. **Territory of the left posterior cerebral artery**
     - supplies the splenium of the corpus callosum and the left visual cortex.
  2. **Occlusion**
     - results in **infarction** of the splenium of the corpus callosum and the left visual cortex; visual input from the right visual cortex cannot reach the parietal language centers of the dominant hemisphere.
     - may cause **alexia without agraphia and aphasia**; because the left inferior parietal lobule and Wernicke speech area are intact, the patient can write and is not dysphasic.

E. **Jacksonian seizures (Jacksonian march)**
  - are unilateral simple partial motor seizures that start with a tonic contraction of the fingers on one hand, the face on one side, or one foot, and progress to clonic contractions of the entire half of the body; they may progress to grand mal seizures.
  - may result from tumors, hematomas, and brain abscesses.
  - may affect the opposite side via the corpus callosum

REVIEW TEST

1. A 55-year-old right-handed veteran received a small shrapnel wound in the head during the Vietnam War. Within 1 year of receiving his wound, the man complained of seizures and was treated with seizure medication. The medication was not effective, and a section of the anterior corpus callosum was performed successfully. Which of the following neurologic deficits is most likely?

(A) Alexia
(B) The inability, with closed eyes, to identify verbally an object held in the left hand
(C) Gait dystaxia
(D) Loss of binocular vision
(E) Sympathetic apraxia in the right hand

2. A 70-year-old hypertensive man suddenly experiences numbness on the right side of his body. When asked to raise his left hand, he raises his right hand. The lesion is most likely in the

(A) right frontal lobe
(B) left parietal lobe
(C) right parietal lobe
(D) left temporal lobe
(E) right internal capsule

3. A 45-year-old farmer complains of headaches. Neurologic examination reveals pronator drift and mild hemiparesis on the right side. The patient's eyes and head are turned to the left side, and papilledema is visible on the left side. The lesion is most likely in which of the following cortices?

(A) Frontal
(B) Insular
(C) Occipital
(D) Parietal
(E) Temporal

4. An 80-year-old microbiologist has a cerebral infarction. His speech is limited to expletives, he cannot write but does respond to questions by shaking his head, and he has lower facial weakness on the right side. The lesion is most likely in the

(A) left frontal lobe
(B) right frontal lobe
(C) left parietal lobe
(D) right parietal lobe
(E) left temporal lobe

5. A lesion resulting in a nonfluent expressive aphasia would most likely be found in the

(A) temporal lobe
(B) parietal lobe
(C) frontal lobe
(D) occipital lobe
(E) limbic lobe

6. Broca aphasia is frequently associated with

(A) auditory hallucinations
(B) finger agnosia
(C) construction apraxia
(D) an UMN lesion
(E) visual field deficits

7. Alexia without agraphia and aphasia would most likely result from occlusion of the

(A) left anterior cerebral artery
(B) right anterior cerebral artery
(C) left middle cerebral artery
(D) left posterior cerebral artery
(E) right posterior cerebral artery

8. Agraphia and dyscalculia would most likely result from a lesion in the

(A) left frontal lobe
(B) left parietal lobe
(C) right occipital lobe
(D) left temporal lobe
(E) splenium of corpus callosum

9. A patient is asked to bisect a horizontal line through the middle, to draw the face of a clock, and to copy a cross. The patient bisected the horizontal line to the left of the midline, placed all of the numerals of the clock on the right side, and did not complete the cross on the left side. The most likely lesion site for this deficit is the

(A) left frontal lobe
(B) right parietal lobe
(C) left parietal lobe
(D) right temporal lobe
(E) left occipital lobe

Questions 10 to 15

Match the descriptions in items 10 to 15 with the appropriate lettered area shown in the figure.

Questions 16 to 20

Match the descriptions in items 16 to 20 with the appropriate lettered area shown in the figure.

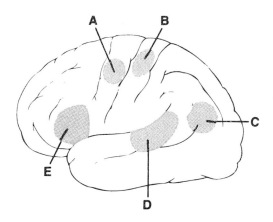

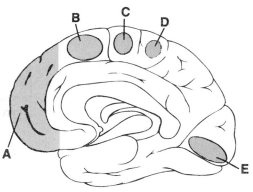

10. Broca speech area

11. Wernicke speech area

12. Lesion in this area results in contralateral astereognosis

13. Infarction in this area results in an UMN lesion

14. Lesion in this area results in contralateral homonymous hemianopia

15. Lesion in this area results in finger agnosia, agraphia, and dyscalculia

16. Supplementary motor area

17. Lesion in this area results in paresthesias and numbness in the contralateral foot

18. Lesion in this area results in contralateral lower homonymous quadrantanopia

19. Lesion in this area results in a contralateral Babinski sign

20. Lesion in this area results in loss of initiative and inappropriate social behavior

ANSWERS AND EXPLANATIONS

1–B. Transection of corpus callosum results in the inability, when blindfolded, to identify verbally an object held in the left hand (dysnomia). The left hemisphere is dominant for language and naming objects. Alexia is found in lesions of the inferior parietal lobule. Gait dystaxia may result from normal pressure hydrocephalus, which also involves dementia and incontinence. The man's visual pathways are not affected. Transection of callosal fibers adjacent to the left premotor cortex produces right hemiparesis, motor (Broca) dysphasia, and sympathetic dyspraxia of the left, nonparalyzed, arm.

2–B. The right hemiparesis points to a lesion on the left side involving the corticospinal tract. Left–right confusion is seen in Gerstmann syndrome along with finger agnosia. This syndrome results from destruction of the left angular gyrus.

3–A. The cortical center for lateral conjugate gaze is located in area 8 of the frontal lobe. Destruction of this area results in turning of the head and eyes toward the side of the lesion. Stimulation of this area results in contralateral turning of the eyes and head; pronator drift and hemiparesis are frontal lobe signs.

4–A. Lower facial weakness is a localizing neighborhood sign. The Broca speech area is located in the posterior part of the inferior frontal gyrus (Brodmann areas 44 and 45).

5–C. Nonfluent, expressive motor aphasia (Broca aphasia) results from a lesion in the posterior inferior frontal gyrus (areas 44 and 45) of the dominant frontal lobe.

6–D. Broca aphasia is frequently associated with an UMN lesion of the contralateral face and arm and occasionally of the leg. Broca speech area lies just anterior to the motor strip; both Broca speech area and the motor strip are irrigated by the superior division of the middle cerebral artery (prerolandic and rolandic arteries). Broca aphasia is frequently associated with sympathetic apraxia, an apraxia of the nonparalyzed left hand.

7–D. Alexia without agraphia and aphasia results from occlusion of the left posterior cerebral artery, which supplies the left visual cortex and callosal fibers (within the splenium) from the right visual association cortex. Interruption of bilateral visual association fibers en route to the left angular gyrus results in alexia. Because the angular gyrus and Wernicke area are spared, the patient will not be agraphic or dysphasic.

8–B. Lesions of the angular gyrus of the dominant hemisphere may result in Gerstmann syndrome, which consists of agraphia, dyscalculia, finger agnosia, and left–right confusion.

9–B. The inability to draw a clock face or bisect a line through the middle is called construction apraxia. Lesions of the right (nondominant) parietal lobe result in construction apraxia, dressing apraxia, anosognosia, and sensory hemineglect.

10–E. Broca speech area (areas 44 and 45) is found in the posterior part of the inferior frontal gyrus of the dominant hemisphere, directly anterior to the premotor and motor cortices.

11–D. Wernicke speech area is located in the posterior part of the superior temporal gyrus (part of Brodmann area 22) of the dominant hemisphere. A lesion of this area results in a fluent sensory (receptive) aphasia.

12–B. A lesion of the left postcentral gyrus results in a right astereognosis (tactile agnosia), the inability to identify objects by touch. Lesions of the superior parietal lobule result in contralateral astereognosis and in sensory neglect.

312

13–A. A lesion in the precentral gyrus is an UMN lesion. The precentral gyrus (motor strip) gives rise to one-third of the pyramidal tract (corticospinal tract) fibers.

14–C. A deep lesion of the angular gyrus could involve the visual radiation, resulting in a contralateral homonymous hemianopia.

15–C. The dominant angular gyrus is the neurologic substrate of Gerstmann syndrome, which consists of right–left confusion, finger agnosia, agraphia, and dyscalculia.

16–B. The supplementary motor cortex (area 6) lies on the medial aspect of the hemisphere, just anterior to the paracentral lobule.

17–D. A lesion in the posterior part of the paracentral lobule would result in loss of joint and position sense (astatognosia) and loss of tactile discrimination (astereognosis) in the contralateral foot.

18–E. A lesion of the superior bank of the calcarine sulcus (cuneus) would result in a contralateral lower homonymous quadrantanopia. A lesion destroying both cunei would produce a lower homonymous altitudinal hemianopia.

19–C. A lesion of the anterior part of the paracentral lobule results in a contralateral paresis of the foot muscles and in Babinski sign (i.e., plantar reflex extensor or extensor toe sign).

20–A. Lesions of the prefrontal cortex may result in personality changes, with disorderly and inappropriate conduct and facetiousness and jocularity (witzelsucht). Lesions interrupt fibers that interconnect the dorsomedial nucleus and the prefrontal cortex (e.g., prefrontal lobotomy or leukotomy).

Apraxia, Aphasia, and Dysprosody

I.   Apraxia

- is the inability to perform motor activities in the presence of intact motor and sensory systems and normal comprehension.

A. Ideomotor apraxia (ideokinetic apraxia)
- is the loss of the ability to perform intransitive or imaginary gestures, resulting in the inability to perform complicated motor tasks (e.g., saluting, blowing a kiss, or making the V-for-victory sign).
- may be typified by **facial apraxia**, which is also known as **buccofacial** or **facial–oral apraxia**, the most common type of apraxia.
- results from a lesion in the Wernicke area.

B. Ideational apraxia (ideatory apraxia)
- is the inability to demonstrate the use of real objects (e.g., smoke a pipe [a multistep complex sequence]).
- is a misuse of objects due to a disturbance of identification (agnosia).
- results from a lesion in the Wernicke area.

C. Construction apraxia
- is the inability to draw or construct a geometric figure (e.g., the face of a clock).
- is called hemineglect if the patient draws only the right half of the clock. The lesion is located in the right inferior parietal lobule (see Figure 23-5).

D. Gait apraxia
- is characterized by diminished cadence, wide base, short steps, and shuffling progression; it is reminiscent of parkinsonian gait.
- is a frontal lobe sign seen in **normal pressure hydrocephalus** with **gait apraxia**, **dementia**, and **incontinence**.

II.   Aphasia

- is impaired or absent communication by speech, writing, or signs (i.e., loss of the capacity for spoken language).
- results from lesions in the dominant hemisphere.
- The following symptoms and signs are associated with certain aphasias (Figure 24-1).

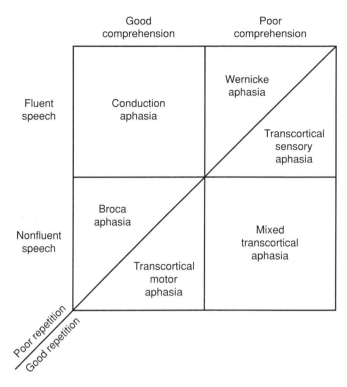

Figure 24-1. The aphasia square makes it easy to differentiate the six most common national board aphasias. Broca, conduction, and Wernicke aphasias are all characterized by poor repetition. (Adapted with permission from Miller J, Fountain N: *Neurology Recall.* Baltimore, Williams & Wilkins, 1997, p. 35.)

A. **Broca (motor) aphasia**
   - is characterized by good comprehension; effortful, dysarthric, telegraphic, nonfluent speech; poor repetition; and contralateral lower facial and upper limb weakness.
   - results from a lesion in the frontal lobe, in the inferior frontal gyrus (Brodmann 44, 45).

B. **Wernicke (sensory) aphasia**
   - is characterized by poor comprehension, fluent speech, poor repetition, and **quadrantanopia**.
   - is also marked by **paraphasic errors** such as **non sequiturs** (Latin, *does not follow*), **neologisms** (words with no meaning), and **driveling speech**.
   - results from a lesion in the posterior temporal lobe, in the superior temporal gyrus (Brodmann 22).

C. **Conduction aphasia**
   - involves the **transection** of the **arcuate fasciculus**; the arcuate fasciculus interconnects Brodmann speech area with Wernicke speech area.
   - is characterized by good comprehension, poor repetition, and fluent speech.

D. **Transcortical motor aphasia**
   - involves good comprehension, good repetition, and nonfluent speech.

E. **Transcortical mixed aphasia**
   - involves poor comprehension, good repetition, and nonfluent speech.

F. **Transcortical sensory aphasia**
   - involves poor comprehension, good repetition, and fluent speech.

G. **Global aphasia**
   - results from a lesion of the perisylvian area, which contains the Broca and Wernicke areas.
   - combines all of the symptoms of Broca and Wernicke aphasias.

H. Thalamic aphasia
- is a dominant thalamic syndrome that closely resembles a thought disorder of patients with schizophrenia and chronic drug-induced psychosis.
- involves fluent paraphasic speech with normal comprehension and repetition.

I. Basal ganglia (caudate nucleus, putamen)
- Diseases of the basal ganglia may cause aphasia.
- Lesions of the anterior basal ganglia result in nonfluent aphasia, and lesions of the posterior basal ganglia result in fluent aphasia.

J. Watershed infarcts
- are areas of infarction in the boundary zones of the anterior, middle, and posterior cerebral arteries. Infarcts cause the motor, mixed, and sensory transcortical aphasias.
- are vulnerable to hypoperfusion and thus may separate the Broca and Wernicke speech areas from the surrounding cortex.

III. Dysprosodies

- are nondominant hemispheric language deficits that affect the emotionality of speech (inflection, melody, emphasis, and gesturing).
- are as common as the dysphasias; they were first "discovered" during World War II.

A. Expressive dysprosody
- results from a lesion that corresponds to the Broca area but is located in the nondominant hemisphere.
- Patients cannot express emotion or inflection in their speech.

B. Receptive dysprosody
- results from a lesion that corresponds to the Wernicke area but is located in the nondominant hemisphere.
- Patients cannot comprehend the emotionality or inflection in the speech they hear.

REVIEW TEST

1. Broca aphasia may result from occlusion of which of the following arteries?

(A) Anterior temporal artery
(B) Anterior choroidal artery
(C) Medial striate artery of Heubner
(D) Operculofrontal artery
(E) Angular artery

2. A patient is given a pipe, tobacco, and matches and is asked to smoke the pipe. The patient rubs the matches on the pipe. Which of the following neurologic diagnoses best describes this behavior?

(A) Construction apraxia
(B) Ideomotor apraxia
(C) Ideational apraxia
(D) Prosopagnosia
(E) Dysprosody

3. A 65-year-old man complains of difficulty walking. He has a history of chronic subdural hematomas. Neurologic examination reveals psychomotor slowing, sphincter incontinence, and enlarged ventricles without convolutional atrophy. The most likely diagnosis is

(A) Huntington disease
(B) normal-pressure hydrocephalus
(C) Parkinson disease
(D) progressive supranuclear palsy
(E) Wilson disease

4. Neurologic examination indicates that a 50-year-old woman with hypertension has left homonymous hemianopia but is not aware of her deficit (anosognosia). When asked to copy a drawing of a clock face, she neglects to draw the numerals on the left side of the clock. Based on this examination, the lesion would most likely be in the

(A) frontal lobe
(B) insula
(C) left parietal lobe
(D) right parietal lobe
(E) right temporal lobe

5. A 48-year-old woman who has had a stroke complains of weakness of her right arm and weakness of her right lower face. Language assessment reveals the following speech deficits: slow, labored speech; dysarthric, telegraphic speech; usually good comprehension; and poor repetition. These neurologic findings best describe which of the following types of aphasia?

(A) Broca aphasia
(B) Conduction aphasia
(C) Transcortical motor aphasia
(D) Transcortical sensory aphasia
(E) Wernicke aphasia

6. A 65-year-old male physician has a cerebrovascular accident. Language assessment reveals the following speech abnormalities: impaired comprehension; impaired repetition; and paraphrasic speech, including non sequiturs and neologisms. Spontaneity and fluency are normal. This evaluation best fits which of the following types of aphasia?

(A) Broca aphasia
(B) Conduction aphasia
(C) Mixed transcortical aphasia
(D) Transcortical motor aphasia
(E) Wernicke aphasia

7. A 50-year-old man has a mass lesion underlying the left frontoparietal operculum. Language assessment reveals good comprehension, fluent speech, poor repetition, anomia, and agraphia. This case best fits which of the following types of aphasia?

(A) Broca aphasia
(B) Conduction aphasia
(C) Global aphasia
(D) Transcortical sensory aphasia
(E) Wernicke aphasia

8. A 45-year-old woman has a stroke. She exhibits weakness in her left arm, and she is unable to show emotion, inflection, and emphasis and gesturing in her propositional language. The lesion responsible for this language difficulty would most likely be in the

(A) left frontal lobe
(B) right frontal lobe
(C) left parietal lobe
(D) left temporal lobe
(E) right temporal lobe

ANSWERS AND EXPLANATIONS

1–D. The Broca speech area, which is located in the lower frontal gyrus of the left hemisphere, is supplied by the operculofrontal artery. This area may also be perfused by the prerolandic artery. Both of these arteries arise from the middle cerebral artery.

2–C. The patient, who is unable to light a match and smoke the pipe in proper sequence on command, has ideational or sensory apraxia, a disorder of a multistep action sequence. Construction apraxia is the inability to draw an entire clock face; patients with nondominant parietal lobe lesions cannot draw the left side of the clock (sensory neglect). Ideomotor apraxia is the inability to follow simple commands (i.e., stick out your tongue or make a fist). Prosopagnosia is the inability to recognize faces. Dysprosody is the difficulty producing or understanding the normal pitch, rhythm, and variation in stress in speech.

3–B. Normal-pressure hydrocephalus is characterized by the triad of gait apraxia (frontal lobe ataxia), incontinence, and dementia. The ventricles are moderately dilated. Huntington disease is a neurodegenerative disorder characterized by choreoathetosis, tremor, and dementia. Parkinson disease is characterized by a pill-rolling resting tremor, cogwheel rigidity, and bradykinesia (slowness in movement). Progressive supranuclear palsy is a movement disorder characterized by paresis of downgaze. Wilson disease (hepatolenticular degeneration) is a disease of copper metabolism characterized by a coarse "wing-beating" tremor. The corneal Kayser-Fleischer ring is pathognomonic.

4–D. Lesions of the nondominant (right) parietal lobe have the following deficits: anosognosia, topographic memory loss, dressing apraxia, sensory neglect, sensory extinction, and left homonymous hemianopia. Frontal lobe signs may include motor abnormalities, impairment of cognitive function, personality changes (disinhibition of behavior), and incontinence. The insula receives olfactory and gustatory input. Temporal lobe signs may include Wernicke aphasia, auditory, visual, olfactory, and gustatory hallucinations, and loss of recent memory.

5–A. Key features that point to Broca aphasia are slow, labored dysarthric telegraphic speech; relatively good speech comprehension; poor repetition; frequent depression; and frequent buccolingual dyspraxia. Broca aphasia is also called motor, expressive, and anterior aphasia. See Figure 24-1.

6–E. Wernicke aphasia is characterized by fluent speech, poor comprehension, poor repetition, and paraphrasic errors (e.g., driveling speech, non sequiturs, and neologisms).

7–B. Conduction aphasia results from a lesion that transects the arcuate fasciculus, thus separating the Broca speech area from the Wernicke speech area. This condition is characterized by markedly impaired repetition, with preserved fluency and comprehension. Conduction aphasia is usually associated with agraphia.

8–B. The center for expressive prosody is located in the posterior part of the inferior frontal gyrus of the nondominant lobe. The center for receptive prosody is located in the posterior part of the superior temporal gyrus of the nondominant hemisphere.

COMPREHENSIVE EXAMINATION

1. The cuneus is separated from the lingual gyrus by the
(A) Rhinal sulcus
(B) Calcarine sulcus
(C) Parietooccipital sulcus
(D) Collateral sulcus
(E) Intraparietal sulcus

2. Which sinus receives drainage from the greatest number of arachnoid granulations?
(A) Straight sinus
(B) Transverse sinus
(C) Sigmoid sinus
(D) Superior sagittal sinus
(E) Cavernous sinus

3. Which of the following statements concerning the Rathke pouch is true?
(A) It is a mesodermal diverticulum
(B) It is derived from the neural tube
(C) It gives rise to the adenohypophysis
(D) It gives rise to the epiphysis
(E) It gives rise to the neurohypophysis

4. Which of the following statements concerning the lateral horn of the spinal cord is true?
(A) It contains preganglionic parasympathetic neurons
(B) It gives rise to a spinocerebellar tract
(C) It is present at all spinal cord levels
(D) It gives rise to preganglionic sympathetic fibers
(E) It is most prominent at sacral levels

5. Which of the following statements concerning the nucleus dorsalis of Clarke is true?
(A) It Is found in the ventral horn
(B) It projects to the cerebellum
(C) It is present at all spinal levels
(D) It is most prominent at upper cervical levels
(E) It is homologous to the cuneate nucleus of the medulla

6. Which of the following groups of cranial nerves is closely related to the corticospinal tract?
(A) CN III, CN IV, and CN V
(B) CN III, CN V, and CN VII
(C) CN III, CN VI, and CN VIII
(D) CN III, CN VI, and CN XII
(E) CN III, CN IX, and CN X

7. The primary auditory cortex is located in the
(A) Frontal operculum
(B) Postcentral gyrus
(C) Superior parietal lobule
(D) Inferior parietal lobule
(E) Transverse temporal gyri

8. The neocerebellum projects to the motor cortex via the
(A) Anterior thalamic nucleus
(B) Ventral anterior nucleus
(C) Ventral lateral nucleus
(D) Lateral dorsal nucleus
(E) Lateral posterior nucleus

9. The dentatothalamic tract decussates in the
(A) Diencephalon
(B) Rostral midbrain
(C) Caudal midbrain
(D) Rostral pons
(E) Caudal pons

10. A pituitary tumor is most frequently associated with
(A) Homonymous hemianopia
(B) Homonymous quadrantanopia
(C) Bitemporal hemianopia
(D) Binasal hemianopia
(E) Altitudinal hemianopia

11. Resection of the anterior portion of the left temporal lobe is most frequently associated with
(A) Left homonymous hemianopia
(B) Right upper homonymous quadrantanopia
(C) Right lower homonymous quadrantanopia
(D) Left upper homonymous quadrantanopia
(E) Left lower homonymous quadrantanopia

12. A 65-year-old farmer has had dull frontal headaches for the last 3 weeks. Neurologic examination reveals spastic hemiparesis on the right side and a pronator drift on the right side. What is the most likely diagnosis?
(A) Brain tumor
(B) Myasthenia gravis
(C) Progressive supranuclear palsy
(D) Pseudotumor cerebri
(E) Subacute combined degeneration

13. An 18-year-old high school student has fractured a cervical vertebra in an automobile accident. Neurologic examination reveals hemiparesis on the right side, Babinski and Hoffmann signs on the right side, loss of pain and temperature sensation on the left side, and normal pallesthesia in all extremities. The spinal cord lesion that would most likely explain the deficits involves the

(A) Dorsal column, left side
(B) Dorsal column, right side
(C) Lateral column, left side
(D) Lateral column, right side
(E) Anterior column, bilateral

14. Light shone into the left eye elicits a direct pupillary reflex but no consensual reflex. A lesion in which of the following structures accounts for this deficit?

(A) Optic nerve, left eye
(B) Optic nerve, right eye
(C) Optic tract, right side
(D) Oculomotor nerve, right side
(E) Oculomotor nerve, left side

15. A 53-year-old housewife has a normal corneal blink reflex on her left side but no consensual blink on her right side. Which of the following neurologic deficits or signs would you expect to find on the right side?

(A) Hyperacusis
(B) Hemianhidrosis
(C) Hemianesthesia
(D) Internal ophthalmoplegia
(E) Severe ptosis

16. A 49-year-old man has a loss of tactile sensation involving the anterior two-thirds of his tongue on the left side. Neurologic examination reveals paralysis of the masseter muscle on the left side and loss of pain and temperature sensation from the teeth of the mandible on the left side. He has a lesion involving which one of the following nerves?

(A) Chorda tympani nerve
(B) Facial nerve
(C) Hypoglossal nerve
(D) Trigeminal nerve, mandibular division
(E) Trigeminal nerve, ophthalmic division

17. A 62-year-old lawyer has a stroke and falls while cutting his lawn. He does not lose consciousness. Neurologic examination reveals loss of pain sensation on the right side of the face and on the left side of the body, falling and past pointing to the right side, difficulty swallowing, horizontal nystagmus to the right side, deviation of the uvula to the left when asked to say ah, and Horner syndrome on the right side. The most likely site of this man's lesion is the

(A) Internal capsule, left side
(B) Midbrain, right side
(C) Pontine tegmentum
(D) Lateral medulla, right side
(E) Medial medulla, right side

18. A 64-year-old pharmacology professor complains of weakness in his right leg and double vision, especially when moving his eyes to the left. Neurologic examination reveals a dilated pupil and ptosis on the left side and a Babinski sign (extensor plantar reflex) on the right side. The most likely site of this patient's lesion is the

(A) Midbrain crus cerebri, right side
(B) Midbrain crus cerebri, left side
(C) Pontine base, left side
(D) Pontine tegmentum, right side
(E) Internal capsule, right side

19. While working in his shop, a 21-year-old machinist is struck by a penetrating metal fragment in the side of the head. Neurologic examination reveals the following language deficits: fluent speech, no ability to read aloud, no ability to repeat what you say, no ability to compensate by writing. The patient understands the problem but cannot resolve it. Where would you expect to find the fragment?

(A) Between the supramarginal gyrus and the inferior frontal gyrus
(B) In the angular gyrus
(C) In the transverse gyri
(D) In the posterior third of the superior temporal gyrus
(E) In the paracentral gyrus

20. The catecholamine norepinephrine is the primary neurotransmitter found in the

(A) Adrenal cortex
(B) Adrenal medulla
(C) Postganglionic parasympathetic neurons to the circular smooth muscle layer of the jejunum
(D) Postganglionic sympathetic neurons to the smooth muscle of the renal arterioles
(E) Postganglionic sympathetic neurons to the sweat glands

21. A 30-year-old man sustains brain damage as the result of an automobile accident. Neurologic examination reveals incomplete retrograde amnesia, severe anterograde amnesia, and inappropriate social behavior, including hyperphagia, hypersexuality, and general disinhibition. The brain injury would most likely involve the

(A) Frontal lobes, lateral convexity
(B) Frontal lobes, medial surface
(C) Temporal lobes, lateral convexity
(D) Temporal lobes, medial surface
(E) Thalami

22. A 55-year-old woman has difficulty reading small print. She most likely has

(A) Astigmatism
(B) Cataracts
(C) Optic atrophy
(D) Macular degeneration
(E) Presbyopia

23. The principal postnatal change in the pyramids is due to

(A) An increase of corticospinal neurons from the paracentral lobule
(B) An increase in the total number of corticospinal axons
(C) A large increase of Schwann cells in the motor cortex
(D) An increase in endoneural tubes to guide sprouting axons
(E) Myelination of preexisting corticospinal axons

24. Special visceral afferent neurons that innervate receptor cells in taste buds synapse in the

(A) Geniculate ganglion
(B) Inferior salivatory nucleus
(C) Nucleus of the solitary tract
(D) Spinal trigeminal nucleus
(E) Ventral posteromedial nucleus

25. A woman receives an injection of a radioisotope to determine regional blood flow in the brain. She has a positron emission tomography scan to visualize variations in cortical blood flow. The examiner asks her to think about flexing her index finger without actually doing it. In which of the following cortical areas would you expect to see increased blood flow?

(A) Broca area
(B) Angular gyrus
(C) Motor strip

(D) Supplementary motor cortex
(E) S-I somatosensory cortex

26. Destruction of the right cuneate nucleus results in which of the following sensory deficits?

(A) Apallesthesia, left hand
(B) Apallesthesia, right hand
(C) Apallesthesia, left foot
(D) Analgesia, left hand
(E) Analgesia, right foot

27. The elaboration of acetylcholine results in which of the following postganglionic sympathetic responses?

(A) Constriction of cutaneous blood vessels
(B) Contraction of arrector pili muscles
(C) Decreased gastrointestinal motility
(D) Increased ventricular contractility
(E) Stimulation of eccrine sweat glands

28. Nausea is mediated by which of the following neural structures?

(A) Celiac ganglion
(B) Greater splanchnic nerve
(C) Superior mesenteric ganglion
(D) Inferior mesenteric ganglion
(E) Vagal nerves

29. Cerebrospinal fluid enters the bloodstream via the

(A) Arachnoid villi
(B) Choroid plexus
(C) Interventricular foramen of Monro
(D) Lateral foramina of Luschka
(E) Median foramen of Magendie

30. Computed tomography of the head of a newborn infant reveals enlargement of the lateral ventricles and the third ventricle. The cause of this hydrocephalus is most likely which of the following?

(A) Aqueductal stenosis
(B) Adhesive arachnoiditis
(C) Choroid plexus papilloma
(D) Calcification of the arachnoid granulations
(E) Stenosis of the median foramen

31. The cellular neuropathology of Alzheimer disease resembles most closely that seen in

(A) Huntington disease
(B) Multi-infarct dementia
(C) Pick disease
(D) Neurosyphilis
(E) Trisomy 21

32. A 40-year-old carpenter visits his general practitioner. He complains of shortness of breath and difficulty in performing his construction work. During the history taking, he tells his physician that he had an attack of gastroenteritis 3 weeks ago. The neurologic examination reveals ascending weakness and tingling in the legs and absence of muscle stretch reflexes in the legs. Cerebrospinal fluid analysis shows elevated protein without significant pleocytosis. The most likely diagnosis is

(A) Amyotrophic lateral sclerosis
(B) Guillain-Barré syndrome
(C) Multiple sclerosis
(D) Myasthenia gravis
(E) Werdnig-Hoffmann syndrome

33. A 25-year-old female high school teacher has had difficulty walking. Five years ago she experienced a loss of vision in her left eye that improved in 3 weeks. Neurologic examination reveals a right afferent pupillary defect, hyperreflexia in both legs, reduced proprioception in both feet, and extensor plantar reflexes. Cerebrospinal fluid analysis shows oligoclonal bands. The most likely diagnosis is

(A) Amyotrophic lateral sclerosis
(B) Guillain-Barré syndrome
(C) Multiple sclerosis
(D) Syringobulbia
(E) Subacute combined degeneration

34. A 48-year-old woman complains of a progressive loss of hearing and a buzzing noise in her right ear. Neurologic examination reveals an absent corneal reflex on the right side and sagging of the right corner of the mouth. Magnetic resonance imaging shows a mass in the right cerebellopontine angle. The neoplasm would most likely arise from proliferation of which of the following cell types?

(A) Fibrous astrocytes
(B) Protoplasmic astrocytes
(C) Microglia
(D) Schwann cells
(E) Oligodendrocytes

35. A 50-year-old plumber complains of weakness in his left leg and a loss of pain and temperature in his right leg. Neurologic examination reveals exaggerated muscle stretch reflexes in the left leg and an extensor plantar reflex on the left side. The lesion would most likely be located in the

(A) Crus cerebri
(B) Internal capsule
(C) Lateral medulla
(D) Medial medulla
(E) Spinal cord

36. A 20-year-old comatose man has sustained massive head injuries in a automobile accident. Ice water injected into the external auditory meatus elicits no ocular response. Head rotation does not result in the doll's-eye phenomenon. The lesion causing the injuries most likely affects the

(A) Cochlear nuclei
(B) Dentate nuclei
(C) Ossicles
(D) Utricles
(E) Vestibular nuclei

37. Which of the following agents may be used as an alternative to L-dopa to alleviate the chemical imbalance found in the striatum of a patient with Parkinson disease?

(A) Aspartate
(B) An anticholinergic agent
(C) Glutamate
(D) A dopamine antagonist
(E) A serotonin reuptake inhibitor

38. Which of the following antidepressants is the most selective inhibitor of serotonin reuptake?

(A) Amitriptyline
(B) Doxepin
(C) Fluoxetine
(D) Nortriptyline
(E) Tranylcypromine

39. A 20-year-old woman suddenly develops double vision. Neurologic examination reveals diplopia when she attempts to look to the left, inability to adduct the right eye, nystagmus in the left eye on attempted lateral conjugate gaze to the left, and convergence of both eyes on a near point. These deficits would result from occlusion of a branch of which of the following arteries?

(A) Anterior cerebral
(B) Basilar
(C) Middle cerebral
(D) Posterior cerebral
(E) Ophthalmic

40. A 50-year old man had a stroke and developed ipsilateral paralysis and atrophy of the tongue, contralateral loss of vibrations sense, contralateral hemiplegia, contralateral Babinski sign. The level of this vascular syndrome is in the

(A) Medial medulla
(B) Lateral medulla
(C) Pontine tegmentum
(D) Pontine base
(E) Midbrain

41. Tritiated proline is injected into the left upper quadrant of the left retina for anterograde transport. Radioactive label would be found in the

(A) Cuneus, left side
(B) Cuneus, right side
(C) Lingual gyrus, left side
(D) Lingual gyrus, right side
(E) Optic nerve, left side

42. Tritiated leucine [(^{3}H)-leucine] is injected into the left inferior olivary nucleus for anterograde transport. Radioactive label would be found in the

(A) Lateral cuneate nucleus, left side
(B) Nuclei of the lateral lemnisci
(C) Dentate nucleus, right side
(D) Nucleus dorsalis of Clarke
(E) Superior olivary nucleus, left side

43. Tritiated proline [(^{3}H)-proline] is injected into the right ventral posterolateral nucleus for retrograde transport. Radioactive label would be found in the

(A) Nucleus ruber, right side
(B) Nucleus gracilis, left side
(C) Nucleus gracilis, right side
(D) Lateral cuneate nucleus, left side
(E) Ventral lateral nucleus

44. Horseradish peroxidase is injected into the nucleus of the inferior colliculus for retrograde transport. Label would be found in which of the following nuclei?

(A) Medial geniculate nucleus
(B) Lateral geniculate nucleus
(C) Superior olivary nucleus
(D) Inferior olivary nucleus
(E) Transverse gyrus of Heschl

45. A 30-year old barber complains of difficulty chewing and weakness in the contralateral extremities and loss of pain and temperature sensation from the ipsilateral face. This lesion would most likely be found in which one of the following choices?

(A) Medulla, medial
(B) Medulla, lateral
(C) Pons, tegmentum
(D) Pons, base
(E) Midbrain, base

46. A 45-year-old carpenter had bilateral paralysis of the tongue. Fasciculations could be seen on the tongue and bilateral loss of deep sensibility (proprioception) in the trunk and limbs. The lesion would most likely be in the

(A) Open medulla, medial lemniscus bilateral, root fibers CN XII, bilateral
(B) Closed medulla pyramidal decussation
(C) Pons, base
(D) Pons, tegmentum
(E) Midbrain, tegmentum

47. A 25-year-old woman has paralysis of the face and lateral rectus muscle, medial rectus palsy on attempted lateral conjugate gaze, nystagmus, normal convergence, miosis, ptosis, and multiple sclerosis. Where would this lesion most likely be found?

(A) Medial medulla
(B) Lateral medulla
(C) Pons, tegmentum
(D) Pons, base
(E) Midbrain, tegmentum

48. A 40-year-old man had a stroke and developed ipsilateral paralysis and atrophy of the tongue, contralateral loss of vibration sense, contralateral hemiplegia, and contralateral Babinski sign. Thrombosis of which artery would result in these neurologic deficits?

(A) Anterior spinal artery
(B) Posterior spinal artery
(C) Posterior inferior cerebellar artery
(D) Anterior inferior cerebellar artery
(E) Labyrinthine artery

49. A 55-year-old right-handed man had abnormal speech and language usage. The psychiatric interview revealed poor comprehension, fluent speech, poor repetition, and the neighborhood signs contralateral quadrantanopia and contralateral hemisensory loss. Match the neurologic deficits to the anatomic substrata.

(A) Precentral gyrus
(B) Superior temporal gyrus
(C) Inferior frontal gyrus
(D) Middle frontal gyrus
(E) Inferior temporal gyrus

50. Which disease is preferentially found in the frontal lobe?

(A) Creutzfeldt-Jakob disease
(B) Pick disease
(C) Down syndrome
(D) Tuberous sclerosis
(E) Sturge-Weber syndrome

51. A 60-year-old right-handed man had abnormal speech and language usage. The psychiatric interview revealed the following speech and language findings: good comprehension of spoken and written language; spontaneous speech fluent but paraphasic; poor repetition; inability to repeat polysyllabic words. A neighborhood sign is contralateral quadrantanopia. Match the neurologic deficits with the anatomic substrata.

(A) Arcuate fasciculus
(B) Arcuate nucleus
(C) Dorsal longitudinal fasciculus
(D) Medial longitudinal fasciculus
(E) Indusium griseum

52. Which of the following structures contains calcium concrements?

(A) Cerebral peduncle
(B) Cerebral aqueduct
(C) Inferior colliculus
(D) Pineal gland
(E) Oculomotor nerve

Questions 53 to 56

The response options for items 53 to 56 are the same. Select one answer for each item in the set.

(A) Abducent nerve
(B) Accessory nerve
(C) Facial nerve
(D) Glossopharyngeal nerve
(E) Hypoglossal nerve
(F) Oculomotor nerve
(G) Olfactory nerve
(H) Optic nerve
(I) Trigeminal nerve
(J) Trochlear nerve
(K) Vagal nerve
(L) Vestibulocochlear nerve

Match each description with the most appropriate cranial nerve.

53. Is derived from the walls of the diencephalic vesicle

54. Is often damaged in the process of transtentorial herniation

55. Mediates the sensory and motor innervation of pharyngeal arches 4 and 6

56. Innervates the muscle that depresses, intorts, and abducts the globe

Questions 57 to 58

The response options for items 57 to 58 are the same. Select one answer for each item in the set.

(A) Basal ganglia
(B) Cerebellum
(C) Frontal lobe
(D) Occipital lobe
(E) Parietal lobe
(F) Temporal lobe
(G) Subthalamic nucleus
(H) Ventral horn

For each patient described, select the most likely involved neurologic substrate.

57. A 50-year-old policeman complains of a tremor in both hands. This tremor is most obvious at rest. While the man is reaching for an object, the tremor disappears.

58. A 35-year-old tennis player is concerned about weakness in his arms and hands, and he notices a loss of muscle mass in the upper limbs. His muscle stretch reflexes are exaggerated in the lower extremities, and he has muscle twitches in the upper limbs.

Questions 59 to 65

The response options for items 59 to 65 are the same. Select one answer for each item in the set.

(A) Diencephalon
(B) Medulla
(C) Midbrain
(D) Pons
(E) Telencephalon

Match each of the following structures with the appropriate part of the brain.

59. Cerebral aqueduct

60. Cranial nerves III and IV

61. Caudate nucleus

62. Optic chiasma

63. Olive and the pyramid

64. Pineal gland

65. Cranial nerves IX, X, XI, and XII

Questions 66 to 70

The response options for items 66 to 70 are the same. Select one answer for each item in the set.

(A) Astrocytes
(B) Ependymal cells
(C) Microglial cells
(D) Oligodendrocytes
(E) Schwann cells

Match each of the following descriptions with the most appropriate type of cell.

66. Are derived from the neural crest

67. May myelinate numerous axons

68. Have filaments that contain glial fibrillary acidic protein

69. Myelinate only one internode

70. Arise from monocytes

Questions 71 to 75

Match the descriptions in items 71 to 75 with the appropriate lettered lesion (*shaded area*) in the diagram of a cross-section of the spinal cord.

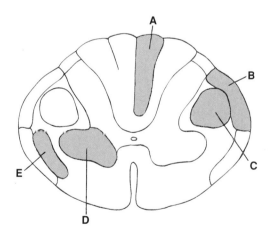

71. Ipsilateral leg dystaxia

72. Ipsilateral flaccid paralysis

73. Contralateral loss of pain and temperature sensation one segment below the lesion

74. Exaggerated muscle stretch reflexes below the lesion

75. Loss of two-point tactile discrimination in the ipsilateral foot

Questions 76 to 81

Match the descriptions in items 76 to 81 with the appropriate lettered lesion (*shaded area*) shown on one of the two cross-sections of the brainstem.

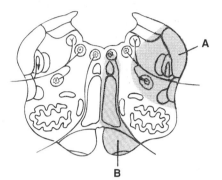

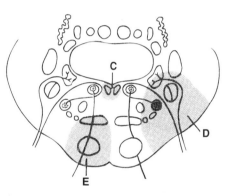

76. Medial rectus palsy on attempted lateral gaze

77. Lateral rectus paralysis; contralateral spastic hemiparesis

78. Occlusion of the posterior inferior cerebellar artery

79. Loss of the corneal reflex; contralateral loss of pain and temperature sensation from the body and extremities

80. Hemiatrophy of the tongue; contralateral hemiparesis; contralateral loss of vibration sensation

81. Hoarseness: Horner syndrome; singultus

Questions 82 to 87

The response options for items 82 to 87 are the same. Select one answer for each item in the set.

(A) Anterior thalamic nucleus
(B) Centromedian nucleus
(C) Ventral lateral nucleus
(D) Ventral posteromedial nucleus
(E) Mediodorsal nucleus

Match each of the following descriptions with the appropriate nucleus.

82. Receives input from the dentate nucleus

83. Receives input of taste sensation from the solitary nucleus

84. Receives input of pain and temperature sensation from the face

85. Receives the mamillothalamic tract

86. Projects to the putamen

87. Has reciprocal connections with the prefrontal cortex

Questions 88 to 93

The response options for items 88 to 93 are the same. Select one answer for each item in the set.

(A) Anterior nucleus
(B) Arcuate nucleus
(C) Mamillary nucleus
(D) Paraventricular nucleus
(E) Suprachiasmatic nucleus

Match each description with the most appropriate hypothalamic nucleus.

88. Receives input from the hippocampal formation

89. Destruction results in hyperthermia

90. Receives input from the retina

91. Projects to the neurohypophysis

92. Regulates the activity of the adenohypophysis

93. Regulates water balance

Questions 94 to 98

The response options for items 94 to 98 are the same. Select one answer for each item in the set.

(A) Caudate nucleus
(B) Globus pallidus
(C) Centromedian nucleus
(D) Substantia nigra
(E) Subthalamic nucleus

Match each description with the most appropriate nucleus.

94. Destruction causes contralateral hemiballism

95. Receives dopaminergic input from the midbrain

96. Gives rise to the ansa lenticularis and the lenticular fasciculus

97. Destruction causes hypokinetic rigid syndrome

98. A loss of cells in this griseum causes greatly dilated lateral ventricles

Questions 99 to 105

The response options for items 99 to 105 are the same. Select one answer for each item in the set.

(A) Acetylcholine
(B) Dopamine
(C) Gamma-aminobutyric acid
(D) Norepinephrine
(E) Serotonin

Match each of the following nuclei or cells with the appropriate neurotransmitter.

99. Raphe nuclei

100. Purkinje cells

101. Nucleus basalis of Meynert

102. Motor cranial nerve nuclei

103. Pars compacta of the substantia nigra

104. Locus ceruleus

105. Globus pallidus

Questions 106 to 110

The response options for items 106 to 110 are the same. Select one answer for each item in the set.

(A) Glutamate
(B) Glycine
(C) β-Endorphin
(D) Enkephalin
(E) Substance P

Match each description with the appropriate neurotransmitter.

106. Neurotransmitter of afferent pain fibers

107. Major inhibitory neurotransmitter of the spinal cord

108. Major neurotransmitter of the corticospinal pathway

109. Located almost exclusively in the hypothalamus

110. Helps inhibit input from afferent pain fibers

Questions 111 to 117

The response options for items 111 to 117 are the same. Select one answer for each item in the set.

(A) Left frontal lobe
(B) Left parietal lobe
(C) Right partial lobe
(D) Left temporal lobe
(E) Right occipital lobe

Match each of the following neurologic deficits with the most likely lesion site.

111. Left upper quadrantanopia

112. Muscle weakness and clumsiness in the right hand; slow, effortful speech

113. Inability to identify a key placed in the left hand with the eyes closed

114. Denial of hemiparesis: patient ignores stimuli from one side of the body

115. Poor comprehension of speech; patient is unaware of the deficit

116. Patient is unable to identify fingers touched by examiner when eyes are closed; is unable to perform simple calculations

117. Babinski sign and ankle clonus

Questions 118 to 122

Match the descriptions in items 118 to 122 with the appropriate lettered structure shown in the magnetic resonance image of the axial section of the brain.

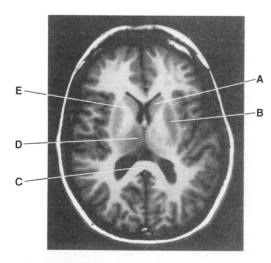

118. Thalamus

119. Internal capsule

120. Putamen

121. Caudate nucleus

122. Splenium

Questions 123 to 127

Match the descriptions in items 123 to 127 with the appropriate lettered structure shown in the magnetic resonance image of the axial section of the brain.

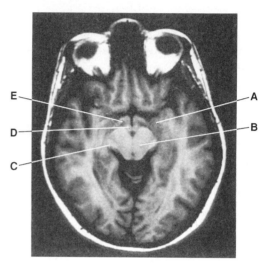

123. Medial geniculate body

124. Mesencephalon

125. Mamillary body

126. Optic tract

127. Amygdala

Questions 128 to 132

Match the descriptions in items 128 to 132 with the appropriate letter shown in the magnetic resonance image of the midsagittal section of the brain.

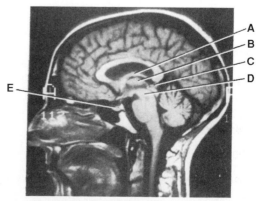

128. Pineal gland

129. Hypophysis

130. Mesencephalon

131. Thalamus

132. Fornix

Questions 133 to 142

Match the descriptions in items 133 to 142 with the appropriate diagnoses shown in the figure.

141. Horner syndrome

142. Retrobulbar neuritis

Questions 143 to 147

The response options for items 143 to 147 are the same. Select one answer for each item in the set.

(A) Diabetes insipidus
(B) Hyperthermia
(C) Hyperphagia and savage behavior
(D) Inability to thermoregulate
(E) Anorexia

Match each defect below with the condition it best describes.

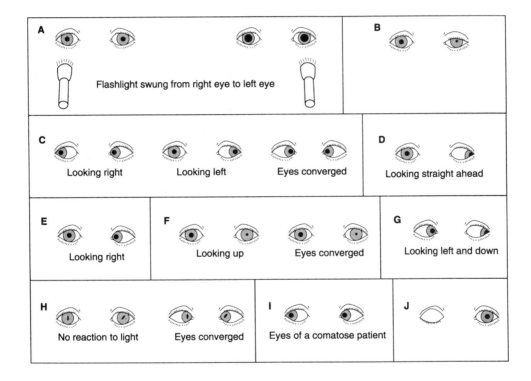

133. Right third-nerve palsy

134. Destructive lesion of the right frontal lobe

135. Argyll Robertson pupil

136. Right fourth-nerve palsy

137. Parinaud syndrome

138. Right sixth-nerve palsy

139. Left third-nerve palsy

140. Internuclear ophthalmoplegia

143. Bilateral lesions of the ventromedial hypothalamic nucleus

144. Bilateral lesions of the posterior hypothalamic nuclei

145. Lesions involving the supraoptic and paraventricular nuclei

146. Destruction of the anterior hypothalamic nuclei

147. Stimulation of the ventromedial nuclei

Questions 148 to 155

Match the descriptions in items 148 to 155 with the appropriate lettered structure in the figure.

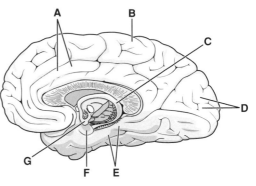

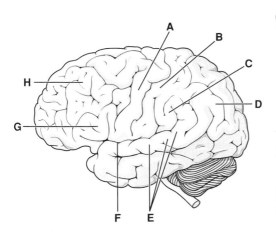

148. Stimulation of this area results in turning the eyes and head to the contralateral side

149. A lesion here results in nonfluent, effortful, telegraphic speech

150. Ablation in this area results in a contralateral upper homonymous quadrantanopia

151. A lesion here results in fluent speech with paraphrasic errors (e.g., non sequiturs, neologisms, driveling speech)

152. A lesion of this area is characterized by finger agnosia, dyscalculia, dysgraphia, and dyslexia

153. Destruction of this area results in an aphasia characterized by fluent speech, good comprehension, and poor repetition

154. Lesions in this gyrus result in contralateral astereognosis

155. Lesions in this gyrus result in contralateral spasticity

Questions 156 to 162

Match the descriptions in items 156 to 162 with the appropriate lettered structure in the figure.

156. In thiamine (vitamin B$_1$) deficiency, hemorrhagic lesions are found in this structure

157. Bilateral lesions in this structure result in hyperphagia, hypersexuality, and psychic blindness (visual agnosia)

158. Infarction (due to cardiac arrest) of this area results in short-term memory loss

159. Lesions of this area result in a lower homonymous quadrantanopia

160. Bilateral transection of this structure may result in the acute amnestic syndrome

161. Lesion of this area results in a contralateral extensor plantar reflex and ankle clonus

162. Ablation of this area may result in akinesia, mutism, apathy, and indifference to pain

163. Which of the following arteries perfuses the medullary pyramid?
(A) Anterior communicating artery
(B) Anterior spinal artery
(C) Anterior choroidal artery
(D) Posterior spinal artery
(E) Posterior inferior cerebellar artery

164. Which artery supplies the intra-axial fibers of the hypoglossal nerve XII?
(A) Basilar artery
(B) Posterior spinal artery
(C) Anterior spinal artery
(D) Anterior inferior cerebellar artery
(E) Vertebral artery

165. A berry aneurysm puts pressure on the optic chiasm in the anteroposterior plane resulting in a bitemporal hemianopia. The aneurysm is most likely found on which one of the following arteries?

(A) Basilar artery
(B) Ophthalmic artery
(C) Anterior spinal artery
(D) Anterior communicating artery
(E) Posterior communicating artery

166. A 10-year-old boy was struck on the side of the head with a golf ball. The middle meningeal artery was lacerated. Blood was found in which space?

(A) Confluence of the sinuses
(B) Subarachnoid space
(C) Subdural space
(D) Subpial space
(E) Epidural space

167. A 25-year-old male student was examined by an ophthalmologist, who found headaches; ptosis; a fixed, dilated pupil; and an eye that looked down and out. An aneurysm was demonstrated with carotid angiogram anteroposterior projection. Which artery harbored the aneurysm?

(A) Anterior cerebral artery
(B) Anterior communicating artery
(C) Internal carotid artery
(D) Ophthalmic artery
(E) Posterior communicating artery

168. Which one of the following arteries irrigates the dentate nucleus?

(A) Vertebral artery
(B) Posterior inferior cerebellar artery
(C) Anterior inferior cerebellar artery
(D) Superior cerebral artery
(E) Posterior cerebral artery

169. A glioma under the facial colliculus results in diplopia and horizontal nystagmus on attempted lateral conjugate gaze. Paralysis of which one of the following muscles would explain the neurologic deficits?

(A) Buccinator
(B) Lateral rectus
(C) Lateral pterygoid
(D) Posterior belly of digastric
(E) Orbicularis oculi

170. Which of following Brodmann areas were not accounted for in his list of cytoarchitectonic regions?

(A) Areas 9, 10, 11
(B) Areas 3, 1, 2
(C) Areas 13-15
(D) Areas 32, 23, 24,
(E) Areas 39, 40

171. In adults the choroid plexus of the lateral ventricle is calcified and can be visualized with plain film or CT. Where within the ventricular system is the calcified glomus of the choroid plexus?

(A) Frontal horn
(B) Trigone
(C) Temporal horn
(D) Occipital horn
(E) Body

172. Which one of the following circumventricular organs has a blood-brain barrier?

(A) Area postrema
(B) Pineal body
(C) Subcommissural organ
(D) Subfornical organ
(E) Median eminence of the tuber cinereum

173. Which artery perfuses the leg area of the motor strip?

(A) Pericallosal artery
(B) Middle cerebral artery
(C) Posterior cerebral artery
(D) Splenial artery
(E) Heubner artery

174. Which one of the following arteries following bilateral hypoperfusion results in Klüver-Bucy syndrome?

(A) Medial striate arteries
(B) Anterior choroidal artery
(C) Anterior communicating artery
(D) Posterior cerebral artery
(E) Posterior choroidal artery

175. Which of the cranial nerves exits the brainstem from the pontomedullary junction?

(A) Abducent nerve
(B) Abducent, facial, and vestibulocochlear nerves
(C) Facial nerve
(D) Intermediate nerve
(E) Vestibulocochlear nerve

176. Which of the following arteries perfuses the medullary pyramid?

(A) Anterior communicating artery
(B) Anterior spinal artery
(C) Anterior choroidal artery
(D) Posterior spinal artery
(E) Posterior inferior cerebellar artery

177. Which artery supplies the intra-axial fibers of the hypoglossal nerve XII?

(A) Basilar artery
(B) Posterior spinal artery
(C) Anterior spinal artery
(D) Anterior inferior cerebellar artery
(E) Vertebral artery

178. A berry aneurysm puts pressure on the optic chiasma in the anteroposterior plane, resulting in a bitemporal hemianopia. The aneurysm is most likely found on which one of the following arteries?

(A) Internal carotid artery
(B) Ophthalmic artery
(C) Anterior communicating artery
(D) Medial striate artery
(E) Posterior communicating artery

179. Which is an abnormal quantity of white cells per microliter in the cerebrospinal fluid?

(A) 2
(B) 3
(C) 4
(D) 5
(E) 8

180. What is the normal value of cerebrospinal fluid protein in milligrams per deciliter?

(A) Less than 25
(B) Less than 35
(C) Less than 45
(D) Less than 55
(E) Less than 65

181. Which is an example of a normal value for cerebrospinal fluid serum glucose in milligrams per deciliter?

(A) 40
(B) 50
(C) 60
(D) 70
(E) 80

182. A 20-year-old female patient was evaluated by a neurologist. The neurologic examination reveals severe headaches, papilledema without mass, elevated cerebrospinal fluid pressure, and deteriorating vision. The diagnosis would most likely be

(A) Normal-pressure hydrocephalus
(B) Hydrocephalus ex vacuo
(C) Pseudotumor cerebri
(D) Arnold Chiari II
(E) Dandy-Walker

183. Cerebrospinal fluid enters the subarachnoid space via which of the following structures?

(A) Arachnoid villi
(B) Cerebral aqueduct
(C) Intraventricular foramina of Monro
(D) Lateral foramina of Luschka
(E) Third ventricle

184. A 40-year old man had a stroke and developed ipsilateral paralysis and atrophy of the tongue, contralateral loss of vibration sense, contralateral hemiplegia, and contralateral Babinski sign. Thrombosis of which artery would result in these neurologic deficits?

(A) Anterior spinal artery
(B) Posterior spinal artery
(C) Posterior inferior cerebellar artery
(D) Anterior inferior cerebellar artery
(E) Labyrinthine artery

185. A 10-year-old boy presents with seizures, olfactory hallucinations, and a right upper quadrantanopia. The most likely causative lesion would be

(A) Aneurysm of the anterior communicating artery
(B) Charcot-Bouchard aneurysm
(C) Temporal lobe astrocytoma
(D) Frontal lobe astrocytoma
(E) Olfactory groove meningioma

186. A 60-year-old high school teacher has up-going toes and spastic paralysis of all limbs and intact sensibility. Where is the corresponding lesion site in this case?

(A) Closed medulla
(B) Open medulla
(C) Base of pons, abducent nucleus
(D) Base of pons, trigeminal nucleus
(E) Midbrain, inferior colliculus

187. The optic cup is an evagination of which of the following?

(A) Telencephalon
(B) Diencephalon
(C) Mesencephalon
(D) Metencephalon
(E) Myelencephalon

188. General somatic afferent fibers are primarily concerned with conveying sensory input

(A) Relating to audition and equilibrium
(B) Relating to information from visceral organs
(C) Relating to vision
(D) Relating to taste and smell
(E) Sensory input from skin, muscle, bone, and joints

189. The spinal cord derives from what part of the neural tube?

(A) Caudal
(B) Cranial
(C) Cavity
(D) Anterior neuropore
(E) Posterior neuropore

190. Which one of the following basal ganglia is derived from the diencephalon?

(A) Amygdaloid nucleus
(B) Head of the caudal nucleus
(C) Tail of the caudal nucleus
(D) Globus pallidus
(E) Putamen

191. Which of the following represents the general somatic efferent column of the pons?

(A) Abducent nucleus
(B) Nucleus ambiguus
(C) Hypoglossal nucleus
(D) Inferior olivary nucleus
(E) Inferior salivatory nucleus

192. Which of the following represents the general visceral efferent column of the pons?

(A) Cerebellum
(B) Spinal trigeminal nucleus
(C) Principal trigeminal nucleus
(D) Superior salivatory nucleus
(E) Pontine nuclei

193. When are the axons of the corticospinal tracts fully myelinated?

(A) In the late embryonic period
(B) In the midfetal period
(C) At birth
(D) By the end of the first postnatal year
(E) By the end of the second postnatal year

194. The cochlear duct contains the spiral organ of Corti and is derived from which of the following?

(A) Both ectoderm and mesoderm
(B) Neural crest
(C) Endoderm
(D) Mesoderm
(E) Ectoderm

195. The stapedius muscle that moves the stapes ossicle is innervated by

(A) CN V
(B) CNXII
(C) CN III
(D) CN VII
(E) Cervical nerves C_2 and C_3.

196. Which one of the following is a classic cerebellar sign?

(A) Athetosis
(B) Chorea
(C) Cogwheel rigidity
(D) Hemiballismus
(E) Intention tremor

197. Which one of the following spinocerebellar tracts shows the phenomenon of doubling?

(A) Cuneocerebellar tract
(B) Ventral spinocerebellar tract
(C) Olivocerebellar tract
(D) Dorsal spinocerebellar tract
(E) Trigeminocerebellar fibers

198. Which of the followings triads of cranial nerves is damaged if the muscles attached to the styloid process are paralyzed?

(A) VII, IX, XII
(B) VII, X, XII
(C) V, IX, X
(D) X, XI, XII
(E) VII, IX, X

199. A 25-year-old male was in a car accident. The emergency department physician noticed clear fluid dribbling from the nose. Rhinorrhea would most likely result from a fracture of which bone?

(A) Ethmoid
(B) Frontal
(C) Lacrimal
(D) Nasal
(E) Palatine

200. Horseradish peroxidase is injected into the circumvallate papillae on the anterior two-thirds of the tongue for retrograde transport labeling. Marker would be found in which of the following way stations?

(A) Geniculate ganglion
(B) Petrosal ganglion
(C) Nodose ganglion
(D) Medial dorsal nucleus of the thalamus
(E) Ventroposterior lateral nucleus of the thalamus

201. Trauma to the foramen rotundum causes damage to which one of the following nerves?

(A) Ophthalmic
(B) Optic
(C) Maxillary
(D) Mandibular
(E) Trochlear

202. An optic glioma is found in the optic canal. Which structures would most likely to be damaged by the invasive tumor?

(A) Optic nerve and ophthalmic artery
(B) Ophthalmic vein and ophthalmic nerve
(C) Ophthalmic nerve and optic nerve
(D) Ophthalmic artery and ophthalmic vein
(E) Optic nerve and ophthalmic vein

203. A 60-year-old hypertensive female complained of facial numbness on the right side including the tongue. A cortical lesion was seen with magnetic resonance imaging. Where would the lesion most likely be found?

(A) Anterior paracentral lobule
(B) Posterior paracentral lobule
(C) Precentral gyrus
(D) Postcentral gyrus
(E) Middle frontal gyrus

204. A 20-year-old female is examined by a neurologist. The patient presents initially with spastic paresthesia and double vision; additional neurologic deficits and signs are optic neuritis, internuclear ophthalmoplegia, urinary urgency, scanning speech, and Lhermitte sign. Match the neurologic deficits and signs to the lettered syndromes.

(A) Multiple sclerosis
(B) Amyotrophic lateral sclerosis
(C) Poliomyelitis
(D) Brown-Séquard syndrome
(E) Syringomyelia

ANSWERS AND EXPLANATIONS

1–B. The calcarine sulcus separates the cuneus from the lingual gyrus. The banks of the calcarine sulcus contain the visual cortex.

2–D. The superior sagittal sinus receives drainage from the greatest number of arachnoid granulations.

3–C. The Rathke pouch is an ectodermal outpocketing of the stomodeum anterior to the buccopharyngeal membrane. It gives rise to the adenohypophysis (pars distalis, pars tuberalis, and pars intermedia).

4–D. The lateral horn (T1–L3) gives rise to preganglionic sympathetic fibers.

5–B. The nucleus dorsalis of Clarke (C8–L3) gives rise to the dorsal spinocerebellar tract, which ascends and enters the cerebellum through the inferior cerebellar peduncle.

6–D. In the midbrain, the pyramidal tract lies in the basis pedunculi; oculomotor fibers of CN III pass through the medial part of the basis pedunculi. In the pons, the pyramidal tract lies in the base of the pons; abducent fibers of CN VI pass through the lateral part of the pyramidal fasciculi. In the medulla, the pyramidal tracts form the medullary pyramids; hypoglossal fibers of CN XII lie just lateral to the pyramids.

7–E. The primary auditory cortex (areas 41 and 42) is located in the transverse temporal gyri of Heschl, a part of the superior temporal gyrus.

8–C. The neocerebellum (the posterior lobe minus the vermis and the paravermis) sends input to the motor cortex through the ventral lateral nucleus of the thalamus. The pathway is the neocerebellar cortex, dentate nucleus, contralateral ventral lateral nucleus of the thalamus, and motor cortex (area 4).

9–C. The dentatothalamic tract decussates in the caudal midbrain tegmentum at the level of the inferior colliculus. This massive decussation of the superior cerebellar peduncles is characteristic of this level.

10–C. Pituitary tumors frequently compress the decussating fibers of the optic chiasm and produce a bitemporal hemianopia. Nasal fibers decussate, and temporal fibers remain ipsilateral.

11–B. Resection of the anterior portion of the temporal lobe transects the fibers of the loop of Meyer and results in a contralateral upper homonymous quadrantanopia. Inferior retinal quadrants are represented in the inferior banks of the calcarine sulcus.

12–A. Headache and papilledema are signs of brain tumor, and pronator drift is a frontal lobe sign due to weakness of the supinator muscle. Tumor pressure on the corticospinal tract results in contralateral spastic hemiparesis. In progressive supranuclear palsy the patient cannot look down. In myasthenia gravis there is weakness of skeletal muscle. In pseudotumor cerebri there are no mass lesions but headache and papilledema. In subacute combined degeneration the posterior columns and the corticospinal tracts are affected.

13–D. The lateral corticospinal tract and the lateral spinothalamic tract are both found in the lateral column. Transection of the corticospinal tract results in ipsilateral paresis, and transection of the spinothalamic tract results in contralateral loss of pain and temperature sensation. Pallesthesia (vibration sense) is normal.

14–D. The contralateral oculomotor nerve is responsible for the consensual reaction.

15–A. Hyperacusis is increased acuity of hearing and undue sensitivity to low tones. It results from paralysis of the stapedius muscle (CN VII). The stapedius reduces the amplitude of sound vibrations of the stapes in the oval window.

16–D. The mandibular division of the trigeminal nerve (CN V-3) innervates the muscles of mastication (e.g., masseter muscle) and mediates the tactile sensation of the anterior two-thirds of the tongue. The glossopharyngeal nerve (CN IX) provides the tactile, nociceptive, and taste innervation of the posterior third of the tongue. The facial nerve (CN VII) provides taste innervation to the anterior two-thirds of the tongue.

17–D. This is the classic lateral medullary syndrome, which is also known as Wallenberg syndrome (see Figure 14-1B).

18–B. This is a classic medial midbrain lesion characteristic of Weber syndrome. It includes the crus cerebri and the exiting intra-axial fibers of the oculomotor nerve (see Figure 14-3C).

19–A. The metal fragment is found between the inferior frontal gyrus and the supramarginal gyrus. The two gyri are connected by the arcuate fasciculus; transection results in conduction aphasia. The arcuate fasciculus interconnects Broca area and Wernicke area. The key deficit is the inability to repeat (see Figure 24-1).

20–D. Norepinephrine is the neurotransmitter of postganglionic sympathetic neurons, with the exception of sweat glands and some blood vessels that receive cholinergic sympathetic innervation. Epinephrine is produced by the chromaffin cells of the adrenal medulla.

21–D. Bilateral damage of the medial temporal gyri, including the amygdalae, may cause severe memory loss (hippocampal formations). Such damage to the amygdalae may lead to inappropriate social behavior (e.g., hyperphagia, hypersexuality, general disinhibition). Bilateral destruction of the amygdalae results in Klüver-Bucy syndrome.

22–E. Presbyopia is progressive loss of the ability to accommodate, the decreased ability to focus on near objects. Astigmatism is the difference in refracting power of the cornea and lens in different meridians. Cataracts are opacities of the lens that appear with aging. Optic atrophy is degeneration of the optic nerve and papillomacular bundle and loss of central vision.

23–E. The corticospinal fibers are not completely myelinated at birth; this does not occur until 18 months to 2 years of age. During this time, the Babinski reflex can be elicited; later it is suppressed.

24–C. The nucleus of the solitary tract receives taste fibers from cranial nerves VII, IX, and X. Neurons of this tract project to the ventral posteromedial nucleus of the thalamus.

25–D. The supplementary motor cortex plans for motor activity. Broca area is a language center. The angular gyrus is concerned with mnemonic constellations. The motor strip gives rise to the corticospinal and corticobulbar tracts. The S-1 somatosensory cortex subserves somatic sensibility.

26–B. Destruction of the right cuneate nucleus results in apallesthesia (loss of vibration sensation) in the right hand. The cuneate nucleus, a way station in the posterior column-medial lemniscus pathway, mediates tactile discrimination and vibration sensation.

27–E. Eccrine sweat glands are innervated by postganglionic sympathetic cholinergic fibers. Apocrine sweat glands are innervated by postganglionic sympathetic norepinephrinergic fibers. (Note: This item is often tested.)

28–E. The vagal nerves mediate the feeling of nausea via general visceral afferent fibers.

29–A. Cerebrospinal fluid enters the bloodstream via the arachnoid villi. Hypertrophied arachnoid villi are called arachnoid granulations or pacchionian bodies.

30–A. Aqueductal stenosis results in enlargement of the third and lateral ventricles. The condition is strongly associated with prenatal infections (e.g., cytomegalovirus infection). Congenital hydrocephalus occurs in 1 in 1000 live births. Mental retardation, spasticity, and tremor are common. Shunting is the treatment of choice; cerebrospinal fluid is shunted from the distended ventricle to the peritoneal cavity.

31–E. Alzheimer disease is commonly seen in trisomy 21, or Down syndrome, after 40 years of age. It is the most common single cause of mental retardation. The neuropathology of Down syndrome is similar to that of Alzheimer disease: reduced choline acetyltransferase activity, cell loss in the nucleus basalis of Meynert, an increase of amyloid β-protein, and Alzheimer neurofibrillary changes and neuritic plaques are always found.

32–B. This describes classic Guillain-Barré syndrome, with prior infection, ascending paralysis, distal paresthesias, and albuminocytologic dissociation.

33–C. This is a classic description of multiple sclerosis. Characteristics of the condition are exacerbations and remissions, involvement (demyelination) of long tracts, blurred vision, and an afferent pupillary defect. Cerebrospinal fluid contains electrophoretically detectable oligoclonal immunoglobulin (oligoclonal bands). In addition, rates of synthesis and concentration of intrathecally generated immunoglobulin G and immunoglobulin M in the cerebrospinal fluid are elevated. Oligoclonal bands are also found in syphilis, meningoencephalitis, subacute sclerosing panencephalitis, and Guillain-Barré syndrome.

34–D. Proliferating Schwann cells may give rise to schwannomas, which are also called acoustic neuromas or neurilemmomas.

35–E. Hemisection of the spinal cord would result in ipsilateral spastic paresis below the lesion and loss of pain and temperature on the contralateral side. The plantar response would be extensor and ipsilateral (Babinski sign).

36–E. A lesion of the vestibular nuclei (lower brainstem) eliminates oculovestibular reflexes.

37–B. An anticholinergic agent (e.g., trihexyphenidyl) may be used as an alternative to L-dopa to alleviate the chemical imbalance found in the striatum of a patient with Parkinson disease.

38–C. Fluoxetine (Prozac) is the most selective inhibitor of serotonin reuptake.

39–B. The paramedian (transverse pontine) branches of the basilar artery supply the medial longitudinal fasciculus of the pons. Destruction of this fasciculus results in medial longitudinal fasciculus syndrome, or internuclear ophthalmoplegia. In addition, the superior cerebellar artery may irrigate the medial longitudinal fasciculus.

40–B. This is a classic national-board lesion, the lateral medullary syndrome, also called Wallenberg syndrome; symptoms include contralateral loss of pain and temperature sensation from the face, loss of gag reflex, hemiataxia and hemisynergia of cerebellar type, Horner's syndrome, ipsilateral nystagmus. The affected structures are the medial and inferior vestibular nuclei, inferior cerebellar peduncle, nucleus ambiguus of CN IX, CN X, and CN XI (somatic visceral efferent), glossopharyngeal nerve roots, vagal nerve roots, spinothalamic tracts, the spinal trigeminal nucleus and tract, and the descending sympathetic tract.

41–A. A lesion of the upper left retinal quadrant in the left eye would show radioactive label in the left cuneus. Lesions of the cuneus result in lower field defects, and lesions of the lingual gyrus result in upper field defects. Remember, upper retinal quadrants project to the upper banks of the calcarine fissure, and lower retinal quadrants project to the lower banks of the calcarine fissure.

42–C. The dentate nucleus receives massive input from the contralateral inferior olivary nucleus; it projects crossed fibers to the ventral lateral nucleus of the thalamus and red nucleus (parvocellular part). The lateral cuneate nucleus gives rise to the cuneocerebellar tract, and the lateral lemniscus and its nuclei are important way stations in the auditory pathway.

43–B. The right ventral posterolateral nucleus receives posterior column modalities via the medial lemniscus from the left side of the body. The nucleus ruber is a midbrain motor nucleus: it plays a role in the control of flexor tone. The lateral cuneate nucleus projects unconscious proprioception to the cerebellum, (e.g., from muscles and tendons). The ventral lateral nucleus receives input from the cerebellum (dentate nucleus).

44–D. The nucleus of the inferior colliculus projects retrogradely to the inferior olivary nucleus of the caudal pons. The medial geniculate nucleus is an auditory way station, the inferior olivary nucleus is a cerebellar relay station, and the transverse gyrus of Heschl is a primary auditory center. Retrograde transport studies show that horseradish peroxidase is picked up by the axon terminals and transported to the perikarya; anterograde studies show that labeled amino acids are taken up by the perikarya and transported anterograde to distant nuclei.

45–D. The base of the pons contains intra-axial root fibers of CN V, corticobulbar fibers to nucleus CN XII, and corticospinal fibers. Spinotrigeminal fibers mediate pain and temperature sensation from the ipsilateral face.

46–A. The open medulla contains the medial lemniscus bilateral and root fibers of CN XII bilateral. Deficits to the medial lemniscus would result in contralateral loss of proprioception, discriminative tactile sensation, and vibration sensation from the trunk and lower extremity. The medulla gives rise to CN IX, CN X, CN XI, and CN XII, and CN XII controls movement of the tongue.

47–C. The pontine tegmentum contains CN VI and CN VII; the medial longitudinal fasciculus (MLF), medial lemniscus, spinotrigeminal nucleus and tract; spinal thalamic tract; and the spinohypothalamic tract (Horner syndrome). Internuclear ophthalmoplegia, also known as MLF syndrome, results from a lesion of the MLF. Lesions occur in the dorsomedial pontine tegmentum and may affect one or both MLFs. This is a frequent sign of multiple sclerosis; it results in medial rectus palsy on attempted lateral gaze and monocular nystagmus in the abducting eye with normal convergence.

48–A. Thrombosis of the anterior spinal artery results in the medial medullary syndrome. Symptoms of medial medullary syndrome include contralateral hemiparesis of the trunk and extremities; contralateral loss of proprioception, discriminative tactile sensation, and vibration sensation from the trunk and extremities; and ipsilateral flaccid paralysis of the tongue.

49–B. Wernicke speech area is in the posterior superior temporal gyrus (Brodmann's area 22). Wernicke aphasia is characterized by faster-than-normal speech, difficulty finding the right words to express ideas, and poor comprehension of the speech of others. Patients appear unaware of the deficit.

50–B. Pick disease, frontotemporal lobar degeneration, shows an extreme degree of atrophy in the temporal and frontal lobes. Creutzfeldt-Jakob is a human prion disease affecting the central nervous system. Down syndrome is a chromosomal anomaly characterized by trisomy 21. Tuberous sclerosis and Sturge-Weber syndrome are neurocutaneous diseases that result in lesions of the skin and neurologic problems (e.g. mental retardation, seizures).

51–A. The arcuate fasciculus (superior longitudinal fasciculus) is a fiber trajectory that interconnects Broca speech area (44, 45) with Wernicke speech area (22). Transection of this fiber bundle results in conduction aphasia with poor repetition of spoken language, relatively good speech comprehension and expression, paraphrasic errors (using incorrect words), and impaired object naming. Patients are aware of the deficit.

52–D. The pineal body is a midline diencephalic structure that contains calcium concrements; it is seen in computed tomographic images. The cerebral peduncles, the superior and inferior colliculi, the oculomotor nerves, and the cerebral aqueduct are found in the midbrain. Stenosis of the aqueduct results in noncommunicating hydrocephalus.

53–H. The optic nerve is derived from the wall of the diencephalic vesicle.

54–F. The oculomotor nerve is often damaged in the process of transtentorial herniation.

55–K. The vagal nerve mediates the sensory and motor innervation of the pharyngeal arches 4 and 6.

56–J. The trochlear nerve innervates the muscle that depresses, intorts, and abducts the globe.

57–A. Parkinson disease is characterized by a symptom triad: pill-rolling tremor, rigidity, and hypokinesia. The substantia nigra (a basal ganglion) bears the brunt of the cell loss. (Other basal ganglia are the caudate nucleus, putamen, and globus pallidus.) Cerebellar disease is characterized by intention tremor, ataxia, and hypotonia. Destruction of the subthalamic nucleus results in contralateral hemiballismus.

58–H. In amyotrophic lateral sclerosis there is loss of both ventral horn cells and cortical pyramidal cells that give rise to the pyramidal tract. This motor system disease consists of an upper motor neuron component and a lower motor neuron component. There are no sensory deficits in amyotrophic lateral sclerosis.

59–C. The cerebral aqueduct is in the midbrain (mesencephalon). It interconnects the third and fourth ventricles.

60–C. The tegmentum of the midbrain contains the nuclei of the oculomotor nerve (CN III) and the trochlear nerve (CN IV). The midbrain also contains the mesencephalic nucleus of the trigeminal nerve (CN V).

61–E. The caudate nucleus, a basal ganglion, is located in the white matter of the telencephalon. It forms the lateral wall of the frontal horn of the lateral ventricle.

62–A. The optic chiasma is in the diencephalon between the anterior commissure and the infundibulum of the pituitary gland (hypophysis).

63–B. The olive and the pyramid are prominent structures on the surface of the medulla. The olive contains the inferior olivary nucleus. The pyramid contains the corticospinal tract.

64–A. The pineal gland (epiphysis cerebri) is part of the epithalamus, which is a subdivision of the diencephalon.

65–B. Cranial nerves IX, X, XI, and XII are located in the medulla.

66–E. Schwann cells of the peripheral nervous system are neural crest derivatives.

67–D. Oligodendrocytes of the central nervous system may myelinate numerous axons. Schwann cells myelinate only one internode.

68–A. The filaments of astrocytes contain fibrillary glial acidic protein, a marker for astrocytes and astrocytic tumor cells. Another biochemical marker is glutamine synthetase found exclusively in astrocytes.

69–E. Schwann cells are myelin-forming cells of the peripheral nervous system. They myelinate only one internode and are derived from the neural crest. Schwann cells function in regeneration and remyelination of severed axons in the peripheral nervous system but may proliferate to form schwannomas, benign tumors of peripheral nerves (e.g. acoustic neuromas of CN VIII).

70–C. Microglial cells arise from monocytes. They are phagocytes of the central nervous system and are also called rod cells, Gitterzellen, histiocytes, and macrocytes.

71–B. Interruption of the dorsal spinocerebellar tract results in ipsilateral leg dystaxia (i.e., inco-ordination). The cerebellum is deprived of its muscle spindle input from the lower extremity.

72–D. Destruction of ventral horn cells (lower motor neurons) results in ipsilateral flaccid paralysis with muscle atrophy and loss of muscle stretch reflexes (areflexia).

73–E. Interruption of the lateral spinothalamic tract results in a contralateral loss of pain and temperature sensation one segment below the lesion. The decussation occurs in the ventral white commissure in the spinal cord.

74–C. Interruption of the lateral corticospinal tract results in an ipsilateral upper motor neuron lesion. It is characterized by exaggerated muscle stretch reflexes (hyperreflexia), spastic paresis, muscle weakness, a loss or diminution of superficial reflexes (i.e., abdominal and cremaster reflexes), and the Babinski sign. The deficits are below the lesion on the same side. The lateral corticospinal tract decussates in the caudal medulla.

75–A. A lesion of the gracile fasciculus results in a loss of two-point tactile discrimination in the ipsilateral foot. The dorsal column–medial lemniscus pathway decussates in the caudal medulla.

76–C. This lesion includes the two medial longitudinal fasciculi. The patient has medial longitudinal fasciculus syndrome and medial rectus palsy on attempted lateral gaze to either side. Convergence remains intact.

77–E. This lesion includes three major structures: the medial lemniscus, corticospinal fibers, and exiting abducent root fibers (CN VI) traversing the corticospinal fibers. Interruption of the abducent fibers causes ipsilateral lateral rectus paralysis with medial strabismus. Damage to the uncrossed corticospinal fibers results in contralateral spastic hemiparesis.

78–A. Occlusion of the posterior inferior cerebellar artery (PICA) infarcts the lateral zone of the medulla, causing PICA syndrome. The major involved structures are the inferior cerebellar peduncle, spinal trigeminal tract and nucleus, spinal lemniscus, nucleus ambiguus, and exiting vagal fibers of CN X.

79–D. This lesion includes the facial motor nucleus of CN VII and its intra-axial fibers, hence the loss of the corneal reflex (efferent limb). The spinal trigeminal tract and nucleus and the spinal lemniscus also are damaged by this lesion. Damage to the spinal trigeminal tract and nucleus causes ipsilateral facial anesthesia, including loss of the corneal reflex (afferent limb). Damage to the spinal lemniscus (lateral spinothalamic tract) causes a contralateral loss of pain and temperature sensation from the body and extremities.

80–B. This lesion damages the hypoglossal nucleus of CN X and exiting root fibers, the medial lemniscus, and the corticospinal tract. Damage to the hypoglossal nerve results in an ipsilateral flaccid paralysis of the tongue, a lower motor neuron lesion. Damage to the medial lemniscus results in a contralateral loss of tactile discrimination and vibration sensation. Damage to the corticospinal (pyramid) tracts results in contralateral spastic hemiparesis. This symptom complex is known as medial medullary syndrome.

81–A. Lateral medullary syndrome (posterior inferior cerebellar artery syndrome) usually includes hoarseness, Horner syndrome, and singultus (hiccups). Damage to the nucleus ambiguus causes flaccid paralysis of the muscle of the larynx with hoarseness (dysphonia and dysarthria). Interruption of descending autonomic fibers to the ciliospinal center at T1 causes sympathetic paralysis of the eye (Horner syndrome). The anatomic causes of singultus are not clear.

82–C. The ventral lateral nucleus receives input from the dentate nucleus of the cerebellum and projects to the motor cortex (area 4). The ventral posterolateral nucleus also receives input from the dentate nucleus and projects to the motor cortex.

83–D. The ventral posteromedial nucleus receives input of taste sensation from the solitary nucleus of the medulla and pons and projects this input to the gustatory cortex of the parietal operculum (area 43).

84–D. The ventral posteromedial nucleus receives general somatic afferent input from the face, including pain and temperature sensation. It also receives special visceral afferent taste sensation) input from the tongue and epiglottis.

85–A. The anterior thalamic nucleus receives input from the mamillary nucleus via the mamillothalamic tract and direct input from the hippocampal formation via the fornix. The anterior nucleus projects, via the anterior limb of the internal capsule, to the cingulate gyrus (areas 23, 24, and 32).

86–B. The centromedian nucleus, the largest of the intralaminar nuclei, projects to the putamen and to the motor cortex. The centromedian nucleus receives input from the globus pallidus and the motor cortex (area 4).

87–E. The mediodorsal nucleus of the thalamus, or the dorsomedial nucleus, has reciprocal connections with the prefrontal cortex (areas 9–12).

88–C. The mamillary nucleus receives input from the hippocampal formation (i.e., subiculum) via the fornix.

89–A. The anterior nucleus of the hypothalamus helps prevent a rise in body temperature by activating processes that favor heat loss (e.g., vasodilation of cutaneous blood vessels, sweating). Lesions of this nucleus result in hyperthermia (hyperpyrexia).

90–E. The suprachiasmatic nucleus receives direct input from the retina; it plays a role in the maintenance of circadian rhythms.

91–D. The neurons of the paraventricular and supraoptic nuclei of the hypothalamus produce antidiuretic hormone (vasopressin) and oxytocin. These peptides are transported via the supraopticohypophyseal tract to the neurohypophysis. Lesions of these nuclei or their hypophyseal tract result in diabetes insipidus.

92–B. The neurons of the arcuate nucleus (infundibular nucleus) produce hypothalamic-releasing and release-inhibiting hormones, which are conveyed to the adenohypophysis through the hypophyseal portal system. These hormones regulate production of adenohypophyseal hormones and their release into the systemic circulation.

93–D. The paraventricular and supraoptic nuclei produce antidiuretic hormone, which helps regulate water balance in the body.

COMPREHENSIVE EXAMINATION

94–E. Hemiballism results from circumscript lesions of the subthalamic nucleus.

95–A. The caudate nucleus and the putamen (caudatoputamen) receive dopaminergic input from the pars compacta of the substantia nigra, the nigrostriatal tract.

96–B. Neurons of the globus pallidus give rise to the ansa lenticularis and the lenticular fasciculus, two pathways that project to the ventral anterior, ventral lateral, and centromedian nuclei of the thalamus.

97–D. Destruction or degeneration of the substantia nigra results in parkinsonism (hypokinetic rigid syndrome).

98–A. In Huntington chorea, there is a loss of neurons in the striatum. Cell loss in the head of the caudate nucleus causes dilation of the frontal horn of the lateral ventricle (hydrocephalus ex vacuo), which is visible on computed tomography and magnetic resonance imaging studies.

99–E. Serotonin (5-HT) is produced by neurons located in the raphe nuclei. This paramidline column of cells extends from the caudal medulla to the rostral midbrain.

100–C. Purkinje neurons are GABA-ergic. GABA-ergic neurons are also found in the striatum, globus pallidus, and pars reticularis of the substantia nigra.

101–A. The nucleus basalis of Meynert contains cholinergic neurons that project to the entire neocortex. This griseum is a ventral forebrain nucleus embedded in the substantia innominata (ventral to the globus pallidus). This nucleus degenerates in Alzheimer disease.

102–A. Acetylcholine is the neurotransmitter of motor cranial nerves (general somatic efferent, special visceral efferent, and general visceral efferent) and anterior horn cells of the spinal cord.

103–B. Neurons of the pars compacta of the substantia nigra contain dopamine. Dopamine also is present in the ventral tegmental area of the midbrain, the superior colliculus, and the arcuate nucleus of the hypothalamus.

104–D. The locus ceruleus is the largest assembly of noradrenergic (norepinephrinergic) neurons in the brain. It is located in the lateral pontine and midbrain tegmenta. Locus ceruleus neurons project to the entire neocortex and cerebellar cortex.

105–C. The globus pallidus contains GABA-ergic neurons that project to the thalamus and subthalamic nucleus.

106–E. Substance P is contained in dorsal root ganglion cells and is the neurotransmitter of afferent pain fibers. Substance P also is produced by striatal neurons, which project to the globus pallidus and substantia nigra.

107–B. Glycine is the major inhibitory neurotransmitter of the spinal cord. The Renshaw interneurons of the spinal cord are glycinergic.

108–A. Glutamate is the major excitatory neurotransmitter of the brain; neocortical glutamatergic neurons project to the caudate nucleus and the putamen (striatum).

109–C. β-Endorphinergic neurons are located almost exclusively in the hypothalamus (arcuate and premamillary nuclei).

110–D. Enkephalinergic neurons in the dorsal horn of the spinal cord presynaptically inhibit the dorsal root ganglion cells that mediate pain impulses.

111–E. A lesion of the lingual gyrus of the right occipital lobe can cause a left upper homonymous quadrantanopia. Lower retinal quadrants are represented in the lower banks of the calcarine sulcus.

112–A. A lesion of the Broca speech area (areas 44 and 45) and the adjacent motor cortex of the precentral gyrus (area 4) can cause Broca expressive aphasia and an upper motor neuron lesion involving the hand area of the motor strip. This territory is supplied by the superior division of the middle cerebral artery (prerolandic and rolandic arteries).

113–C. A parietal lesion in the left postcentral gyrus (areas 3, 1, and 2) or in the left superior parietal lobule (areas 5 and 7) can cause astereognosis, the deficit in which a patient with eyes closed cannot identify a familiar object placed in the right hand. This territory is supplied by the superior division of the middle cerebral artery (the rolandic and anterior parietal arteries). The dorsal aspect of the superior parietal lobule on the convex surface is also supplied by the anterior cerebral artery.

114–C. Characteristic signs of damage to the nondominant hemisphere include hemineglect, topographic memory loss, denial of deficit (anosognosia), and construction and dressing apraxia. A lesion in the right inferior parietal lobule could account for these deficits. This territory is supplied by the inferior division of the middle cerebral artery (posterior parietal and angular arteries).

115–D. Wernicke receptive aphasia is characterized by poor comprehension of speech, unawareness of the deficit, and difficulty finding the correct words to express a thought. The Wernicke speech area is found in the posterior part of the left superior temporal gyrus (area 22). This territory is supplied by the inferior division of the middle cerebral artery (posterior temporal branches).

116–B. Gerstmann syndrome includes left-right confusion, finger agnosia, dysgraphia, and dyscalculia. This syndrome results from a lesion of the left angular gyrus of the inferior parietal lobule. This territory is supplied by branches from the inferior division of the middle cerebral artery (angular and posterior parietal arteries).

117–A. A lesion of the anterior paracentral lobule results in an upper motor neuron lesion (spastic paresis) involving the contralateral foot. Ankle clonus, exaggerated muscle stretch reflexes, and the Babinski sign are common.

118–D. The thalamus.

119–E. The anterior limb of the internal capsule.

120–B. The putamen.

121–A. The head of the caudate nucleus.

122–C. The splenium of the corpus callosum.

123–C. The medial geniculate body.

124–B. The mesencephalon.

125–D. The mamillary body.

126–E. The optic tract.

127–A. The amygdala (amygdaloid nuclear complex).

128–C. The pineal gland (epiphysis).

129–E. The hypophysis (pituitary gland).

130–D. The mesencephalon (midbrain).

131–B. The thalamus.

132–A. The fornix.

133–J. A right third-nerve palsy with complete ptosis. The ptosis results from paralysis of the levator palpebrae muscle.

134–I. A destructive lesion of the frontal eye fields results in a deviation of the eyes toward the lesion. An irritative lesion results in deviation of the eyes away from the lesion.

135–H. The Argyll Robertson pupil is characterized by irregular miotic pupils that do not respond to light but do converge in response to accommodation. It is a sign of tertiary syphilis.

136–G. A right fourth-nerve palsy is characterized by the inability of the patient to depress the glove from the adducted position.

137–F. Parinaud syndrome is characterized by inability to perform upward or downward conjugate gaze and may be associated with ptosis and pupillary abnormalities.

138–E. A right sixth-nerve palsy is characterized by inability to abduct the eye.

139–D. A third-nerve palsy is characterized by a down-and-out eye, complete ptosis, and a dilated (blown) pupil. The lid was retracted to view the pupil.

140–C. Internuclear ophthalmoplegia results from a lesion of one or both medial longitudinal fasciculi. Transection of the right medial longitudinal fasciculus results in medial rectus palsy on attempted lateral gaze to the left. Convergence is normal, and nystagmus is seen in the abducting eye.

141–B. Horner syndrome consists of miosis, mild ptosis, hemianhidrosis, and enophthalmos. It results from a loss of sympathetic input to the head.

142–A. Retrobulbar neuritis is an inflammation of the optic nerve that reduces the light-carrying ability of the nerve. This condition can be diagnosed by the swinging flashlight test. Light shown into the normal eye results in constriction of both pupils. Swinging the flashlight to the affected eye results in a dilated pupil in both eyes. This pupil is called an afferent, or Marcus Gunn, pupil.

143–C. A bilateral lesion of the ventromedial hypothalamic nucleus results in hyperphagia and savage behavior.

144–D. A bilateral lesion of the posterior hypothalamic nucleus results in the inability to thermoregulate (poikilothermia). Bilateral destruction of only the posterior aspect of the lateral hypothalamic nucleus results in anorexia and emaciation.

145–A. Lesions involving the supraoptic and paraventricular nuclei or the supraopticohypophyseal tract result in diabetes insipidus with polydipsia and polyuria.

146–B. Destruction of the anterior hypothalamic nuclei results in hyperthermia.

147–E. Stimulation of the ventromedial nuclei inhibits the urge to eat, resulting in emaciation (cachexia). Destruction of the ventromedial nuclei results in hyperphagia and savage behavior.

148–H. Stimulation of the frontal eye field (Brodmann area 8) results in turning of the eyes and head to the contralateral side.

149–G. A lesion of the Broca speech area (Brodmann areas 44, 45) results in nonfluent, effortful, and telegraphic speech, as well as Broca aphasia.

150–F. Ablation of the anterior third of the temporal lobe interrupts the loop of Meyer, which projects to the lingual gyrus (the lower bank of the calcarine fissure). The lower bank of the calcarine fissure represents the upper visual field. This lesion results in a contralateral upper homonymous quadrantanopia—pie in the sky.

151–E. A lesion destroying the Wernicke area (Brodmann 22) is Wernicke aphasia, which is characterized by poor comprehension, fluent speech, poor repetition, and paraphasic errors (non sequiturs, neologisms, and driveling speech [meaningless double talk]).

152–D. This constellation of dominant hemispheric deficits results from destruction of the angular gyrus (Brodmann area 39). Called Gerstmann syndrome, it is characterized by left-right confusion, finger agnosia, dyslexia, dysgraphia, dyscalculia, and a homonymous contralateral lower quadrantanopia.

153–C. A lesion of the supramarginal gyrus (Brodmann area 40) or of the arcuate fasciculus results in conduction aphasia characterized by fluent speech, good comprehension, poor repetition, and paraphrasic speech (fluently spoken jargon-like Wernicke aphasia) and writing.

154–B. Lesions of the postcentral gyrus, sensory strip (Brodmann area 3, 1, 2) result in contralateral astereognosia, hemihypesthesia, and agraphesthesia.

155–A. Lesions of the precentral gyrus, motor strip (Brodmann area 4) result in contralateral spastic hemiparesis with pyramidal signs.

156–G. In thiamine (vitamin B1) deficiency, hemorrhagic lesions are found in the mamillary bodies.

157–F. Bilateral lesions of the amygdala result in Klüver-Bucy syndrome, with hyperphagia, hypersexuality, and psychic blindness (visual agnosia).

158–E. Bilateral damage to the parahippocampal gyri and the underlying hippocampal formation results in severe loss of short-term memory (e.g., hypoxia, hypoxemia, and herpes simplex virus encephalitis).

159–D. Lesions of the cuneus interrupt the visual radiations en route to the upper bank of the calcarine fissure, which represents the inferior visual field quadrants.

160–C. The fornix (a limbic structure) interconnects the septal area and the hippocampal formation. Bilateral transection of this structure may result in an acute amnestic syndrome.

161–B. The motor strip for the foot is in the anterior paracentral lobule on the medial aspect of the hemisphere. A lesion here results in a contralateral hemiparesis of the foot and leg with pyramidal signs.

COMPREHENSIVE EXAMINATION **345**

162–A. Ablation of the cingulate gyrus (cingulectomies) has been used to treat psychotic and neurotic patients. The cingulate gyrus is part of the limbic lobe; lesions may result in akinesia, mutism, apathy, and indifference to pain.

163–B. The anterior spinal artery supplies the pyramids, medial lemniscus, and intra-axial fibers of the hypoglossal nerve (CN XII) in the medulla. The anterior communicating artery connects the two anterior cerebral arteries and is a common site for berry (saccular) aneurysms. The anterior choroidal artery supplies the choroid plexus of the temporal horn, the hippocampus, amygdala, optic tract, lateral geniculate body and globus pallidus. The posterior spinal artery supplies the gracile and cuneate fasciculi and their posterior relay nuclei. The posterior inferior cerebellar artery supplies the dorsolateral zone of the medulla.

164–C. The anterior spinal artery perfuses the intra-axial fibers of the anterior horn. The basilar artery gives rise to the pontine arteries. The posterior spinal artery irrigates the posterior (dorsal) columns. The vertebral artery is a branch of the subclavian artery. The anterior inferior cerebellar artery supplies the facial and trigeminal nuclei, the vestibular and cochlear nuclei.

165–D. The anterior communicating artery is a common site for berry aneurysms; berry aneurysms of the anterior communicating artery frequently pressure the optic chiasm and cause a bitemporal lower quadrantanopia. The basilar artery gives rise to the pontine arteries. The ophthalmic artery branches into the central artery of the retina. The anterior cerebral artery supplies the anterior limb of the internal capsule via the medial striate artery (Heubner's artery). The posterior communicating artery irrigates the optic chiasm, optic tract, hypothalamus, subthalamus, and anterior half of the ventral portion of thalamus. Berry aneurysms of the posterior communicating artery frequently cause third nerve palsy.

166–E. Laceration of the middle meningeal artery results in epidural hemorrhage. The middle meningeal artery lies between the periosteal and meningeal dura, below the temporal and parietal bones and supplies most of the dura and almost its entire calvarial portion.

167–E. The aneurysm was on the posterior communicating artery; pressure on the occulomotor nerve results in a complete third nerve palsy with the following signs: dilated fixed pupil, ptosis, and eye looking down and out. The anterior cerebral anterior supplies part of the caudate nucleus, putamen, and anterior limb of the internal capsule via the medial striate artery of Heubner. The anterior communicating artery supplies the leg and foot areas of the motor and sensory cortices (paracentral lobule). The internal carotid artery provides direct branches to the optic nerve, optic chiasm, hypothalamus, and genu of the internal capsule. The ophthalmic artery branches into the central artery of the retina.

168–D. The superior cerebellar artery supplies the dentate nucleus, the largest efferent nucleus of the cerebellum. Damage to this nucleus results in cerebellar signs: dystaxia, dysmetria, and intention tremor. The vertebral artery gives rise to the posterior inferior cerebellar artery, which supplies the medial and inferior vestibular nuclei, inferior cerebellar peduncle, nucleus ambiguus, intra-axial fibers of the glossopharyngeal nerve (CN IX) and vagal nerve (CN X), spinothalamic tract, and spinal trigeminal nucleus and tract. The anterior inferior cerebellar artery irrigates the dorsal lateral pons—CNN, V, VII, VIII. The posterior cerebral artery supplies the posterior half of the thalamus, the medial and lateral geniculate bodies, the occipital lobe, visual cortex, and inferior surface of the temporal lobe, including the hippocampal formation.

169–B. A lesion of the lateral rectus muscle results in diplopia and horizontal nystagmus on attempted lateral conjugated gaze. It is innervated by CN VI. The buccinator muscle (facial expression), the posterior belly of the digastric muscle (facial expression), and the orbicularis oculi (corneal reflex) are innervated by the facial nerve (CN VII). The pterygoid muscle (mouth movement) is innervated by the mandibular division of the trigeminal nerve (CN V3).

170–C. Areas 13 to 15 were omitted by Brodmann.

171–B. The trigone contains a calcified globus of choroid plexus. In axial computed tomographic sections the adult calcified pineal body is also visualized, lying halfway between the two trigona.

172–C. The subcommissural organ lies in the roof of the cerebral aqueduct near the posterior commissure; it has a blood-brain barrier. All circumventricular organs except the subcommissural organ have fenestrated capillaries and thus lack a blood-brain barrier.

173–A. The pericallosal artery, a branch of the anterior cerebral artery, irrigates the leg area of the paracentral lobule. The middle cerebral artery supplies the trunk, arm, and face areas of the motor and sensory cortices. The posterior cerebral artery supplies the occipital lobe, visual cortex, and inferior surface of the temporal lobe, including the hippocampal formation. The splenial artery supplies the spleen. Heubner's medial striate artery irrigates the anterior limb of the internal capsule.

174–B. The anterior choroidal artery is a branch of the middle cerebral artery. It supplies the amygdaloid nucleus, the posterior limb of the internal capsule, the globus pallidus, and the optic tract. Klüver-Bucy syndrome results in placidity, hypersexuality, hyperphagia, and psychic blindness (visual agnosia). Lesion of internal capsule results in Babinski sign. Lesion of globus pallidus results in contralateral reduction of rigidity in Parkinson disease.

175–B. Three cranial nerves, the abducent, facial and vestibulocochlear nerves, exit from the pontomedullary sulcus. The facial nerve has two divisions, the cranial nerve proper (motor) and the intermediate division (sensory). The intermediate division contains general somatic afferent and special visceral afferent fibers.

176–B. The anterior spinal artery supplies the pyramid and the medial lemniscus. The anterior communicating artery connects the two anterior cerebral arteries and is a common site for berry (saccular) aneurysms. The anterior choroidal artery supplies the choroid plexus of the temporal horn, the hippocampus, amygdala, optic tract, lateral geniculate body, and globus pallidus. The posterior spinal artery supplies the gracile and cuneate fasciculi and their posterior relay nuclei. The posterior inferior cerebellar artery supplies the dorsolateral zone of the medulla (Wallenberg).

177–C. The anterior spinal artery perfuses the intra-axial fibers of the anterior horn. The basilar artery gives rise to the pontine arteries. The posterior spinal artery irrigates the posterior (dorsal) columns. The vertebral artery is a branch of the subclavian artery. The anterior inferior cerebellar artery supplies the facial and trigeminal nuclei, the vestibular nuclei, and the cochlear nuclei.

178–C. The anterior communicating artery connects the two anterior cerebral arteries. Berry (saccular) aneurysms may impinge upon the optic chiasm and produce a bitemporal hemianopia. The posterior communicating artery is also the site of berry aneurisms which may pressure the oculomotor nerve causing a third nerve palsy: the eyes look "down and out".

179–E. Cerebrospinal fluid typically contains no more than 5 lymphocytes per microliter (see Table 2-1).

180–C. The normal total protein value for cerebrospinal fluid is less than 45 mg/dl in the lumbar cistern (see Table 2-1).

181–E. Normal serum glucose levels in cerebrospinal fluid are 66% of blood, which is 80 to 120 mg/dl.

182–C. Pseudotumor cerebri, or benign intracranial hypertension, is characterized by papilledema without mass, elevated cerebrospinal fluid pressure, and deteriorating vision. Normal-pressure hydrocephalus is characterized clinically by the triad of progressive dementia, ataxic gait, urinary incontinence, (wacky, wobbly, and wet). Hydrocephalus ex vacuo results from a loss of neurons in the caudate nucleus (e.g., Huntington disease). Arnold Chiari II is a cerebellomedullary malformation in which the caudal vermis, cerebellar tonsils, and medulla herniate through the foramen magnum, resulting in an obstructive hydrocephalus. Dandy-Walker consists of a huge cyst of the posterior fossa associated with atresia of the outlet foramina of Luschka and Magendie.

183–D. Cerebrospinal fluid enters the subarachnoid space via the outlet foramina of the fourth ventricle (foramina of Luschka and Magendie).

184–A. Thrombosis of the anterior spinal artery results in the medial medullary syndrome (see Figure 14-1). Deficits include contralateral hemiparesis of the trunk and extremities; contralateral loss of proprioception, discriminative tactile sensation, and vibration sensation from the trunk and extremities; and ipsilateral flaccid paralysis of the tongue.

185–C. Seizures have the highest incidence in the temporal lobe. Astrocytoma is the most common glioma in the temporal lobe. Charcot-Bouchard microaneurysms are found in the lenticulostriate arteries. They rupture most frequently in the basal ganglia. They are the most common cause of nontraumatic intraparenchymal hemorrhage. The olfactory groove meningioma impinges on the olfactory tract and optic nerve, causing ipsilateral anosmia, ipsilateral optic atrophy, and contralateral papilledema. The astrocytoma transected Meyer loop and produced the contralateral quadrantanopia.

186–A. The lesion is found in the lower closed medulla at the spinomedullary junction. The term *closed* means not covered by the fourth ventricle. A lesion of the decussation of the pyramids results in spastic paralysis of all limbs and intact sensibility. The location of the cranial nerve nuclei of the brainstem reveals where the lesion is in the neuraxis: midbrain, CN III and CN IV; pons, CN V, CN VI, CN VII, and CN VIII; medulla, CN VIII, CN IX, CN X, and CN XI.

187–B. The optic cup and its derivatives, the retina and optic nerve, develop from the diencephalon.

188–E. General somatic afferent fibers are one of four functional components of spinal nerves (see Figure 6-3). They convey sensory input from skin, muscle, bone, and joints to the central nervous system. General visceral afferent fibers convey sensory input from visceral organs to the central nervous system. Special somatic afferent fibers convey sensory information related to vision, audition and equilibrium, while special visceral afferent fibers convey sensory information related to taste and smell.

189–A. The spinal cord derives from the caudal part of the neural tube. The cranial part becomes the brain. The cavity gives rise to the central canal of the spinal cord and ventricles of the brain. The anterior neuropore is an opening in the neural tube that in the fourth week becomes the lamina terminalis. The posterior neuropore is a second opening in the neural tube that closes in the forth week.

190–D. The globus pallidus originates in the diencephalon. Neuroblasts from the subthalamus migrate into the telencephalic white matter to form the globus pallidus.

191–A. The abducent nucleus is the general somatic efferent column of the pons.

192–D. The superior salivatory nucleus is the general visceral efferent column of the pons. All somatic and visceral motor nuclei are derived from the basal plate. The cerebellum and pontine nuclei and the sensory nuclei of cranial nerves are derivatives of the alar plate.

193–E. Axons of the corticospinal tracts are not fully myelinated until the end of the second postnatal year. Babinski sign (extensor plantar reflex) can be elicited in infants for this reason.

194–E. The cochlear duct is derived from a thickening of the surface ectoderm called the otic placode.

195–D. The stapes is innervated by CN VII.

196–E. Intention tremor is a deficit in coordination of voluntary movements caused by lesions in the lateral cerebellum (e.g., finger-to-nose test). Athetosis is slow, writhing movements representative of basal ganglia damage. Chorea is involuntary movements caused by overactivity of dopamine and is a classic symptom of Huntington's disease. Cogwheel rigidity is a classic rigidity seen in Parkinson disease due to lack of dopamine. Hemiballismus is large, flinging movements of the limbs due to a lesion in the subthalamic nucleus.

197–B. The ventral spinocerebellar tract crosses the midline via the anterior commissure and crosses the dorsal aspect of the superior cerebellar peduncle to terminate in the anterior cerebellar vermis.

198–A. The stylohyoid, stylopharyngeus, and styloglossus muscles are attached to the styloid process. The stylohyoid muscle is innervated by the somatic visceral efferent component of CN VII. The stylopharyngeus is innervated by the somatic visceral efferent component of CN IX. The styloglossus is innervated by CN XII.

199–A. Rhinorrhea would most likely result from a fracture of the cribriform plate of the ethmoid bone, which could tear the arachnoid membrane and result in a leakage of cerebrospinal fluid into the nasal cavity.

200–A. The facial nerve (CN VII) innervates the taste buds from the anterior two-thirds of the tongue, providing input to the solitary tract and solitary nucleus via the geniculate ganglion (see gustatory pathway, Figure 20-2).

201–C. The maxillary nerve passes through the foramen rotundum. The mandibular nerve passes through the foramen ovale. The ophthalmic nerve passes through the superior orbital fissure. The optic nerve passes through the optic canal. The trochlear nerve passes thru the cavernous sinus. A fracture of the foramen rotundum causes damage to the maxillary nerve.

202–A. The optic canal transmits the optic nerve (CN II) and the ophthalmic artery.

203–D. The postcentral gyrus is the sensory strip, the somatosensory cortex (areas 3,1,2). Sensation to the face and tongue areas is on the inferior aspect of the postcentral gyrus (see the sensory homunculus, Chapter 23). The anterior paracentral lobule subserves motor innervation to the feet. The posterior paracentral lobule subserves sensory innervation to the feet. The precentral gyrus is the motor cortex. The middle frontal gyrus contains the frontal eye field (area 8).

204–A. Multiple sclerosis is a demyelinating disease characterized by exacerbations and remissions. In multiple sclerosis patients, cerebral spinal fluid contains oligoclonal immunoglobulin G bands, indicating chronic inflammation. Amyotrophic lateral sclerosis is a motor neuron disease. Poliomyelitis is an enterovirus. Brown-Séquard syndrome is spinal cord hemisection. Syringomyelia is central cavitation of the cervical spinal cord.

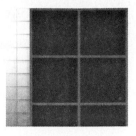

Appendix

TABLE A–1	*Appendix: Table of Cranial Nerves*			
Cranial Nerve	**Type**	**Origin**	**Function**	**Course**
I—Olfactory	SVA	Bipolar olfactory neurons (in olfactory epithelium in roof of nasal cavity)	Smell (olfaction)	Central axons project to the olfactory bulb via the cribriform plate of the ethmoid bone.
II—Optic	SSA	Retinal ganglion cells	Vision	Central axons converge at the optic disk and form the optic nerve, which enters the skull via the optic canal. Optic nerve axons terminate in the lateral geniculate bodies.
III—Oculomotor				
Parasympathetic	GVE	Edinger-Westphal nucleus (rostral midbrain)	Sphincter muscle of iris; ciliary muscle	Axons exit the midbrain; the interpeduncular fossa, traverse the cavernous sinus, and enter the orbit via the superior orbital fissure.
Motor	GSE	Oculomotor nucleus (rostral midbrain)	Superior, inferior, and medial recti muscles; inferior oblique muscle; levator palpebrae muscle	
IV—Trochlear	GSE	Trochlear nucleus (caudal midbrain)	Superior oblique muscle	Axons decussate in superior medullary velum, exit dorsally inferior to the inferior colliculi, encircle the midbrain, traverse the cavernous sinus, and enter the orbit via the superior orbital fissure.

(Continue)

349

TABLE A-1	Appendix: Table of Cranial Nerves (continued)

Cranial Nerve	Type	Origin	Function	Course
V—Trigeminal				
Motor	SVE	Motor nucleus CN V (mid pons)	Muscles of mastication and tensor tympani muscle	Ophthalmic nerve exits via the superior orbital fissure; maxillary nerve exits via the foramen rotundum; mandibular nerve exits via the foramen ovale; ophthalmic and maxillary nerves traverse the cavernous sinus; GSA fibers enter the spinal trigeminal tract of CN V.
Sensory	GSA	Trigeminal ganglion and mesencephalic nucleus CN V (rostal pons and midbrain)	Tactile, pain, and thermal sensation from the face; the oral and nasal cavities and the supratentorial dura	
VI—Abducent	GSE	Abducent nucleus (caudal pons)	Lateral rectus muscle	Axons exit the pons from the inferior pontine sulcus, traverse the cavernous sinus, and enter the orbit via the superior orbital fissure.
VII—Facial				
Parasympathetic	GVE	Superior salivatory nucleus (caudal pons)	Lacrimal gland (via sphenopalatine ganglion); submandibular and sublingual glands (via submandibular ganglion)	Axons exit the pons in the cerebellar pontine angle and enter the internal auditory meatus; motor fibers traverse the facial canal of the temporal bone and exit via the stylomastoid foramen; taste fibers traverse the chorda tympani and lingual nerve; GSA fibers enter the spinal trigeminal tract of CN V; SVA fibers enter the solitary tract.
Motor	SVE	Facial nucleus (caudal pons)	Muscles of facial expression; stapedius muscle	
Sensory	GSA	Geniculate ganglion (temporal bone)	Tactile sensation to skin of ear	
Sensory	SVA	Geniculate ganglion	Taste sensation from the anterior two-thirds of tongue (via chorda tympani)	

TABLE A-1		*Appendix: Table of Cranial Nerves (continued)*		
Cranial Nerve	**Type**	**Origin**	**Function**	**Course**
VIII—Vestibulocochlear Vestibular nerve	SSA	Vestibular ganglion (internal auditory meatus)	Equilibrium (innervates hair cells of semicircular ducts, saccule, and utricle)	Vestibular and cochlear nerves join in the internal auditory meatus and enter the brain stem in the cerebellopontine angle; vestibular nerve projects to the vestibular nuclei and the flocculonodular lobe of the cerebellum; cochlear nerve projects to the cochlear nuclei.
Cochlear nerve		Spiral ganglion (modiolus of temporal bone)	Hearing (innervates hair cells of the organ of Corti)	
IX—Glossopharyngeal Parasympathetic	GVE	Inferior salivatory nucleus (rostral medulla)	Parotid gland (via the otic ganglion)	Axons exit (motor) and enter (sensory) medulla from the postolivary sulcus; axons exit and enter the skull via jugular foramen; GSA fibers enter the spinal trigeminal tract of CN V; GVA and SVA fibers enter the solitary tract.
Motor	SVE	Nucleus ambigus (rostral medulla)	Stylopharyngeus muscle	
Sensory	GSA	Superior ganglion (jugular foramen)	Tactile sensation to external ear	
Sensory	GVA	Inferior (petrosal) ganglion (in jugular foramen)	Tactile sensation to posterior third of tongue, pharynx, middle ear, and auditory tube; input from carotid sinus and carotid body	
Sensory	SVA	Inferior (petrosal) ganglion (in jugular foramen)	Taste from posterior third of the tongue	
X—Vagal Parasympathetic	GVE	Dorsal nucleus of CN X (medulla)	Viscera of the thoracic and abdominal cavities to the left colic flexure [via terminal (mural) ganglia]	Axons exit (motor) and enter (sensory) medulla from the postolivary sulcus; axons exit and enter the skull via the jugular foramen; GSA fibers enter the spinal trigeminal tract of CN V; GVA and SVA fibers enter the solitary tract.

(Continue)

TABLE A–1	**Appendix: Table of Cranial Nerves (continued)**

Cranial Nerve	Type	Origin	Function	Course
Motor	SVE	Nucleus ambigus (mid-medulla)	Muscles of the larynx and pharynx	
Sensory	GSA	Superior ganglion (jugular foramen)	Tactile sensation to the external ear	
Sensory	GVA	Inferior (nodose) ganglion (in jugular foramen)	Mucous membranes of the pharynx, larynx, esophagus, trachea, and thoracic and abdominal viscera to the left colic flexure	
Sensory	SVA	Inferior (nodose) ganglion (in jugular foramen)	Taste from the epiglottis	
XI—Accessory				
Motor (cranial)	SVE	Nucleus ambiguus (medulla)	Intrinsic muscles of the larynx (except the cricothyroid muscle) via recurrent laryngeal nerve	Axons from the cranial division exit the medulla from the postolivary sulcus and join the vagal nerve; axons from spinal division exit the spinal cord, ascend through the foramen magnum, and exit the skull via the jugular foramen.
Motor (spinal)		Ventral horn neurons C1–C6	Sternocleidomastoid and trapezius muscles	
XII—Hypoglossal	GSE	Hypoglossal nucleus (medulla)	Intrinsic and extrinsic muscles of the tongue (except the palatoglossus muscle)	Axons exit from the preolivary sulcus of the medulla and exit the skull via the hypoglossal canal.

SVA = special visceral afferent; SSA = special somatic afferent; GVE = general visceral efferent; GSE = general somatic efferent; SVE = special visceral efferent; GSA = general somatic afferent; GVA = general visceral afferent; CN = cranial nerve.

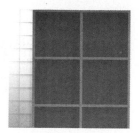

Glossary

abasia—Inability to walk.

abulia—Inability to perform voluntary actions or to make decisions; seen in bilateral frontal lobe disease.

accommodation—Increase in thickness of the lens needed to focus a near external object on the retina.

adenohypophysis—Anterior lobe of the pituitary gland, derived from Rathke pouch.

adenoma sebaceum—Cutaneous lesion seen in tuberous sclerosis.

Adie pupil—Myotonic pupil; a tonic pupil, usually large, that constricts very slowly to light and convergence; generally unilateral and frequently occurs in young women with absent knee or ankle reflexes.

afferent pupil (Marcus Gunn pupil)—A pupil that reacts sluggishly to direct light stimulation; caused by a lesion of the afferent pathway (e.g., multiple sclerosis involving the optic nerve).

agenesis—Failure of a structure to develop (e.g., agenesis of the corpus callosum).

ageusia—Loss of the sensation of taste (gustation).

agnosia—Lack of the sensory-perceptional ability to recognize objects; visual, auditory, and tactile.

agraphesthesia—Inability to recognize figures written on the skin.

agraphia—Inability to write; seen in Gerstmann syndrome.

akathisia—Acathisia, the inability to remain in a sitting position; motor restlessness; may appear after the withdrawal of neuroleptic drugs.

akinesia—Absence or loss of the power of voluntary motion; seen in Parkinson disease.

akinetic mutism—State in which patient can move and speak but cannot be prompted to do so; due to bilateral occlusion of the anterior cerebral artery or midbrain lesions.

alar plate—Division of the mantle zone that gives rise to sensory neurons; receives sensory input from the dorsal root ganglia.

albuminocytologic dissociation—Elevated cerebrospinal fluid (CSF) protein with a normal CSF cell count; seen in Guillain-Barré syndrome.

alexia—Visual aphasia; word or text blindness; loss of the ability to grasp the meaning of written or printed words; seen in Gerstmann syndrome.

Alzheimer disease—Condition characterized pathologically by the presence of senile plaques, neurofibrillary tangles, granulovacuolar degeneration, Hirano bodies, and amyloid deposition; patients are demented, with severe memory loss.

alternating hemianesthesia—Ipsilateral facial anesthesia and a contralateral body anesthesia; results from a pontine or medullary lesion involving the spinal trigeminal tract and the spinothalamic tract.

alternating hemiparesis—Ipsilateral cranial nerve palsy and a contralateral hemiparesis (e.g., alternating abducent hemiparesis).

altitudinal hemianopia—Defect in which the upper or lower half of the visual field is lost.

amaurosis fugax—Transient monocular blindness usually related to carotid artery stenosis or less often to embolism of retinal arterioles.

amnesia—Disturbance or loss of memory; seen with bilateral medial temporal lobe lesions.

amusia—Form of aphasia characterized by the loss of ability to express or recognize simple musical tones.

amyotrophic lateral sclerosis (ALS)—A nonhereditary motor neuron disease affecting both upper and lower motor neurons; characterized by muscle weakness, fasciculations, fibrillations and giant motor units on electromyelography. There are no sensory deficits in ALS. It is also called Lou Gehrig's disease.

amyotrophy—Muscle wasting or atrophy.

analgesia—Insensibility to painful stimuli.

anencephaly—Failure of the cerebral and cerebellar hemispheres to develop; results from failure of the anterior neuropore to close.

anesthesia—State characterized by the loss of sensation.

aneurysm—Circumscribed dilation of an artery (e.g., berry aneurysm).

anhidrosis—Absence of sweating; found in Horner syndrome.

anisocoria—Pupils that are unequal in size; found in third-nerve palsy and Horner syndrome.

anomia—Anomic aphasia; the inability to name objects; may result from a lesion of the angular gyrus.

anosmia—Olfactory anesthesia; loss of the sense of smell.

anosognosia—Ignorance of the presence of disease.

Anton syndrome (visual anosognosia)—Lack of awareness of being cortically blind; bilateral occipital lesions affecting the visual association cortex.

aphasia—Impaired or absent communication by speech, writing, or signs; loss of the capacity for spoken language.

aphonia—Loss of the voice.

apparent enophthalmos—Ptosis seen in Horner syndrome that makes the eye appear as if it is sunk back into the orbit.

apraxia—Disorder of voluntary movement; the inability to execute purposeful movements; the inability to properly use an object (e.g., a tool.)

aprosodia (aprosody)—Absence of normal pitch, rhythm, and the variation of stress in speech.

area postrema—Chemoreceptor zone in the medulla that responds to circulating emetic substances; it has no blood-brain barrier.

areflexia—Absence of reflexes.

Argyll Robertson pupil—Pupil that responds to convergence but not to light (near light dissociation); seen in neurosyphilis and lesions of the pineal region.

arrhinencephaly—Characterized by agenesis of the olfactory bulbs; results from malformation of the forebrain; associated with trisomy 13 to 15 and holoprosencephaly.

Arnold-Chiari malformation—Characterized by herniation of the caudal cerebellar vermis and cerebellar tonsils through the foramen magnum; associated with lumbar myelomeningocele, dysgenesis of the corpus callosum, and obstructive hydrocephalus.

ash-leaf spots—Hypopigmented patches typically seen in tuberous sclerosis.

astasia-abasia—Inability to stand or walk.

astatognosia—Position agnosia; the inability to recognize the position or disposition of an extremity or digit in space.

astereognosis (stereoanesthesia)—Tactile amnesia; the inability to judge the form of an object by touch.

asterixis—Flapping tremor of the outstretched arms seen in hepatic encephalopathy and Wilson disease.

ataxia (incoordination)—Inability to coordinate muscles during the execution of voluntary movement (e.g., cerebellar and posterior column ataxia).

athetosis—Slow, writhing, involuntary purposeless movements seen in Huntington disease (chorea).

atresia—Absence of one or more normal openings (e.g., atresia of the outlet foramina of the fourth ventricle, which results in Dandy-Walker syndrome).

atrophy—Muscle wasting; seen in lower motor neuron disease.

auditory agnosia—Inability to interpret the significance of sound; seen in Wernicke dysphasia/aphasia.

autotopagnosia (somatotopagnosia)—Inability to recognize parts of the body; seen with parietal lobe lesions.

Babinski sign—Extension of the great toe in response to plantar stimulation (S-I); indicates corticospinal (pyramidal) tract involvement.

Balint syndrome (optic ataxia)—Condition characterized by a failure to direct oculomotor function in the exploration of space; failure to follow a moving object in all quadrants of the field once the eyes are fixed on the object.

ballism—Dyskinesia resulting from damage to the subthalamic nucleus; consists in violent flailing and flinging of the contralateral extremities.

basal plate—Division of the mantle zone that gives rise to lower motor neurons.

Bell palsy—Idiopathic facial nerve paralysis.

Benedikt syndrome—Condition characterized by a lesion of the midbrain affecting the intra-axial oculomotor fibers, medial lemniscus, and cerebellothalamic fibers.

berry aneurysm—Small saccular dilation of a cerebral artery; ruptured berry aneurysms are the most common cause of nontraumatic subarachnoid hemorrhage.

blepharospasm—Involuntary recurrent spasm of both eyelids; effective treatment is injections of botulinum toxin into the orbicularis oculi muscles.

blood–brain barrier—Tight junctions (zonulae occludentes) of the capillary endothelial cells.

blood–cerebrospinal fluid barrier—Tight junctions (zonulae occludentes) of the choroid plexus.

bradykinesia—Extreme slowness in movement; seen in Parkinson disease.

Broca aphasia—Difficulty in articulating or speaking language; found in the dominant inferior frontal gyrus; also called expressive, anterior, motor, or nonfluent aphasia.

bulbar palsy—Progressive bulbar palsy; a lower motor neuron paralysis affecting primarily the motor nuclei of the medulla; the prototypic disease is amyotrophic lateral sclerosis, characterized by dysphagia, dysarthria, and dysphonia.

caloric nystagmus—Nystagmus induced by irrigating the external auditory meatus with either cold or warm water; remember COWS mnemonic: cold, opposite; warm, same.

cauda equina—Sensory and motor nerve rootlets found below the vertebral level L2; lesions of the cauda equina result in motor and sensory defects of the leg.

cerebral edema—Abnormal accumulation of fluid in the brain; associated with volumetric enlargement of brain tissue and ventricles; may be vasogenic, cytotoxic, or both.

cerebral palsy—Defect of motor power and coordination resulting from brain damage; the most common cause is hypoxia and asphyxia manifested during parturition.

Charcot-Bouchard aneurysm—Miliary aneurysm; microaneurysm; rupture of this type of aneurysm is the most common cause of intraparenchymal hemorrhage; most commonly found in the basal ganglia.

Charcot-Marie-Tooth disease—Most commonly inherited neuropathy affecting lower motor neurons and dorsal root ganglion cells; also called peroneal muscular atrophy.

cherry-red spot (macula)—seen in Tay-Sachs disease; resembles a normal-looking retina; the retinal ganglion cells surrounding the fovea are packed with lysosomes and no longer appear red.

chorea—Irregular, spasmodic, purposeless, involuntary movements of the limbs and facial muscles; seen in Huntington disease.

choreiform—Resembling chorea.

choreoathetosis—Abnormal body movements of combined choreic and athetoid patterns.

chromatolysis—Disintegration of Nissl substance following transection of an axon (axotomy).

clasp-knife spasticity—When a joint is moved briskly, resistance is felt initially and then fades like the opening of a pocket knife; seen with corticospinal lesions.

clonus—Contractions and relaxations of a muscle (e.g., ankle or wrist clonus); seen with corticospinal tract lesions.

cogwheel rigidity—Rigidity characteristic of Parkinson disease. Bending a limb results in ratchet-like movements.

conduction aphasia—Aphasia in which patient has relatively normal comprehension and spontaneous speech but difficulty with repetition; results from a lesion of the arcuate fasciculus, which interconnects the Broca area and the Wernicke area.

confabulation—Making bizarre and incorrect responses; seen in Wernicke-Korsakoff psychosis.

construction apraxia—Inability to draw or construct geometric figures; frequently seen in non-dominant parietal lobe lesions.

conus medullaris syndrome—Condition characterized by paralytic bladder, fecal incontinence, impotence, and perianogenital sensory loss; involves segments S3–Co.

Corti organ (spiral organ)—Structure containing hair cells responding to sounds that induce vibrations of the basilar membrane.

COWS (mnemonic)—**Cold, opposite; warm, same.** Cold water injected into the external auditory meatus results in nystagmus to the opposite side; warm water injected into the external auditory meatus results in nystagmus to the ipsilateral or same side.

Creutzfeldt-Jakob disease—Rapidly progressing dementia, supposedly caused by an infectious prion; histologic picture is that of a spongiform encephalopathy; classic triad is dementia, myoclonic jerks, and typical electroencephalograph findings; similar spongiform encephalopathies are scrapie (in sheep), kuru, and Gerstmann-Straüssler-Scheinker disease, which is characterized by cerebellar ataxia and dementia.

crocodile tears syndrome—Lacrimation during eating; results from a facial nerve injury proximal to the geniculate ganglion; regenerating preganglionic salivatory fibers are misdirected to the pterygopalatine ganglion, which projects to the lacrimal gland.

cupulolithiasis—Dislocation of the otoliths of the utricular macula that causes benign positional vertigo.

cycloplegia—Paralysis of accommodation (CN III) (i.e., paralysis of the ciliary muscle).

Dandy-Walker malformation—Characterized by congenital atresia of the foramina of Luschka and Magendie, hydrocephalus, posterior fossa cyst, and dilatation of the fourth ventricle; associated with agenesis of the corpus callosum.

decerebrate posture (rigidity)—posture in comatose patients in which the arms are overextended, the legs are extended, the hands are flexed, and the head is extended; the causal lesion is in the rostral midbrain.

decorticate posture (rigidity)—posture in comatose patients in which the arms are flexed and the legs are extended; the causal lesion (anoxia) involves both hemispheres.

dementia pugilistica (punch-drunk syndrome)—Condition characterized by dysarthria, parkinsonism, and dementia; ventricular enlargement and fenestration of the septum pellucidum are common; most common cause of death is subdural hematoma.

diabetes insipidus—Condition characterized by excretion of large amounts of pale urine; results from inadequate output of the antidiuretic hormone from the hypothalamus.

diplegia—Paralysis of the corresponding parts on both sides of the body.

diplopia—Double vision.

doll's-eyes maneuver (oculocephalic reflex)—Moving the head of a comatose patient with intact brainstem; results in a deviation of the eyes to the opposite direction.

Down syndrome—Condition that results from a chromosomal abnormality (trisomy 21); Alzheimer disease is common in Down syndrome after age 40 years.

dressing apraxia—Loss of the ability to dress oneself; frequently seen in nondominant parietal lobe lesions.

Duret hemorrhages—Midbrain and pontine hemorrhages due to transtentorial (uncal) herniation.

dysarthria—Disturbance of articulation (e.g., vagal nerve paralysis).

dyscalculia—Difficulty in performing calculations; seen in lesions of the dominant parietal lobule.

dysdiadochokinesia—Inability to perform rapid alternating movements (e.g., supination and pronation of the hand); seen in cerebellar disease.

dysesthesia—Impairment of sensation; disagreeable sensation produced by normal stimulation.

dyskinesias—Movement disorders attributed to pathologic states of the striatal (extrapyramidal) system; movements are generally characterized as insuppressible, stereotyped, and automatic.

dysmetria—Past pointing; a form of dystaxia seen in cerebellar disease.

dysnomia—Dysnomic (nominal) aphasia; difficulty in naming objects or persons; seen with some degree in all aphasias.

dysphagia—Difficulty in swallowing; dysaglutition.

dysphonia—Difficulty in speaking; hoarseness.

dyspnea—Difficulty in breathing.

dysprosodia—Dysprosody; difficulty of speech in producing or understanding the normal pitch, rhythm, and variation in stress; lesions are found in the nondominant hemisphere.

dyssynergia—Incoordination of motor acts; seen in cerebellar disease.

dystaxia—Difficulty in coordinating voluntary muscle activity; seen in posterior column and cerebellar disease.

dystonia (torsion dystonia)—Sustained involuntary contractions of agonists and antagonists (e.g., torticollis); may be caused by the use of neuroleptics.

dystrophy—Progressive changes possibly related to nutrition. When applied to muscle disease, it implies abnormal development and genetic determination.

edrophonium (Tensilon)—Diagnostic test for myasthenia gravis.

embolus—Plug formed by a detached thrombus.

emetic—Agent that causes vomiting; see **area postrema**.

encephalocele—Result of herniation of meninges and brain tissue through an osseous defect in the cranial vault.

encephalopathy—Any disease of the brain.

enophthalmos—Recession of the globe (eyeball) with the orbit.

epicritic sensation—Discriminative sensation; posterior column-medial lemniscus modalities.

epilepsy—Chronic disorder characterized by paroxysmal brain dysfunction caused by excessive neuronal discharge (seizure); usually associated with some alteration of consciousness; may be associated with a reduction of gamma-aminobutyric acid.

epiloia—Tuberous sclerosis, a neurocutaneous disorder; characterized by dementia, seizures, and adenoma sebaceum.

epiphora—Tear flow due to lower eyelid palsy (CN VII).

exencephaly—Congenital condition in which the skull is defective with the brain exposed; seen in anencephaly.

extrapyramidal (motor) system—Motor system including the striatum (caudate nucleus and putamen), globus pallidus, subthalamic nucleus, and substantia nigra; also called the striatal (motor) system.

facial apraxia—Inability to perform facial movements on command.

fasciculations—Visible twitching of muscle fibers seen in lower motor neuron disease.

festination—Acceleration of a shuffling gait seen in Parkinson disease.

fibrillations—Nonvisible contractions of muscle fibers found in lower motor neuron disease.

flaccid paralysis—Complete loss of muscle power or tone resulting from a lower motor neuron disease.

folic acid deficiency—Common cause of megaloblastic anemia; may also cause fetal neural tube defects (e.g., spina bifida).

gait apraxia—Diminished capacity to walk or stand; frequently seen with bilateral frontal lobe disease.

gegenhalten—Paratonia; a special type of resistance to passive stretching of muscles; seen with frontal lobe disease.

Gerstmann syndrome—Condition characterized by right-left confusion, finger agnosia, dysgraphia, and dyscalculia; results from a lesion of the dominant inferior parietal lobule.

glioma—Tumor (neoplasm) derived from glial cells.

global aphasia—Difficulty with comprehension, repetition, and speech.

graphesthesia—Ability to recognize figures written on the skin.

hallucination—False sensory perception with localizing value.

hematoma—Localized mass of extravasated blood; a contained hemorrhage (e.g., subdural or epidural).

hemianopia—Hemianopsia; loss of vision in one half of the visual field of one or both eyes.

hemiballism—Dyskinesia resulting from damage to the subthalamic nucleus; consists of violent flinging and flailing movements of the contralateral extremities.

hemianhidrosis—Absence of sweating on half of the body or face; seen in Horner syndrome.

hemiparesis—Slight paralysis affecting one side of the body; seen in stroke involving the internal capsule.

hemiplegia—Paralysis of one side of the body.

herniation—Pressure-induced protrusion of brain tissue into an adjacent compartment; may be transtentorial (uncal), subfalcine (subfalcial), or transforaminal (tonsillar).

heteronymous—Referring to noncorresponding halves or quadrants of the visual fields (e.g., binasal hemianopia).

herpes simplex encephalitis—Disorder characterized by headache, behavioral changes (memory), and seizures; the most common cause of encephalitis in the central nervous system; the temporal lobes are preferentially the target of hemorrhagic necrosis.

hidrosis—Sweating, perspiration, and diaphoresis.

Hirano bodies—Eosinophilic rodlike structures (inclusions) found in the hippocampus in Alzheimer disease.

holoprosencephaly—Failure of the prosencephalon to diverticulate and form two hemispheres.

homonymous—Referring to corresponding halves or quadrants of the visual fields (e.g., left homonymous hemianopia).

Horner syndrome—Oculosympathetic paralysis consisting of miosis, hemianhidrosis, mild ptosis, and apparent enophthalmos.

hydranencephaly—Condition in which the cerebral cortex and white matter are replaced by membranous sacs; believed to be the result of circulatory disease.

hydrocephalus—Condition marked by excessive accumulation of cerebrospinal fluid and dilated ventricles.

hygroma—Collection of cerebrospinal fluid in the subdural space.

hypacusis—Hearing impairment.

hypalgesia—Decreased sensibility to pain.

hyperacusis—Abnormal acuteness of hearing; the result of a facial nerve paralysis (e.g., Bell palsy).

hyperphagia—Gluttony; overeating as seen in hypothalamic lesions.

hyperpyrexia—High fever as seen in hypothalamic lesions.

hyperreflexia—An exaggeration of muscle stretch reflexes as seen with upper motor neuron lesions; a sign of spasticity.

hyperthermia—Increased body temperature; seen with hypothalamic lesions.

hypertonia—Increased muscle tone; seen with upper motor neuron lesions.

hypesthesia—Hypoesthesia; diminished sensitivity to stimulation.

hypokinesia—Diminished or slow movement; seen in Parkinson disease.

hypophysis—Pituitary gland.

hypothermia—Reduced body temperature; seen in hypothalamic lesions.

hypotonia—Reduced muscle tone; seen in cerebellar disease.

ideational or sensory apraxia—Characterized by the inability to formulate the ideational plan for executing the several components of a complex multistep act; patient cannot go through the steps of lighting a cigarette when asked to; occurs most frequently in diffuse cerebral degenerating disease (e.g., Alzheimer disease, multi-infarct dementia).

ideomotor or "classic" apraxia (ideokinetic apraxia)—Inability to button one's clothes when asked; inability to comb one's hair when asked; inability to manipulate tools (e.g., hammer or screwdriver), although patient can explain their use; and inability to pantomime actions on request.

idiopathic—Denoting a condition of an unknown cause (e.g., idiopathic Parkinson disease).

infarction—Sudden insufficiency of blood supply caused by vascular occlusion (e.g., emboli or thrombi), resulting in tissue necrosis (death).

intention tremor—Tremor that occurs when a voluntary movement is made; a cerebellar tremor.

internal ophthalmoplegia—Paralysis of the iris and ciliary body caused by a lesion of the oculomotor nerve.

internuclear ophthalmoplegia (INO)—Medial rectus palsy on attempted conjugate lateral gaze caused by a lesion of the medial longitudinal fasciculus.

intra-axial—Refers to structures found within the neuraxis; within the brain or spinal cord.

ischemia—Local anemia caused by mechanical obstruction of the blood supply.

junction scotoma—results from a lesion of decussating fibers from the inferior nasal retinal quadrant, which loop into the posterior part of the contralateral optic nerve; in the contralateral upper temporal quadrant.

Kayser-Fleischer ring—Visible deposition of copper in Descemet membrane of the corneoscleral margin; seen in Wilson disease (hepatolenticular degeneration).

Kernig sign—Test for meningitis. Subject lies on back with thigh flexed to a right angle, then tries to extend the leg; this movement is impossible with meningitis.

kinesthesia—Sensory perception of movement, muscle sense; mediated by the posterior column-medial lemniscus system.

Klüver-Bucy syndrome—Characterized by psychic blindness, hyperphagia, and hypersexuality; results from bilateral temporal lobe ablation including the amygdaloid nuclei.

labyrinthine hydrops—Excess of endolymphatic fluid in the membranous labyrinth; cause of **Ménière disease.**

lacunae—Small infarcts associated with hypertensive vascular disease.

Lambert-Eaton myasthenic syndrome—Condition that results from a defect in presynaptic acetylcholine release; 50% of the patients have a malignancy (e.g., lung or breast tumor).

lead-pipe rigidity—Rigidity characteristic of Parkinson disease.

Lewy bodies—Eosinophilic, intracytoplasmic inclusions found in the neurons of the substantia nigra in Parkinson disease.

Lhermitte sign—Electric-like shocks extending down the spine caused by flexing the head; due to damage of the posterior columns.

lipofuscin (ceroid)—Normal inclusion of many neurons and glial cells; increases as the brain ages.

Lish nodules—Pigmented hamartomas of the iris seen in neurofibromatosis type 1.

lissencephaly—Agyria: results from failure of the germinal matrix neuroblasts to reach the cortical mantle and form the gyri; the surface of the brain remains smooth.

locked-in syndrome—Results from infarction of the base of the pons; infarcted structures include the corticobulbar and corticospinal tracts, leading to quadriplegia and paralysis of the lower cranial nerves; patients can communicate only by blinking or moving their eyes vertically.

locus ceruleus—Pigmented (neuromelanin) nucleus found in the pons and midbrain; contains the largest collection of norepinephrinergic neurons in the brain.

macrographia (megalographia)—Large handwriting seen in cerebellar disease.

magnetic gait—Patient walks as if feet were stuck to the floor; seen in normal-pressure hydrocephalus.

medial longitudinal fasciculus (MLF)—Fiber bundle found in the dorsomedial tegmentum of the brainstem just under the fourth ventricle; it carries vestibular and ocular motor axons, which mediate vestibulo-ocular reflexes (e.g., nystagmus); severance of this tract results in internuclear ophthalmoplegia.

Mees lines—Transverse lines on fingernails and toenails; due to arsenic poisoning.

megalencephaly—Large brain weighing more than 1800 g.

meningocele—Protrusion of the meninges of the brain or spinal cord through an osseous defect in the skull or vertebral canal.

meningoencephalocele—Protrusion of the meninges and the brain through a defect in the occipital bone.

meroanencephaly—Less severe form of anencephaly in which the brain is present in rudimentary form.

microencephaly (micrencephaly)—a small brain weighing less than 900 g. The adult brain weighs about 1400 g.

micrographia—Small handwriting seen in Parkinson disease.

microgyria (polymicrogyria)—Small gyri; the cortical lamination pattern is not normal; seen in Arnold-Chiari syndrome.

Millard-Gubler syndrome—Alternating abducent and facial hemiparesis; an ipsilateral sixth and seventh nerve palsy and a contralateral hemiparesis.

mimetic muscles—Muscles of facial expression; innervated by facial nerve (CN VII).

miosis—Constriction of the pupil; seen in Horner syndrome.

Möbius syndrome—Congenital oculofacial palsy; consists of a congenital facial diplegia (CN VII) and a convergent strabismus (CN VI).

mononeuritis multiplex—Vasculitic inflammation of several different nerves (e.g., polyarteritis nodosa).

MPTP (1-methyl-4-phenyl-1,3,3,6-tetrahydropyridine) **poisoning**—Toxic destruction of the dopaminergic neurons in the substantia nigra, resulting in parkinsonism.

multi-infarct dementia—Dementia due to the cumulative effect of repetitive infarcts; strokes characterized by cortical sensory, pyramidal, and bulbar and cerebellar signs, which result in permanent damage; primarily seen in hypertensive patients.

multiple sclerosis—Classic myelinoclastic disease in which the myelin sheath is destroyed, with the axon remaining intact; characterized by exacerbations and remissions, with paresthesias, double vision, ataxia, and incontinence; cerebrospinal fluid findings include increased gamma globulin, increased beta globulin, presence of oligoclonal bands, and increased myelin basic protein.

muscular dystrophy—X-linked myopathy characterized by progressive weakness, fiber necrosis, and loss of muscle cells; two most common types are Duchenne and myotonic muscular dystrophy.

mydriasis—Dilation of the pupil; seen in oculomotor paralysis.

myelopathy—Disease of the spinal cord.

myeloschisis—Cleft spinal cord resulting from failure of the neural folds to close or from failure of the posterior neuropore to close.

myoclonus—Clonic spasm or twitching of a muscle or group of muscles as seen in juvenile myoclonic epilepsy; composed of single jerks.

myopathy—Disease of the muscle.

myotatic reflex—Monosynaptic muscle stretch reflex.

neglect syndrome—Result of a unilateral parietal lobe lesion; neglect of one-half of the body and of extracorporal space; simultaneous stimulation results in extinction of one of the stimuli; loss of optokinetic nystagmus on one side.

Negri bodies—Intracytoplasmic inclusions observed in rabies; commonly found in the hippocampus and cerebellum.

neuraxis—Unpaired part of the central nervous system: spinal cord, rhombencephalon, and diencephalon.

neurilemma—Neurolemma; the sheath of Schwann; Schwann cells (neurilemmal cells) produce the myelin sheath in the peripheral nervous system.

neurofibrillary tangles—Abnormal double helical structures found in the neurons of Alzheimer patients.

neurofibromatosis (von Recklinghausen disease)—A neurocutaneous disorder. Neurofibromatosis type 1 consists predominately of peripheral lesions (e.g., café au lait spots, neurofibromas, Lish nodules, schwannomas). Type 2 consists primarily of intracranial lesions (e.g., bilateral acoustic schwannomas and gliomas).

neurohypophysis—Posterior lobe of the pituitary gland; derived from the downward extension of the hypothalamus, the infundibulum.

neuropathy—Disorder of the nervous system.

Nissl bodies/substance—Rough endoplasmic reticulum found in the nerve cell body and dendrites but not in the axon.

nociceptive—Capable of appreciation or transmission of pain.

normal-pressure hydrocephalus—Hydrocephalus characterized by normal cerebrospinal fluid pressure and the clinical triad of dementia, gait dystaxia (magnetic gait), and urinary incontinence; shunting is effective; mnemonic is **W**acky, **W**obbly, **W**et.

nucleus basalis of Meynert—Contains the largest collection of cholinergic neurons in the brain; located in the forebrain between the anterior perforated substance and the globus pallidus; neurons degenerate in Alzheimer disease.

nystagmus—Oscillations of the eyeballs; named after the fast component; seen in vestibular and cerebellar disease.

obex—Caudal apex of the rhomboid fossa; marks the beginning of the open medulla.

Ondine curse—Inability of patient to breathe while sleeping; results from damage to the respiratory centers of the medulla.

optokinetic nystagmus—Nystagmus induced by looking at moving stimuli (targets); also called railroad nystagmus.

otitis media—Infection of the middle ear, which may cause conduction deafness; may also cause Horner syndrome.

otorrhea—Discharge of cerebrospinal fluid via the ear canal.

otosclerosis—New bone formation in the middle ear resulting in fixation of the stapes; the most frequent cause of progressive conduction deafness.

palsy—Paralysis; often used to connote partial paralysis or paresis.

papilledema—Choked disk; edema of the optic disk; caused by increased intracranial pressure (e.g., tumor, epidural or subdural hematoma).

paracusis—Impaired hearing; an auditory illusion or hallucination.

paralysis—Loss of muscle power due to denervation; results from a lower motor neuron lesion.

paraphrasia (paraphasia)—A form of aphasia in which a person substitutes one word for another, resulting in unintelligible speech.

paraplegia—Paralysis of both lower extremities.

paresis—Partial or incomplete paralysis.

paresthesia—Abnormal sensation such as tingling, pricking, or numbness; seen with posterior column disease (e.g., tabes dorsalis).

Parinaud syndrome—Lesion of the midbrain tegmentum resulting from pressure of a germinima, a tumor of the pineal region; the patient has a paralysis of upward gaze.

Pick disease—Dementia affecting primarily the frontal lobes; always spares the posterior third of the superior temporal gyrus; clinically indistinguishable from Alzheimer disease.

pill-rolling tremor—Tremor at rest; seen in Parkinson disease.

planum temporale—Auditory association cortex found posterior to the transverse gyri of Heschl on the inferior bank of the lateral sulcus; a part of Wernicke area; larger on the left side in males.

poikilothermia—Inability to thermoregulate; seen with lesions of the posterior hypothalamus.

polydipsia—Frequent drinking; seen in lesions of the hypothalamus (diabetes insipidus).

polyuria—Frequent micturition; seen with hypothalamic lesions (diabetes insipidus).

porencephaly—Cerebral cavitation caused by localized agenesis of the cortical mantle; the cyst is lined with ependyma.

presbycusis (presbyacusia)—The inability to perceive or discriminate sounds as part of the aging process; due to atrophy of the organ of Corti.

progressive supranuclear palsy—Characterized by supranuclear ophthalmoplegia, primarily a downgaze paresis followed by paresis of other eye movements; as the disease progresses, the remainder of the motor cranial nerves becomes involved.

proprioception—Reception of stimuli originating from muscles, tendons, and other internal tissues; conscious proprioception is mediated by the dorsal column–medial lemniscus system.

prosopagnosia—Difficulty in recognizing familiar faces.

protopathic sensation—Pain, temperature, and light (crude) touch sensation; the modalities mediated by the spinothalamic tracts.

pseudobulbar palsy (pseudobulbar supranuclear palsy)—Upper motor neuron syndrome resulting from bilateral lesions that interrupt the corticobulbar tracts; symptoms include difficulties with articulation, mastication, and deglutition; results from repeated bilateral vascular lesions.

psychic blindness—Type of visual agnosia seen in the Klüver-Bucy syndrome.

psychosis—Severe mental thought disorder.

ptosis—Drooping of the upper eyelid; seen in Horner syndrome and oculomotor nerve paralysis (CN III).

pyramidal (motor) system—Voluntary motor system consisting of upper motor neurons in the corticobulbar and corticospinal tracts.

quadrantanopia—Loss of vision in one quadrant of the visual field in one or both eyes.

quadriplegia—Tetraplegia; paralysis of all four limbs.

rachischisis—Spondyloschisis; failure of the vertebral arches to develop and fuse and form the neural tube.

raphe nuclei—Paramedian nuclei of the brainstem that contain serotonergic neurons.

Rathke pouch—Ectodermal outpocketing of the stomodeum; gives rise to the adenohypophysis (anterior lobe of the pituitary gland).

retrobulbar neuritis—Optic neuritis frequently caused by the demyelinating disease multiple sclerosis.

rhinorrhea—Leakage of cerebrospinal fluid via the nose.

rigidity—Increased muscle tone in both extensors and flexors; seen in Parkinson disease; cogwheel rigidity and lead-pipe rigidity.

Romberg sign—Loss of balance when the subject stands with feet together and closes the eyes; a sign of dorsal column ataxia.

saccadic movement—Quick jump of the eyes from one fixation point to another; impaired saccades are seen in Huntington disease.

scanning speech—Scanning dysarthria; words are broken up into syllables; typical of cerebellar disease and multiple sclerosis; example: I DID not GIVE any TOYS TO my son FOR CHRISTmas.

schizophrenia—Psychosis characterized by a disorder in the thinking processes (e.g., delusions and hallucinations); associated with dopaminergic hyperactivity.

scotoma—Blind spot in the visual field.

senile (neuritic) plaques—Swollen dendrites and axons, neurofibrillary tangles, and a core of amyloid; found in Alzheimer disease.

shagreen spots—Cutaneous lesions found in tuberous sclerosis.

shaken baby syndrome—Syndrome with three major physical findings: retinal hemorrhages, large head circumference, and bulging fontanelle; 80% of the subdural hemorrhages are bilateral.

sialorrhea (ptyalism)—Excess of saliva (e.g., drooling); seen in Parkinson disease.

singultus—Hiccups; frequently seen in the posterior inferior cerebellar artery syndrome.

simultanagnosia—Inability to understand the meaning of an entire picture even though some parts may be recognized; the inability to perceive more than one stimulus at a time.

somatesthesia—Somesthesia; bodily sensations that include touch, pain, and temperature.

spastic paresis—Partial paralysis with hyperreflexia resulting from transection of the corticospinal tract.

spasticity—Increased muscle tone (hypertonia) and hyperreflexia (exaggerated muscle stretch reflexes); seen in upper motor neuron lesions.

spina bifida—Neural tube defect with the variants: spina bifida occulta, spina bifida with meningocele, spina bifida with meningomyelocele, and rachischisis; results from failure of the vertebral laminae to close in the midline.

status marmoratus—Hypermyelination in the putamen and thalamus; results from perinatal asphyxia; clinically presents as double athetosis.

stereoanesthesia—Astereognosis; inability to judge the form of an object by touch.

Stiff-man syndrome—Myopathy characterized by progressive and permanent stiffness of the muscles of the back, neck, and spreading to involve the proximal muscles of the extremities; caused by a disturbance of the inhibitory action of Renshaw cells in the spinal cord.

strabismus—Lack of parallelism of the visual axes of the eyes; squint; heterotropia.

striae medullares (of the rhombencephalon)—Fiber bundles that divide the rhomboid fossa into a rostral pontine part and a caudal medullary part.

stria medullaris (of the thalamus)—Fiber bundle extending from the septal area to the habenular nuclei.

stria terminalis—Semicircular fiber bundle extending from the amygdala to the hypothalamus and septal area.

Sturge-Weber syndrome—Neurocutaneous congenital disorder including a port-wine stain (venous angioma) and calcified leptomeningeal angiomatoses (railroad track images seen on plain film); seizures occur in up to 90% of patients.

subclavian steal syndrome—Occlusion of the subclavian artery, proximal to the vertebral artery, resulting in a shunting of blood down the vertebral and into ipsilateral subclavian artery; physical activity of the ipsilateral arm may cause signs of vertebrobasilar insufficiency (dizziness or vertigo).

sulcus limitans—Groove separating the sensory alar plate from the motor basal plate; extends from the spinal cord to the mesencephalon.

sunset sign—Downward look by eyes; the sclerae are above the irides and the upper eye lids are retracted; seen in congenital hydrocephalus and in progressive supranuclear palsy.

swinging flashlight sign—Test to diagnose a relevant afferent pupil; light shone into the afferent pupil results in a small change in pupil size bilaterally, and light shone into the normal pupil results in a decrease in pupil size in both eyes.

sympathetic apraxia—Motor apraxia in the left hand; seen in lesions of the dominant frontal lobe.

syringomyelia—Cavitation of the cervical spinal cord resulting in bilateral loss of pain and temperature sensation and wasting of the intrinsic muscles of the hands; syringes may be found in the medulla (syringobulbia) and pons (syringopontia) and in Arnold-Chiari malformation.

tabes dorsalis—Locomotor ataxia; progressive demyelination and sclerosis of the dorsal columns and roots; seen in neurosyphilis.

tactile agnosia—Inability to recognize objects by touch.

tardive dyskinesia—Syndrome of repetitive, choreoathetoid movements frequently affecting the face; results from treatment with antipsychotic agents.

Tay-Sachs disease (GM$_2$ gangliosidosis)—Best-known inherited metabolic disease of the central nervous system; characterized by motor seizures, dementia, and blindness; a cherry-red spot (macula) occurs in 90% of cases; is caused by a deficiency of hexosaminidase A; primarily affects Ashkenazi Jews.

tethered cord syndrome (filum terminale syndrome)—Syndrome characterized by numbness of the legs and feet, foot drop, loss of bladder control, and impotence.

thrombus—Clot in an artery that is formed from blood constituents; gives rise to an embolus.

tic douloureux—Trigeminal neuralgia.

tinnitus—Ringing in the ear(s); seen with irritative lesions of the cochlear nerve (e.g., acoustic neuroma).

titubation—A head tremor in the anterior–posterior direction, often accompanying midline cerebellar lesions; is also a staggering gait.

tremor—Involuntary, rhythmic, oscillatory movement.

tuberous sclerosis (Bourneville disease)—Neurocutaneous disorder characterized by the trilogy of mental retardation, seizures, and adenoma sebaceum; cutaneous lesions include periungual fibromas, shagreen patches, and ash-leaf spots.

uncinate fit—Form of psychomotor epilepsy, including hallucinations of smell and taste; results from lesions of the parahippocampal gyrus (uncus).

upper motor neurons (UMNs)—Cortical neurons that give rise to the corticospinal and corticobulbar tracts; destruction of UMNs or their axons results in a spastic paresis; some authorities include brainstem neurons that synapse on lower motor neurons (i.e., neurons from the red nucleus).

vertigo—Sensation of whirling motion due to vestibular disease.

visual agnosia—Inability to recognize objects by sight.

von Hippel-Lindau disease—Disorder characterized by lesions of the retina and cerebellum; retinal and cerebellar hemangioblastomata; non–central nervous system lesions may include renal, epididymal, and pancreatic cysts, as well as renal carcinoma.

Wallenberg syndrome—Condition characterized by hoarseness, cerebellar ataxia, anesthesia of the ipsilateral face and contralateral body, and cranial nerve signs of dysarthria, dysphagia, dysphonia, vertigo, and nystagmus; results from infarction of the lateral medulla due to occlusion of the vertebral artery or its major branch, the posterior inferior cerebellar artery; Horner syndrome is frequently found on the ipsilateral side

Wallerian degeneration—Anterograde degeneration of an axon and its myelin sheath after axonal transection.

Weber syndrome—Lesion of the midbrain basis pedunculi involving the root fibers of the oculomotor nerve and the corticobulbar and the cortospinal tracts.

Werdnig-Hoffman syndrome (spinal muscular atrophy)—Early childhood disease of the anterior horn cells (lower motor neuron disease).

Wernicke aphasia—Difficulty in comprehending spoken language; also called receptive, posterior, sensory, or fluent aphasia.

witzelsucht—Inappropriate facetiousness and silly joking; seen with frontal lobe lesions.

Index

Note: Page numbers followed by f indicate illustrations; those followed by t indicate tables; and those followed by Q indicate end-of-chapter Question and Answer sections.

A